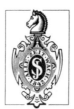

Karl Lennert and Alfred C. Feller

Histopathology of Non-Hodgkin's Lymphomas
(Based on the Updated Kiel Classification)

With a Section on Clinical Therapy
by M. Engelhard and G. Brittinger

Translated by M. Soehring

Second Completely Revised Edition
With 161 Figures, Some in Colour

Springer-Verlag
Berlin Heidelberg New York London Paris
Tokyo Hong Kong Barcelona Budapest

Prof. Dr. Dr. h.c. mult. KARL LENNERT
Zentrum für Pathologie und angewandte Krebsforschung,
Niemannsweg 11, 2300 Kiel, FRG

Prof. Dr. ALFRED CHRISTIAN FELLER
Pathologisches Institut der Universität Würzburg,
Luitpoldkrankenhaus, Josef-Schneider-Straße 2,
8700 Würzburg, FRG

Translator:
MARTHA SOEHRING
Deutsch-Nienhof, 2301 Westensee, FRG

Title of the German Edition
K. LENNERT und A. C. FELLER, Histopathologie der Non-Hodgkin-Lymphome
© Springer-Verlag Berlin Heidelberg 1981, 1990

ISBN-13:978-3-642-97189-1   e-ISBN-13:978-3-642-97187-7
DOI:10.1007/978-3-642-97187-7

Library of Congress Cataloging-in-Publication Data. Lennert, Karl. Histopathology of non-Hodgkin-Lymphomas / Karl Lennert and Alfred C. Feller. 2nd completely rev. ed., Translation of: Histopathologie der Non-Hodgkin-Lymphome. Includes Bibliographical references and index. 1. Lymphoma-Histopathology. I. Feller, Alfred C. II. Title. [DNLM: 1. Lymphoma-classification. 2. Lymphoma-pathology. QZ 350 L 567h] RC 280.L9L4613   1992   616.99′446-dc20   DNLM/DLC

© Springer-Verlag Berlin Heidelberg 1981, 1992
Softcover reprint of the hardcover 2nd edition 1992

Typesetting, printing and bookbinding by Konrad Triltsch GmbH, Würzburg
21/3130-5 4 3 2 1   – Printed on acid-free paper

Preface to the Second Edition

The 1st Edition of *Histopathology of Non-Hodgkin's Lymphomas*, written in collaboration with Professor H. STEIN and published in 1981, was received well and is now out of print. In the meantime, there has been an explosion of data that not only have made the definitions of various entities more precise but, above all, have confirmed the main entities originally delineated in the Kiel classification. The development of monoclonal antibodies and molecular cytogenetics has also made it possible to identify T-cell lymphomas more accurately. For example, many of the malignant lymphomas that were previously considered to be unclassifiable can now be included in a classification scheme that places the T-cell lymphomas alongside of the list of B-cell lymphomas. In 1988 the European Lymphoma Club published an "updated Kiel classification" (STANSFELD et al. 1988) based on this new knowledge. It includes a number of previously undefined types of T-cell lymphoma. Studies done in Japan (T. SUCHI et al.) and China (L. Y. TU) have contributed to the understanding of these lymphoma types.

When we wrote the 1st Edition of *Histopathology of Non-Hodgkin's Lymphomas* (1981) we could take advantage of the experience we had already presented at length in the handbook *Malignant Lymphomas Other than Hodgkin's Disease* (1978). Since then there have been so many advances that the 2nd Edition of *Histopathology of Non-Hodgkin's Lymphomas* has become larger than a "booklet". We were compelled to describe and document a number of new cytological findings and a few entities in more detail than in the 1st Edition. This has led to a certain degree of imbalance from chapter to chapter for the sake of clarity.

The 2nd Edition of *Histopathology of Non-Hodgkin's Lymphomas* is based on the updated Kiel classification. The English version of the 2nd Edition appears 2 years after the German Edition, during which there has been another significant improvement in our understanding of certain entities. We have had to make a few additions to the updated Kiel classification in order to accommodate the newest data.

The reader will notice that a few terms have been adapted to international usage. For example, instead of "reticulum cell" we now say "follicular dendritic cell" etc. We see no reason to stick to a term just for the sake of semantics, since common comprehension is more important.

The present book is intended chiefly for use by pathologists in everyday diagnostics. Although the complex results of molecular genetics and virus research evoke ever greater interest, they go far beyond the scope of this book. Hence we include them only so far as they have to do with a diagnosis.

Another quality of this book is the concentration on malignant lymphomas of the lymph nodes (and thymus). We have chosen to leave out most primary extranodal lymphomas, including those of mucosa-associated lymphoid tissue (MALT). Nevertheless, we could not avoid mentioning MALT lymphomas in the chapter on monocytoid B-cell lymphoma. Malignant neoplasms of macrophages, dendritic cells or interdigitating cells are not discussed at all, since they do not represent genuine lymphomas and are still in need of clarification. This is especially true of malignant histiocytosis, which has become extremely rare.

Dr. M. ENGELHARD and Professor G. BRITTINGER kindly agreed to write a brief chapter on Therapeutic Principles. It illustrates the clinical relevance of the Kiel classification and also lays out the current scope of lymphoma therapy.

Again, we are grateful for the help of many others. Valuable contributions to certain chapters were made by the following colleagues: Dr. B. COGLIATTI, Dr. H. GRIESSER, Dr. S. NIZZE, Dr. J. PAULSEN, Dr. C. VON SCHILLING and Dr. T. SUCHI. Mrs. K. MÜLLER was responsible for the excellent technical quality of the histological slides. Mrs. I. HORN and Mrs. E. PFLUG performed the immunohistochemical stainings. Mrs. H. BLESSMANN and Mrs. R. KÖPKE prepared high-quality photographs. Mr. W. VATER executed the graphics with great precision. Mr. J. HEDDERICH of the Department of Medical Statistics and Documentation (Director: Professor K. SAUTER) did the groundwork for compiling and computing the statistical data. Mrs. K. DEGE, who worked under a grant from the Kind-Philipp-Stiftung, assisted with the translation of the chapters on T-cell lymphomas. Mrs. M. SOEHRING deserves special mention for both the English translation and word processing, which were done with great precision and care. Mrs. D. SCHMÖE was responsible for the exact bibliography.

It was also a pleasure to work with Mr. B. LEWERICH, Dr. M. WILSON, Mr. A. GÖSLING and Dr. U. HEILMANN of Springer-Verlag, who helped to transpose the manuscript into this fine-looking book.

Kiel and Würzburg, Spring 1992   KARL LENNERT
                                                       ALFRED C. FELLER

Preface to the First Edition

Soon after publication of our handbook "Malignant Lymphomas Other than Hodgkin's Disease", there were calls for a small, handy synopsis for the diagnosis of lymphoma. The members of the European Lymphoma Club (Professor J. DIEBOLD, Paris, Dr. R. GÉRARD-MARCHANT, Villejuif, Professor Y. KAPANCI, Geneva, Professor G. KELÉNYI, Pécs, Dr. H. NOEL, Brussels, Professor F. RILKE, Milan, Dr. A. G. STANSFELD, London, and Professor J. A. M. VAN UNNIK, Utrecht) also urged me to write such a manual for routine diagnostic work. They even identified themselves with this plan and offered to translate the text into several other languages. It is a special pleasure to thank Professor DIEBOLD, Dr. GÉRARD-MARCHANT, Professor RILKE and Dr. STANSFELD for the prompt translation from German into French, Italian and English. Professor RILKE took the initiative and also wrote a chapter on the "Working Formulation for Clinical Usage". My thanks are also due to the former co-workers and close colleagues who kindly agreed to translate the text into other languages – Professor A. LLOMBART BOSCH (Spanish), Dr. IRENE LORAND and Professor J. M. MACHADO (Portuguese), and Professor N. MOHRI (Japanese). The publication of this manual in various languages, including my native German, should facilitate its use in routine work.

The brief description of non-Hodgkin's lymphomas is based exclusively on the Kiel classification, which aims at a synthesis of morphology and immunology. Professor H. STEIN thus contributed the most important immunological data on each type of lymphoma. A detailed description of clinical features is not included, as it is being prepared by Professor G. BRITTINGER and the members of the Kiel Lymphoma Study Group. Also for reasons of brevity, rare entities, such as heavy chain diseases, are given only very minor attention. Furthermore, only the most important and recent literature is cited.

Many people have been involved in the preparation of this manual. My thanks are due especially to the members of the European Lymphoma Club and the Kiel Lymphoma Study Group and to all the people who work with me at the Institute of Pathology. I thank particularly Mrs. M. SOEHRING, who did all the secretarial work with great care and without tiring and who prepared the English manuscript. Mrs. D. SCHMIDT was responsible for the precise bibliography.

The publishers, foremost Dr. H. GÖTZE and Mr. B. LEWERICH, have proved again their understanding and efficiency with this little book, for which I am very grateful.

Kiel, Spring 1981   KARL LENNERT

Contents

Abbreviations

AILD	Angioimmunoblastic lymphadenopathy with dysproteinaemia
ALL	Acute lymphoblastic leukaemia
APAAP	Alkaline phosphatase–anti-alkaline phosphatase
ATLL	Adult T-cell leukaemia/lymphoma
BL	Burkitt's lymphoma
CALLA	Common ALL antigen
CD	Leucocyte differentiation cluster
cIg	Cytoplasmic immunoglobulin
CLL	Chronic lymphocytic leukaemia
CS	Clinical staging
DAB	Diaminobenzidine
DPPIV	Dipeptidyl peptidase IV
EBV	Epstein-Barr virus
ECLg	Epithelioid cellular lymphogranulomatosis
EMA	Epithelial membrane antigen
ESR	Erythrocyte sedimentation rate
FCC	Follicular centre cell
H & E	Haematoxylin and eosin
HCL	Hairy cell leukaemia
HPF	High power field
HTLV	Human T-lymphocyte virus
IBL	Immunoblastic lymphadenopathy
Ig	Immunoglobulin
IL-2	Interleukin-2
IPSID	Immunoproliferative small intestinal disease
LCA	Leucocyte common antigen
LCAL	Large cell anaplastic lymphoma
LeL	Lymphoepithelioid lymphoma (Lennert's lymphoma)
LgX	Lymphogranulomatosis X
MALT	Mucosa-associated lymphoid tissue
ML	Malignant lymphoma
NHL	Non-Hodgkin's lymphoma
NK	Natural killer
PAP	Peroxidase–anti-peroxidase
PAS	Periodic acid–Schiff
PCR	Polymerase chain reaction
PLL	Prolymphocytic leukaemia
PS	Pathological staging

sIg	Surface immunoglobulin
TcR	T-cell receptor
TdT	Terminal deoxynucleotidyl transferase
VCA	Viral capsid antigen
WF	Working Formulation

1 The Diagnosis of Lymphoma

1.1 Practical Tips[1]

1. The diagnosis of lymphoma begins with the biopsy excision. The surgeon must avoid squeezing the tissue and must obtain a specimen of adequate size. If possible, an experienced assistant should prepare imprints from the freshly cut surface of the node by carefully touching it on well-degreased glass slides and should then immediately place the node in fixative.

2. As a rule, fixation for 6–12 h in diluted (1:4) buffered formalin is sufficient. Sections of especially high cytological quality are obtained from tissue fixed in special solutions such as that composed of 750 ml absolute alcohol, 200 ml undiluted formalin and 50 ml acetic acid. Bouin's fixative is not recommended.

3. The most common fault in the processing of lymph nodes is *embedding* the tissue improperly. *Good* embedding in paraffin (Paraplast) is sufficient for routine diagnoses. For an analysis of the cytological details, lymph nodes must be embedded more carefully than non-lymphoid tissue. Hence it is *essential* to embed lymph nodes separately, preferably with a separate machine or by hand. When the paraffin embedding is insufficient, the biopsy can be saved by re-embedding in resin[2] (cf. Addendum, p. 264). The improvement in quality is often so dramatic that it is hard to believe that one is looking at the same tissue (Fig. 1). Re-embedding in resin is also very helpful for studying cytological details. Primary resin embedding is not necessary for routine diagnoses, nor is it practical, because the sections are too thin and thus lacking in contrast. When such sections are viewed at a low magnification, it is difficult to recognize the lymph node structure and the basic pattern of a neoplasm. These sections require a laborious and time-consuming analysis at higher magnifications. Moreover, the results of immunohistological staining are not satisfactory when resin-embedded tissue is used.

4. When the lymph node has been properly embedded, it is easy to prepare 4 μm thick sections. Stretching or drying of the sections at too high temperatures (> 45 °C; cf. Addendum, p. 263) must be avoided. Figure 2 shows examples of poorly (a) and well-cut (b) sections from the same paraffin block.

5. In the diagnosis of lymph node lesions *Giemsa staining* is the most useful. It is the only method that allows a precise cytological diagnosis according to the rules of haematology. The staining must be of high quality, however. A poor Giemsa stain is worse than none at all. The stock solution should be purchased

---

[1] Cf. Banks 1985.
[2] J. D. Elema, personal communication 1979; Poppema 1984.

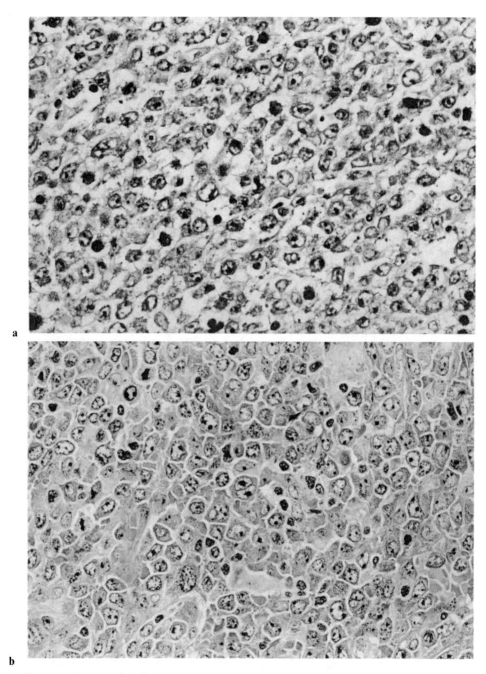

a

b

Fig. 1a, b. Poor results of paraffin embedding (**a**) are improved by re-embedding in resin (**b**). Polymorphic centroblastic lymphoma. Giemsa. 440 : 1

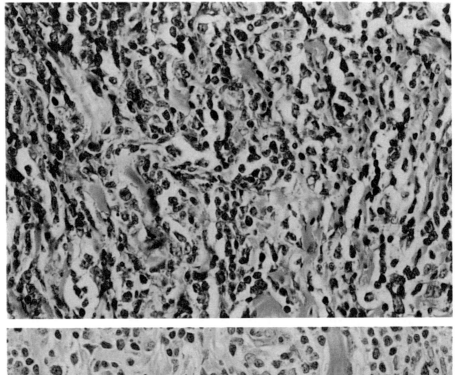

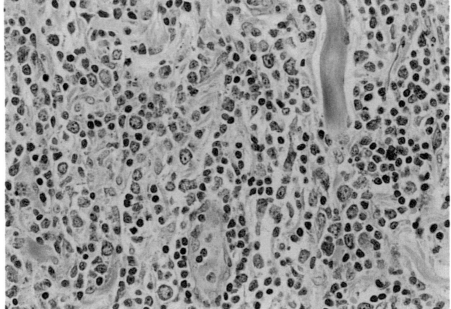

Fig. 2a, b. Giemsa-stained sections of poor (**a**) and good quality (**b**) prepared from the same block. **a** Presented at a lymphoma workshop. This section is of no use for making a diagnosis. **b** This section reveals a diffuse centroblastic-centrocytic lymphoma. Skin biopsy. 440:1

from Merck (*Darmstadt,* Fed. Rep. Germany); the results obtained with all other Giemsa solutions are, as a rule, poor and often worthless. In addition to the Giemsa-stained slides, one should always examine sections stained by silver impregnation (e.g. Gomori's method), with periodic acid–Schiff (PAS) and with haematoxylin and eosin (H & E). It is also advisable to prepare an unstained section to be kept for subsequent special staining (e.g. chloroacetate esterase) if the need should arise.

6. Imprints are very useful in cytological analysis. For this purpose, we stain them with Pappenheim (May-Grünwald-Giemsa) no earlier and, if possible, not much later than 1 day after biopsy. We also apply at least acid phosphatase and acid non-specific esterase (α-naphthyl acetate esterase, pH 5.8) stains to imprints. A diffuse esterase reaction is still one of the most reliable criteria for identifying cells of the macrophage system. An acid phosphatase reaction can appear in various patterns and is of variable diagnostic value (cf. T-lymphoblastic lymphoma [p. 246], hairy cell leukaemia [p. 64], large cell anaplastic lymphoma [p. 241]). When lymphoid cells are stained with dipeptidyl peptidase IV (DPPIV) a positive reaction is specific to T cells.[3] It is possible to identify myeloid cells with the help of the peroxidase and chloroacetate esterase stains. Although other cytochemical reactions may be of scientific interest, they do not provide any additional information of significant diagnostic value.

7. One should examine lymph node sections (and imprints) *before* looking at the clinical data. Not until a preliminary diagnosis has been made should the clinical data be checked to see whether they agree with the morphological picture. The reverse procedure often puts the pathologist on the wrong track, or at least precludes an objective, independent evaluation. The most important clinical information is the age of the patient.

8. In the evaluation of lymph nodes, microscopic examination at a low magnification is of less significance than it is in the histopathological diagnosis of other organs and tissues, because the diagnosis of lymph node lesions is chiefly *cellular* and only to a lesser extent structural. Nevertheless, every histological examination of a lymph node begins with a low magnification in order to determine whether the lymph node architecture is effaced or intact. It is generally effaced in malignant neoplasms. One should be cautious, however, because it may also be effaced in reactive processes and at least partially intact in malignant neoplasms. At a low magnification, it is also possible to recognize focal lesions, metastatic tumours and lesions in the tissue surrounding the lymph node. A nodular pattern is of particular diagnostic significance.

9. When the lymph node architecture is effaced, i.e. when follicles or sinuses are not recognizable, cytological analysis at a higher, or the highest, magnification must be performed to determine the nature of the process. First, Giemsa-stained sections are examined to see whether the process is made up of a "monotonous" (uniform) or of a mixed population of cells. If the process is monotonous looking, one then determines whether the cells are small, medium sized or large.

---

[3]   Lojda 1977; Feller et al. 1982a,b, 1984; Mentlein et al. 1984.

Other criteria for defining the type of cell are: nuclear shape; number, size and location of the nucleoli; and amount and staining of the cytoplasm. Imprints are examined to find out more about the chromatin structure; they also reveal the staining properties and presence or absence of granules in the cytoplasm. Pathologists with less experience should use oil immersion for a good cytological analysis of sections as well.

10. With silver impregnation it is particularly easy to survey the lymph node architecture and to recognize a nodular or follicular growth pattern. Moreover, the number and arrangement of small vessels (capillaries and venules) can be more clearly determined with silver impregnation than with any other stain. An increase in the number of capillaries may be an indication of a histiocytic or monocytic neoplasm; an increase in the number of epithelioid venules may be a sign of a low-grade malignant T-cell neoplasm. The *amount* of reticulin fibres is not, in general, a useful criterion. Although a marked increase in the number of reticulin fibres *and capillaries* in monocytic and histiocytic neoplasms is not specific, it is of some diagnostic significance. The fibre *pattern* also helps in making a distinction between tumour metastases and malignant lymphomas (ML). Finally, silver impregnation of sections of totally necrotic lymph nodes makes the underlying architecture and, in many cases, even the tumour cells visible; this prevents a false diagnosis of a lymph node infarction and sometimes even makes it possible to determine the nature of a tumour (e.g. follicular lymphoma!).

11. When Giemsa staining reveals a monotonous looking proliferation of medium-sized cells ("lymphoblastic" proliferation), we apply chloroacetate esterase staining to exclude the possibility of a myeloid neoplasm. In addition, we always try to investigate imprints with cytochemical methods to recognize T-lymphoblastic lymphoma. When the blood picture is leukaemic, blood smears may also be used for a cytochemical characterization of the blast cells.

12. Electron microscopy seldom provides more diagnostic information than does a technically good light microscopic preparation.

13. In 10%–15% of the cases of ML it is necessary to apply immunohistochemical methods to make a diagnosis. As a rule, these methods can be used in ambiguous cases to distinguish between T-cell and B-cell lymphomas and between lymphomas and non-lymphoid undifferentiated tumours. The monoclonality of a B-cell proliferation can be recognized by demonstrating light chain restriction. In order to verify the clonal nature of a T-cell lymphoma, however, one has to use molecular genetic techniques. It is already possible to make most immunohistochemical diagnoses by examining paraffin sections. Only about 5%, at most, of the cases of non-Hodgkin's lymphoma (NHL) require an immunohistochemical analysis of cryostat sections for a definitive classification.

Even though one may have high expectations of immunohistochemistry, it is still possible to misinterpret the results. Consistent, useful results can be obtained only by regular application of the methods. An antibody may show a considerable number of "cross-reactions"; these must always be taken into consideration, especially in the interpretation of the expression of a single antigen. In a few cases it is impossible to reconcile the immunohistochemical and morphological findings. When the actively proliferating cells are labelled clearly, we favour the immunohistochemical results. In all other cases of discrepancy we rely on the morphological findings.

14. When the morphological and immunohistochemical results are contradictory and the clonality of a T-cell proliferation has to be proved, it is sensible to perform a molecular genetic analysis to determine the rearrangement of characteristic gene segments of the T-cell receptor. So far, this is the only method available for identifying the clonality of a T-cell process. The method can also be used to determine the clonality of a B-cell proliferation in which there is no expression of immunoglobulin (Ig) light chains. By applying molecular genetic techniques as an ancillary measure, it is possible to clarify nearly all cases, at least with respect to their clonality and cellular origin. We are aware that the introduction of the polymerase chain reaction (PCR) technique has opened up a whole new horizon. At present, however, there are still some unsolved problems when interpreting clonality in lymphoproliferative diseases.

15. The diagnostic report should be clear and brief. In cases in which it is not possible to determine the exact type of lymphoma, the right treatment can often be chosen if the pathologist states whether the lymphoma is of low-grade or high-grade malignancy. The pathologist should endeavour to provide this information in all cases, even if it means obtaining another biopsy.

1.2 Immunohistochemistry and Molecular Genetics as Ancillary Diagnostic Measures

The diagnostic use of immunohistochemical methods[4] can be restricted to the relatively small number (10%–15%) of lymphoproliferative processes in which the morphological findings are inconclusive. An immunohistochemical analysis in such cases has three aims:

1. Determining the cellular origin and distinguishing a lymphoma from non-lymphomatous neoplasms
2. Classification of the ML
3. Demonstration of clonality of a lymphoproliferative process

To 1: In addition to stainings for Ig, there are now a large number of antibodies that react with formalin-resistant antigens, i.e. that can be applied to *paraffin* sections. The availability of these antibodies makes it possible to determine whether a neoplasm is a T-cell or B-cell lymphoma in about 90% of the ambiguous cases. Moreover, non-lymphoid tumours can be recognized. This is especially important in the distinction of large cell undifferentiated tumours. About 80%–90% of those cases in which it is impossible to decide between an undifferentiated carcinoma and a lymphoma by morphology alone can be classified

---

[4] Reviews: Stein 1978; Taylor and Chandor 1981; Knowles II et al. 1983, 1985; Jones 1983; Van der Valk et al. 1983; Delsol et al. 1984; Pallesen et al. 1984; Stein et al. 1984b; Picker et al. 1987; Chan et al. 1988; Pallesen 1988.

Table 1. Monoclonal and polyclonal antibodies reacting in formalin-fixed, paraffin-embedded tissue. (Based on NORTON et al. 1987; DAVEY et al. 1990)

Cluster	Antibody	Lymphoid specificity [a]	LR [b]
CD15 [c]	Leu-M1, TÜ9	Myeloid cells, Sternberg-Reed cells	−
CD20-like	L26	B cells, follicular dendritic cells	+
CD30	BerH2	Activated T, B and histiocytic cells	−
CD43	MT1	T cells, B-cell subpopulation, myelomonocytic cells	+
CD45	2B11+PD7/26	Leucocyte common antigen	+
CD45R	4KB5, MB1	B cells, T-cell subpopulation	+
CD45RA	MT2	B cells, T cells	+
CD45RO	UCHL1	T cells, myelomonocytic cells	+
CD45 related	Ki-B3	B cells, T-cell subpopulation, myelomonocytic cells	+
CD68	KP1	Macrophages, monocytes, some B cells	−
CDw75	LN1	B cells, germinal centre cells, some macrophages	−
−	IgM, G, A, E	Ig heavy chains	+
−	Igϰ, λ	Ig light chains	+
−	Ki-M1p	Monocytes, macrophages, sinusoidal B cells	?
−	Ki-M4p	Follicular dendritic cells	−
−	Lysozyme	Macrophages, myeloid cells, monocytes	+
−	MB2	B cells, monocytes, macrophages	−
−	Poly CD3	T cells	−
19A2	Anti-PCNA/Cyclin	Proliferating cell nuclear antigen	−

[a] The main specificity is mentioned first.
[b] LR = leucocyte restriction.
[c] CD = leucocyte differentiation cluster.

immunohistochemically as ML, often as so-called large cell anaplastic lymphoma. Only a few antibodies are of high specificity, however. Hence several antibodies have to be used to draw up an antigen profile. Furthermore the cells of some large cell anaplastic lymphomas may express epithelial membrane antigens and occasionally even cytokeratins.[5] In such cases one also has to determine the antigen profile in order to draw reliable conclusions about the origin of the tumour cells.

Table 1 is a list of monoclonal antibodies that are suitable for diagnoses on formalin-fixed tissue. Systematic analysis of monoclonal antibodies on formalin-fixed tissue[6] is resulting in a steadily growing number of useful reagents. A relatively large number of these reagents recognize epitopes of the leucocyte common antigen (CD45), but each one also shows a certain specificity within the B- or T-cell system (CD45RA, CD45RB, CD45RO). When using these antibodies, or ones that have not yet been fully "clustered" or immunohistochemically defined, such as MT2 (CD45RA), MB2, LN1 (CDw75) or LN2 (CD74), one must remember that they have only limited cell line specificity. By including them in the making of an antigen profile, however, one can draw conclusions about the cellular origin of a lymphoid neoplasm. Introduction of the monoclonal antibody L26 (reacts with an antigen resembling CD20) has provided a B-cell reagent that

[5]   Gustmann et al. 1991.
[6]   Mason and Gatter 1987; Norton and Isaacson 1987; Poppema et al. 1987; Chittal et al. 1988; Van der Valk et al. 1989.

makes it possible to recognize more than 80% of the B-cell lymphomas and to distinguish them to a large extent from T-cell lymphomas.[7] This reaction pattern can be supplemented by demonstrating HLA class II antigens in formalin-fixed tissue[8] and the activation antigen CD30 (BcrH2). There are still only a limited number of antibodies available for demonstrating the complete macrophage system in formalin-fixed tissue. Polyclonal antibodies against muramidase (lysozyme) and monoclonal antibodies such as MAC387 or KP1 (CD68) may be considered reliable reagents, although the latter do not recognize the whole spectrum of macrophages in the lymphoreticular system. In conclusion, the availability of a steadily growing collection of monoclonal antibodies will soon make it possible to completely understand the cellular origin of ML for diagnostic purposes.

The benign or malignant nature and the cellular origin of only a small number (about 5%) of lymphoproliferative processes cannot be clarified by examining paraffin sections stained with immunohistochemical methods. In such cases it is necessary to use fresh, unfixed tissue. The tissue should be either snap-frozen (in liquid nitrogen) immediately after removal or processed within 8–10 h. Cryostat sections are then examined after staining with the indirect peroxidase or the alkaline phosphatase–anti-alkaline phosphatase (APAAP) method (cf. Addendum, p. 271). Other investigators prefer the avidin-biotin method.[9] For demonstrating Ig in paraffin sections the streptavidin method is evidently most helpful.[10] Excellent results can also be obtained by visualization of mRNA.[10a]

An antigen profile of an infiltrate showing a partial antigen loss in comparison with normal lymphoid cells is an indication of a neoplastic, non-reactive proliferation. This is especially helpful in the diagnosis of T-cell lymphomas.[11] Viral infections in lymph nodes, however, may also result in a partial antigen loss in blast cells.

Another advantage of examining fresh tissue is the possibility of using the Ki-67 antibody. The proliferative activity of tumour cells can be determined quickly and reliably with this antibody.[12] Recently the PCNA/cyclin method was introduced for determining the proliferation index in paraffin sections.[12a] The results obtained with this method, however, are not always directly comparable with those obtained with Ki-67.

With fresh tissue it is also possible to demonstrate clonality and the cellular origin of the proliferating cells by doing molecular genetic analyses by DNA and RNA extraction.

Table 2 is a selected list of currently available monoclonal antibodies that we consider to be suitable for immunohistochemical diagnoses on fresh tissue. The antibodies are listed next to defined clusters, allowing a comparative analysis when various antibodies are used. The clusters are defined by the antigens whose

---

[7]   Cartun et al. 1987; Hamilton-Dutoit and Pallesen 1989.
[8]   Sorg et al. 1985.
[9]   Hsu et al. 1981; Norton and Isaacson 1987.
[10] P. Isaacson, personal communication.
[10a] Pringle et al. 1990
[11] Hastrup et al. 1989.
[12] Gerdes et al. 1984.
[12a] Hall et al. 1990; Dierendonck et al. 1991; Kamel et al. 1991.

molecular weight has been determined and that react in the same manner with certain cell populations (including cell lines).

To 2: The antigen profiles given in Tables 3–5 are characteristic immunohisto-chemical reaction patterns of ML. One must bear in mind, however, that there are no absolute criteria. Hence a deviation from the characteristic antigen profile must be considered possible in each case. Only the use of a combination of antibodies makes it possible to classify a lymphoma as a defined entity with a high probability. It is not permissible to interpret the expression of a single antigen by itself.[13]

To 3: The clonality of a lymphoproliferative process still serves as an important criterion for determining its benign or malignant nature. Although biclonal B-cell lymphomas, polyclonal EBV-induced B-cell lymphomas[14] and monoclonal be-nign tumours (e.g. meningioma[15]) have been described, in ambiguous cases clon-ality is still the most important diagnostic criterion of malignancy in addition to the histological and clinical pictures.

In the B-cell system clonality is usually quite easy to prove in about two-thirds of the lymphomas. In paraffin or cryostat sections the Ig must belong to only *one* class, i.e. one must find sole, or at least predominant (10:1 or higher), expression of only *one* light chain type. It is usually possible to demonstrate light chain restriction on paraffin sections, especially when cytoplasmic Ig (cIg) is present in some of the tumour cells. When only surface Ig (sIg) is expressed, the demonstration of light chain restriction is not always successful; in such cases frozen tissue has to be examined. Occasionally, even sIg is lacking, in which case one has to depend on a molecular genetic analysis of Ig genes.

It is now possible to determine the clonality of T cells with DNA probes for T-cell receptor (TcR) genes. Such analyses use DNA probes that code for defined segments of the TcR gene complex ($\alpha, \beta, \gamma, \delta$). Ig genes can also be recognized with DNA probes for joining or constant regions.

During the differentiation of a cell in the B-cell or T-cell system the various segments of the TcR genes and Ig genes are rearranged. This means that the gene segments (dispersed over the chromosome within the gene locus) are first rear-ranged in order to form a functional gene that can then be transcribed. The rearranged gene segments or those that have remained in the germ line are frag-mented by restriction enzymes and then electrophoretically separated. In a *poly-clonal* lymphoproliferative process this results in fragments of multiple sizes. Since these fragments are present in small amounts in each localization, they cannot be visualized with the corresponding radioactively labelled DNA probe. In contrast, a *monoclonal* lymphoproliferative process is characterized by identi-cal rearrangement of the gene segments of one cell clone. Hence fragments of the same size can be separated by electrophoresis to the same point. The labelling of these fragments can be made visible by autoradiography because of their greater quantity. Such a molecular genetic analysis makes it possible to recognize mono-clonal proliferations that make up at least 3%–5% of a cell population.

---

[13] Pallesen 1988.
[14] Frizzera 1987.
[15] Zankl et al. 1979.

Table 2. Recognizable antigens and antibodies suitable for the diagnosis of malignant lymphoma, lymphoid leukaemia and myelomonocytic leukaemia. (Based on KNAPP et al. 1989)

Cluster	Antibody	Lymphohistiocytic specificity
CD1[a]	T6, VIT6, Leu-6, NA1/34	Thymic cortex, Langerhans cells, interdigitating cells
CD2	Lyt3, T11, Leu-5, 9.6	Sheep erythrocyte receptor
CD3	OKT3, Leu-4, UCHT1	All T cells
CD4	T4, Leu-3a	Helper/inducer T cells
CD5	Leu-1, T1, T101	T lymphocytes, B-cell subpopulation
CD6	T12, T411	T lymphocytes, B-cell subpopulation
CD7	TÜ14, 3A1, Leu-9	85% of peripheral T lymphocytes, thymic cortex
CD8	T8, Leu-2a	Suppressor/cytotoxic T cells
CD9	FMC8, BA2	Immature cells, monocytes, thrombocytes
CD10	VIL-A1, J5, BA3	Common ALL antigen
CD11a	OKM1, Leu-15	Monocytes, granulocytes, NK[b] cells
CD11b	VIM12, Mo1	Monocytes, granulocytes, C3bi receptor
CD11c	Ki-M1, SHC-L3, Leu-M5	Monocytes, granulocytes
CD13	MY7	Monocytes, granulocytes, NK cells
CD14	Leu-M3, UCHM1, VIM13	Monocytes, granulocytes, follicular dendritic cells
CD15	VIM-D5, Leu-M1, 3C4	Granulocytes, Hodgkin cells, X-hapten
CD16	Leu-11	Granulocytes, NK cells, FcIgG receptor
CD19	B4, HD37	B cells
CD20	B1, 2H7, L26	B-cell subpopulation, follicular dendritic cells
CD21	B2, HB5, BL-14	B-cell subpopulation, a few cases of T-ALL, follicular dendritic cells, C3d/EBV receptor
CD22	To15, HD39, HD6	All B cells
CD23	PL13, Ki-B1, TÜ1	"Follicular mantle" cells, follicular dendritic cells
CD24	BA-1, VIBC5, HB8	All B cells, granulocytes
CD25	TAC, 2A3	IL-2 receptor-α-chain, activated T and B cells
CD26	Anti-DPPIV, TS145	Activated T cells (diaminopeptidase IV)
CD28	9.3, KOLT2	T-cell subpopulation
CD29	4B4	T-cell subpopulation
CD30	Ki-1, HRS-1, BerH2	Activation antigen, Hodgkin cells, Sternberg-Reed cells
CDw32	2E1	Monocytes, granulocytes, thrombocytes, B-cells, Fc receptor
CD33	MY9	Myelomonocytic cells
CD34	MY10	B-cell precursors, myeloid precursors
CD35	To5, CR1	C3b receptor, granulocytes, monocytes, follicular dendritic cells
CD37	HD28	B cells
CD38	T10, HB7	Immature bone marrow cells, plasma cells, activated T cells
CD39	G28-10	Follicular mantle cells, follicular dendritic cells, extrafollicular B cells
CD43	MT1	T cells, B-cell subpopulation, myelomonocytic cells
CD45	T200, T29/33	Common leucocyte antigen
CD45RA	F8-11-13	Common leucocyte antigen
CD45RB	PD7/26/16	Common leucocyte antigen

Table 2. (continued)

Cluster	Antibody	Lymphohistiocytic specificity
CD45RO	UCHL1	Common leucocyte antigen (mostly T cells)
CD57	Leu-7	NK cells, T-cell and B-cell subpopulation
CD68	Ki-M6	Monocytes, macrophages
CD72	S-HCL2	B cells
CD74	LN2	B cells, monocytes, macrophages
CDw75	LN1	B cells, T-cell subpopulation
CD77	38.13	B-cell subpopulation (in germinal centres)

[a] CD = leucocyte differentiation cluster.
[b] NK = natural killer.

Table 3. Characteristic antigen expression in low-grade malignant B-cell lymphomas

	sIg	cIg	CD22	CD10	CD5	CD23	CD11c
B-CLL	+	−	+	−	+	+	−
B-PLL	+	−	+	−	+	−	−
Hairy cell leukaemia	+	−	+	−	−	−	+
Immunocytoma	+	+	+	−	+/−	+	−
Plasmacytoma	+	+	−	−	−	−	−
ML centroblastic-centrocytic	+	−	+	+	−	−	−
ML centrocytic	+	−	+	−	+	−	−

Table 4. Characteristic antigen expression in high-grade malignant B-cell lymphomas

	sIg	cIg	CD21	CD22	CD10	CD30
ML centroblastic	+	−/+	−/+	+	+/−	−
ML immunoblastic	+	+/−	−/+	+	−	−
ML lymphoblastic	−/+	−	−/+	+	+/−	−
Burkitt's lymphoma	+	−	−	+	+	−
cIg + Burkitt's lymphoma	+	+	−	+	−	−
ML large cell anaplastic	−	−	NA[a]	+	−	+

[a] NA = not analysed.

Table 5. Antigen expression in low-grade and high-grade malignant T-cell lymphomas

	CD1	CD2	CD3	CD4	CD5	CD7	CD8	CD30
T-CLL	−	+	+	+/−	+	+/−	−/+	−
T-PLL	−	+	+	+/−	+	+	−/+	−
Mycosis fungoides	−	+	+	+	+	−/+	−	−/+
LeL	−	+	+	+	+	−/+	−	−
AILD (LgX) type	−	+	+	+	+	−/+	−/+	−
T-zone lymphoma	−	+	+	+	+	+/−	−	−
ML pleomorphic	−	+	+	+/−	+	+/−	−/+	−/+
ML immunoblastic	−	+/−	+	+/−	+	+/−	−/+	−/+
ML large cell anaplastic	−	+/−	−/+	+/−	−/+	−	−/+	+
ML lymphoblastic	+/−	+/−	+/−	+/−	+/−	+	−/+	−

The demonstration of TcR gene rearrangement is an additional indication of the T-cell origin of a cell proliferation. Correspondingly, the demonstration of rearrangement of the heavy and light Ig chain genes can be considered proof of the B-cell nature of a cell proliferation. Immature cells (lymphoblasts) that have not yet gone through a final determination sometimes show simultaneous rearrangement of both the β chain of the TcR gene and the Ig heavy chain genes.[16] Clonality can also be proven by PCR in a number of cases.[16a]

Immunophenotyping and molecular genetic rearrangement studies now make it possible to place a vast majority of the lymphomas in the B-cell or T-cell system.[17] So-called null cell lymphomas are probably extremely rare exceptions.[18]

[16] Waldmann et al. 1985; Griesser et al. 1986; O'Connor 1987.
[16a] E.g. Trainor et al. 1990.
[17] Pelicci et al. 1985.
[18] Knowles II et al. 1985.

2 The Kiel Classification

2.1 Principles

The old simple classification[19] used in Germany until the introduction of the Kiel classification differed from the classification recommended by RAPPAPORT,[20] which has been widely accepted in Western countries because of its apparent clinical relevance. Since neither the old German classification nor RAPPAPORT's classification is compatible with the knowledge gained from modern research in immunology, it was clearly necessary to apply the results of this research to neoplasms of lymphocytes and their variants. This required taking three steps: (1) the various cell types of lymphoid tissue (and lymphoid neoplasms) had to be defined by haematological and cytochemical methods; (2) the immunological characteristics ("markers") of the morphologically identified cells had to be determined; and (3) lymphoma cells had to be morphologically and immunologically matched with their normal counterparts. These investigations led to a new understanding of ML. By taking the criteria of general pathology and haematology and the clinical behaviour of ML into consideration, it was then possible to propose a new classification. The so-called Kiel classification[21] (Table 6) is based on that proposition.

LUKES and COLLINS[22] followed a similar course. First, they used the shape of the nuclei to characterize lymphoid cells. They distinguished follicular centre cells (FCC) with cleaved nuclei from those with non-cleaved nuclei, and lymphoid cells with convoluted nuclei. At the same time, their diagnostic labels indicated whether a lymphoma is composed of B cells, T cells or "undefined" cells. In contrast, the main terms used in the Kiel classification were originally morphological ones; "B" and "T" were found only in the names of some of the subtypes. The main terms for many B-cell lymphomas indicate that they are derived from the B-cell system (e.g. immunocytoma, plasmacytoma and all germinal centre cell tumours), even without the "B" prefix.

Other guiding principles of the Kiel classification are:

1. The cellular composition is of primary importance. This distinguishes the Kiel classification from most other classifications, whose first criterion is the growth pattern of the lymphoma (diffuse or nodular).

---

[19] Lennert 1967, 1969.
[20] 1966.
[21] Gérard-Marchant et al. 1974; Lennert et al. 1975; Lennert 1976.
[22] 1974a,b, 1975a,b; Collins et al. 1976; Lukes et al. 1978a.

2. A distinction is made between low-grade and high-grade ML. The low-grade
ML consist of "-cytes", but may also contain a certain number of "-blasts"; the
high-grade ML consist of "-blasts". In other words, low-grade ML are usually
composed of small cells, which are sometimes interspersed with large cells. High-
grade ML are mainly composed of medium-sized to large cells.
3. Since practically all types of ML may be associated with a leukaemic blood
picture, and since it is often impossible to predict this histologically, leukaemias
and "solid" lymphomas have been placed together in the Kiel classification.
4. Because paraproteinaemia (e.g. macroglobulinaemia) is a facultative phenomenon in Ig-producing lymphomas, the disease is defined by its underlying
morphological characteristics alone (e.g. immunocytoma).
5. All types of high-grade ML, with the exception of lymphoblastic lymphoma,
can be either primary or secondary. A secondary high-grade ML develops out of
a low-grade ML of the same cell class. This transformation represents evolution
and not the development of a different neoplasm. Hence we avoid using the term
"composite lymphoma". Secondary high-grade ML is diagnosed as soon as the
cells in at least one circumscribed area of a low-grade ML show homogeneous
transformation into large cells of the same class.

Publication of the Kiel classification was soon followed by numerous favourable
reports of both its applicability in histopathological diagnosis[23] and its clinical
relevance.[24] There have also been several monographs and reviews based on the
Kiel classification.[25] The new classification was also positively rated in textbooks
and handbooks on (lymph node) pathology.[26] Some of the reactions to the
classification, however, were critical. These will be discussed in Sect. 2.2.
    Even we were not completely satisfied with our classification, especially be-
cause a relatively high percentage (12%[27]) of lymphomas still could not be
classified. Hence we strove for an increasingly detailed immunohistochemical
definition of the various lymphoma types.[28] We also applied molecular genetic
methods[29] and re-embedded tissue in synthetics[30] in order to achieve a description of the cytological details as exact and as reproducible as possible, especially
in cases of T-cell lymphoma and high-grade malignant B-cell lymphoma. As a
result, we had to re-evaluate the existing, "tried and true" Kiel classification,
revise and add to it, and use more precise terms where necessary. In particular,

[23] Gérard-Marchant 1974a,b; Robb-Smith 1975; Dühmke 1976; Sandritter and Grimm 1977;
    Becker 1978; Fischer 1978; Heimann et al. 1978; Kelényi 1978; Georgii et al. 1979; Vanden
    Heule et al. 1979; Shtern 1980.
[24] Musshoff et al. 1976; Bremer et al. 1977; Brittinger et al. 1977, 1978; Mandard et al. 1977;
    Braun-Falco et al. 1978; Delbrück et al. 1978; Garwicz et al. 1978; Machado et al. 1978;
    Meugé et al. 1978; Takácsi-Nagy et al. 1978; Diehl et al. 1979; Musshoff 1979; Glimelius et
    al. 1983; Porwit-Ksiazek and Mioduszewska 1983; Leonard et al. 1983; Lieberman et al.
    1986.
[25] Rilke et al. 1978a, 1980; Rivas and Oliva 1980; Plank et al. 1983; Wright and Isaacson 1983;
    Pileri 1985; Stansfeld 1985; Fischer 1986.
[26] E.g. Symmers 1978; Robb-Smith and Taylor 1981.
[27] Lennert et al. 1975.
[28] Stein et al. 1984a.
[29] O'Connor et al. 1985; Griesser et al. 1986a, 1987, 1989; Tkachuk et al. 1988.
[30] Hui et al. 1988.

Table 6. Kiel classification of non-Hodgkin's lymphomas (originally published in 1974; modification of the version published in 1978)

Low-grade malignant lymphomas

Lymphocytic
  B-CLL
  T-CLL
  Hairy cell leukaemia
  Mycosis fungoides and Sézary's syndrome
  T-zone lymphoma

Lymphoplasmacytic/-cytoid (immunocytoma)

Plasmacytic

Centrocytic

Centroblastic-centrocytic
  follicular ± diffuse
  diffuse
  ± sclerosis

High-grade malignant lymphomas

Centroblastic

Lymphoblastic
  Burkitt type
  convoluted-cell type
  unclassified

Immunoblastic

---

it had become possible to classify the relatively rare T-cell lymphomas and to add new entities that were previously not, or not definitely, considered to be NHL (e.g. lymphoepithelioid lymphoma, AILD/LgX type). Moreover, we had to include large cell anaplastic lymphoma (LCAL), which had been identified with the monoclonal antibody Ki-1 (CD30). Finally, the B-cell lymphomas of high-grade malignancy that were difficult to distinguish morphologically from one another were reclassified.

In 1988 the European Lymphoma Club decided to introduce an updated Kiel classification, with separate columns for B-cell and T-cell types (Table 7). The B-cell lymphoma column differs in only two major respects from the previous Kiel classification. First, LCAL has been added. Second, Burkitt's lymphoma has been separated from the lymphoblastic lymphomas, because it can be clearly defined morphologically and it shows hardly any immunohistochemical relationships to the lymphoblastic lymphomas of the B-cell series; even the chromosomal abnormalities found in Burkitt's lymphoma may differ somewhat from those observed in lymphoblastic lymphoma.[31] Another, minor difference is the placement of monocytoid B-cell lymphoma, which has been moved from the list of *rare types* to the main entities. Table 7 reveals that the separation into low-grade and high-grade ML has been kept in the updated classification, even though the greater morphological variability of T-cell lymphomas makes it diffi-

---

[31] Rowley 1984; Fletcher et al. 1991; Pui et al. 1991.

Table 7. Updated Kiel classification of non-Hodgkin's lymphomas (1988) with a few additions

B	T
Low-grade malignant lymphomas	
Lymphocytic	Lymphocytic
Chronic lymphocytic leukaemia	Chronic lymphocytic leukaemia
Prolymphocytic leukaemia	Prolymphocytic leukaemia
Hairy-cell leukaemia	
	Small cell, cerebriform
	Mycosis fungoides, Sézary's syndrome
Lymphoplasmacytic/-cytoid (immunocytoma)	Lymphoepithelioid (Lennert's lymphoma)
Plasmacytic	Angioimmunoblastic (AILD, LgX)
Centroblastic-centrocytic	T-zone lymphoma
follicular ± diffuse	
diffuse	
Centrocytic (mantle cell)	Pleomorphic, small cell (HTLV-1 ±)
Monocytoid, including marginal zone cell	
High-grade malignant lymphomas	
Centroblastic	Pleomorphic, medium-sized and large cell (HTLV-1 ±)
Immunoblastic	Immunoblastic (HTLV-1 ±)
Burkitt's lymphoma	
Large cell anaplastic (Ki-1 +)	Large cell anaplastic (Ki-1 +)
Lymphoblastic	Lymphoblastic
Rare types	*Rare types*

cult to draw strict lines. In the table it is also evident that several types of ML occur in both the B-cell and the T-cell system with the same or similar morphological appearances (chronic lymphocytic leukaemia, prolymphocytic leukaemia, immunoblastic lymphoma, LCAL, and lymphoblastic lymphoma). Follicular centroblastic-centrocytic lymphoma has an equivalent in the T-cell column, namely T-zone lymphoma. Functional activity of B-cell lymphoma cells leads to Ig secretion; examples of this are immunocytoma and plasmacytoma. Functional activity of T-cell lymphoma cells leads to the production of lymphokines; examples of this are lymphoepithelioid lymphoma and the AILD (LgX) type. Hence there are a number of parallels in morphology and signs of function between the B-cell and T-cell lymphomas. We have taken these parallels into account in the table by placing corresponding B-cell and T-cell lymphomas opposite each other. This should make it easier to remember the classification.

By moving lymphoblastic lymphoma to the end of the table and separating it with a broken line, we wish to point out the special status of these lymphomas, which represent neoplasms of precursor cells. All other lymphoma types, perhaps with the exception of LCAL, are derived from peripheral lymphocytes and their activation or proliferation forms.

We have added a category called "rare types". In the B-cell series it originally contained monocytoid B-cell lymphoma and large cell sclerosing B-cell lymphoma of the mediastinum. After publication of the updated Kiel classification, however, we realized that monocytoid B-cell lymphoma is not as rare as it appeared to be at first. Hence we have now included monocytoid B-cell lymphoma as the last category in the group of low-grade malignant B-cell lymphomas. We have added two other types to the "rare types" category, viz. microvillous, large cell lymphoma and high-grade malignant B-cell lymphomas with a high content of T cells.

The "rare types" in the T-cell series include hairy cell leukaemia of T type, the large cell multilobated type of PINKUS,[32] erythrophagocytic Tγ lymphoma, ML of plasmacytoid T cells, lymphohistiocytic lymphoma, peripheral T-cell lymphoma associated with haemophagocytic syndrome, signet-ring cell lymphoma of T-cell type, Liebow's lymphomatoid granulomatosis and angiocentric lymphoma. With some of these "rare" lymphomas there is dispute as to their existence or nature or as to the justification for recognizing them as separate entities.

When the updated Kiel classification was first made public,[33] we were criticized for leaving out polymorphic immunocytoma. The reasons for not including this subtype in the table were as follows.

1. Subgroups of the lymphoma types were excluded wherever possible in order to maintain clarity. This was done with other entities as well, such as centroblastic-centrocytic lymphoma and centroblastic lymphoma.
2. Polymorphic immunocytoma is diagnosed more often than it actually occurs. Including it in the table would just further this tendency.

Table 7 is not supposed to imply that all ML are classifiable. There are still a small number of cases (approx. 1%) that cannot be classified even with the best morphological and immunological techniques. In most "unclassified" cases, however, the reason for the imprecise diagnosis is shortcomings in the biopsy excision or processing techniques. Nevertheless, even poorly prepared slides usually allow the pathologist to say whether it is a case of low-grade or high-grade ML. This gives the clinician at least one criterion on which to base treatment.

The updated Kiel classification of nodal lymphomas, including thymic lymphomas (and covering most cutaneous lymphomas), presented here reflects the current limits of classification that can be reached with the morphological and immunohistochemical methods available at present. Further studies may result in minor variations or reveal rare special types. It is unlikely, however, that any of the basic entities of the classification will have to undergo significant changes. If a change should actually become necessary—we are thinking of and hoping especially for a simplification—this would result only from systematic application of new methods such as those of classic and molecular cytogenetics. It would

---

[32] Pinkus et al. 1979.
[33] Meeting of the European Association for Haematopathology in Geneva, March 1988.

certainly be necessary to expand the Kiel classification if we were to include all the extranodal lymphomas, especially those of the mucosa-associated lymphoid tissue (MALT). On the other hand, it might be more sensible to ascertain whether different systems of organs develop different types of lymphomas, which would necessitate separate classifications.

2.2 Pros and Cons

The main *advantages* of the Kiel classification are the following.

1. The Kiel classification makes it possible to apply experience gained in experimental immunology to neoplasms of cells of the immune system. This holds true not only for the separation of tumours into B-cell and T-cell types. Most lymphomas can be associated with various phases of development or functional activity of lymphocytes. The Kiel classification is not an abstract, purely descriptive construct. On the contrary, it is guided by physiological models and their morphological appearances. It can be understood and learned accordingly.

2. It is possible to roughly separate ML into low-grade and high-grade categories by looking at routine sections, without immunohistochemical or other special stainings. This is of great practical significance, because in cases of high-grade ML the clinician can start treatment immediately, without having to wait for a detailed report.

The principle of separating ML into low-grade and high-grade categories has also proved to be correct in relation to survival. Patients with low-grade ML in stages III and IV, with the possible exception of centroblastic-centrocytic lymphoma patients in stage III, show a steady mortality rate and are not curable with presently available treatment regimens. In contrast, long-term full remission can be achieved in a considerable number of patients with high-grade ML in the same stages. This is evident as a plateau in the survival curve (see Fig. 17).

A biological justification for distinguishing low-grade and high-grade ML has been provided by analyses of the percentage of proliferating cells. GERDES et al.[34] showed that, in spite of individual variations, there is a relatively sharp line between low-grade and high-grade ML, which can be drawn by comparing the percentages of Ki-67-positive cells in the various entities (Fig. 3).

3. The morphologically defined entities prove in part to be distinguishable as entities with immunocytochemical methods. Sometimes a morphological classification is more exact; sometimes immunocytochemistry has to be applied in order to classify a lymphoma as belonging to the B-cell or T-cell system. Contradictions between good morphological slides and immunocytochemical data are rare. In such cases, all the criteria have to be considered with scrupulous care.

4. In 80 % of the cases of ML immunocytochemical analyses are unnecessary for a diagnosis. In approximately 15 % of cases it is currently easy to make a diagnosis on paraffin sections stained with immunological methods. Only the

---

[34] 1984.

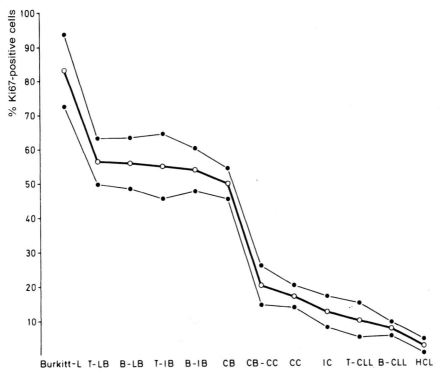

Fig. 3. Growth fractions in various types of non-Hodgkin's lymphoma, expressed in terms of the percentage of Ki-67-positive cells in frozen sections. The *bold line* represents the median values, the two *thin lines* show the standard deviations. *Burkitt-L* = Burkitt's lymphoma. *T-LB* = lymphoblastic lymphoma of T-cell type. *B-LB* = lymphoblastic lymphoma of B-cell type. *T-IB* = immunoblastic lymphoma of T-cell type. *B-IB* = immunoblastic lymphoma of B-cell type. *CB* = centroblastic lymphoma. *CB-CC* = centroblastic-centrocytic lymphoma. *CC* = centrocytic lymphoma. *IC* = immunocytoma. *T-CLL* = chronic lymphocytic leukaemia of T-cell type. *B-CLL* = chronic lymphocytic leukaemia of B-cell type. *HCL* = hairy cell leukaemia. (Based on data from GERDES et al. 1984)

remaining 5 % still require an immunocytochemical analysis of cryostat sections. It is likely that in a few years the cryostat technique will be unnecessary for diagnostic purposes, and all diagnostically important information will be obtainable from paraffin sections. It is important, however, to be aware of the increasing evidence that viral infections are involved in the multistep development of ML. At present we still need snap-frozen tissue to identify such tumours.

5. The entities of the Kiel classification were defined on the basis of sections stained with the Giemsa method customarily used in haematology. This makes it possible to apply the Kiel classification to smears or imprints of clinical cytologists and haematologists.[35] Hence many clinical haematologists prefer our classification.[36]

---

[35] Schwarze 1986.
[36] E.g. Lopes Cardozo 1976; Orell and Skinner 1982; D. A. G. Galton, personal communication; F. G. J. Hayhoe, personal communication.

6. The subtle morphological and immunocytochemical analysis of lymphomas provides a solid basis on which to perform classic cytogenetic and molecular genetic studies of ML.

7. With the help of an immunologically defined classification it is possible to understand the nature of the lymphomas that develop secondarily in certain diseases (e.g. immune disorders) or as a result of exposure to a pathogen.

8. The term "composite lymphoma" is for the most part unnecessary. In almost all such cases the tumours are high-grade malignant variants of the same cell class that develop out of a low-grade malignant variant (analogous to the blast crisis in chronic myeloid leukaemia; cf. p. 14).

The most important *arguments against* the Kiel classification can be summarized according to the criteria that RAPPAPORT[37] considers to be essential for the approval of new classifications.

1. The Kiel classification is too complicated and cannot be learned by a non-specialized pathologist.

Contra: It is not surprising that the classification of lymphomas is complicated. The immunological lymphocyte system is functionally and, to some extent, morphologically so differentiated and diverse that the tumours derived from these cells must reflect this diversity. Moreover, morphological differences, especially those between small lymphoid cells, are very subtle and can be made out only with the best morphological techniques or with immunohistological methods. Why get upset over the diversity of ML when there is full acceptance of the diversity of soft tissue tumours?[38] Likewise, the FAB classification of acute myeloid leukaemia recognizes considerable diversity: the most recent "working classification"[39] distinguishes no less than ten subtypes. Nothing is to be achieved by simplification at any price.

The question whether the Kiel classification can be learned by a non-specialized pathologist cannot be answered with a simple no. It is true, however, that learning the Kiel classification requires a concentrated effort and a minimum of adequate techniques (good paraffin embedding, a few antibodies suitable for paraffin sections). As a matter of fact, the Kiel classification is practised successfully by several hundred pathologists, particularly in Europe but also in other parts of the world. A prerequisite for proficiency in making diagnoses according to the Kiel classification has been attendance at one or more of our tutorials or workshops. These meetings have also resulted in the establishment of new study groups, which meet together regularly to discuss their cases.

We think that the two fundamental distinctions drawn in the updated Kiel classification, i.e. between low-grade and high-grade malignancy and between B-cell and T-cell lymphomas, make this classification relatively easy to learn. The lymphoma types in the four main groups are arranged so that morphologically

---

[37] Presented at numerous meetings and tutorials.
[38] Enzinger and Weiss 1988.
[39] Second MIC Cooperative Study Group 1988.

and functionally equivalent or similar entities are listed opposite each other in the B-cell and T-cell columns. The precursor cell lymphomas are placed in a separate group and listed as the last high-grade malignant variant (see Table 7).

It must be openly admitted, however, that a general pathologist who sees a lymphoma *once* a week, who does not use special techniques and who gets his knowledge only from books will hardly be able to gain the skill required to make a diagnosis that is up-to-date and widely expected by clinicians. A pathologist who does not want, or is not able, to take the trouble to learn modern lymphoma diagnostics and use the appropriate methods may send his cases to an experienced colleague or a specialized institution. Optimum care of the patient should not be jeopardized by an inaccurate or uncertain initial diagnosis.

2. The Kiel classification is not reproducible, or at least not more so than other classifications.

Contra: This argument is based on the results of a National Cancer Institute (NCI) study[40] (see p. 23). It is true that the rate of reproducibility varied for various reasons and was by no means encouraging. DORFMAN,[41] however, has already justly pointed out that the results of the NCI study were of only very limited use because the factor of fatigue played a significant role. In our opinion, the poor reproducibility was due more to the quality and type of the histological slides. When only H & E stainings are available and the slides are not prepared in one's own laboratory, one cannot be as confident in making a diagnosis as with one's own material. Every pathologist lives on his own artefacts!

Recently, a study of the reproducibility of our classification of T-cell lymphomas was published[42] in which the authors concluded that the reproducibility was inadequate. In a Letter to the Editor[43] we commented at some length on this and pointed out that such a study cannot be done without controlling the quality of the histological material or without sufficient training of the panelists. It is foolish to think that one can learn and employ a difficult classification like that of T-cell lymphomas just by reading a short summary of it. This became obvious during the NCI study.

If we want to talk about self-reproducibility, we should not limit ourselves to something as difficult as lymphoma diagnostics. There are innumerable statistics on supposedly much simpler tumours of all different types that often show a reproducibility rate of 50% or less.

3. It has not been proven that the Kiel classification is more clinically relevant than other, simpler classifications.[44]

---

[40] The Non-Hodgkin's Lymphoma Pathologic Classification Project 1982.
[41] 1983.
[42] Hastrup et al. 1991.
[43] Feller et al. 1991.
[44] The Non-Hodgkin's Lymphoma Pathologic Classification Project 1982; Rosenberg 1983 and many others.

Contra: This may be true for survival curves; but other important data, such as blood leucocyte counts or blood protein values, were not evaluated in the NCI study. In contrast, the retrospective and prospective evaluations of two large series by the Kiel Lymphoma Study Group (under the direction of G. BRIT-TINGER) provided innumerable details that verify the relevance of the Kiel classification on the basis of numerous clinical parameters.[45]

4. So far as we know, our classification has not been called scientifically incorrect, even though suggestions for improvement have been made at various times.[46] We take such suggestions into consideration in the following description of each entity, or we explain why they were not followed.

2.3 Comparison with Other Lymphoma Classifications, Including the Working Formulation[47]

In the early 1970s, several purely morphologically oriented classifications of NHL were suggested in view of new classificatons based on the current immunological concepts (Lukes-Collins classification,[48] Kiel classification[49]). The classification of DORFMAN[50] was a variant of the Rappaport classification. The latter was proposed by RAPPAPORT[51] in 1956, finalized in the AFIP Fascicle "Tumors of the Hematopoietic System" in 1966[52] and then revised in 1976.[53] The classification of the British National Lymphoma Investigation,[54] the WHO classification[55] and the classification of the Japanese Lymphoma Study Group[56] were independently proposed at about the same time.

In fact, in the United States a dispute developed on the widely used Rappaport classification versus the two new immunologically oriented classifications. Whereas it was almost impossible to translate from the Rappaport classification into the Kiel classification and vice versa[57] (see Table 8), it was relatively easy to translate back and forth between the Lukes-Collins classification and the Kiel classification.[58] The Rappaport classification was simple to use and had proved to be prognostically relevant in numerous clinical studies in the 1960s. The differ-

---

[45] Brittinger et al. 1979a,b, 1984.
[46] Lieberman et al. 1986.
[47] This chapter was written with the authoritative assistance of F. Rilke.
[48] Lukes and Collins 1974a,b; Lukes et al. 1978b.
[49] Gérard-Marchant et al. 1974; Lennert et al. 1975; Lennert 1976, 1978.
[50] 1974.
[51] Rappaport et al. 1956.
[52] Rappaport 1966.
[53] Nathwani et al. 1976.
[54] Bennett et al. 1974.
[55] Mathé et al. 1976.
[56] Suchi et al. 1979; cf. The T- and B-Cell Malignancy Study Group 1981.
[57] Krüger et al. 1981.
[58] Lennert et al. 1983.

Table 8. Entities of the Kiel classification (1974, 1978) and their equivalents in the classification of RAPPAPORT (1966)

Kiel classification	Rappaport classification
Low-grade malignant lymphomas	
Lymphocytic	ML, lymphocytic, well differentiated, diffuse
B-CLL	
T-CLL	
Hairy cell leukaemia	
Mycosis fungoides and Sézary's syndrome	
T-zone lymphoma	
Lymphoplasmacytic/-cytoid (immunocytoma)	ML, lymphocytic with dysproteinemia
Plasmacytic	
Centrocytic	⎰ ML, lymphocytic, well differentiated, nodular or diffuse ⎱ ML, lymphocytic, poorly differentiated, nodular or diffuse
Centroblastic-centrocytic follicular ± diffuse diffuse ± sclerosis	ML, lymphocytic, well differentiated, nodular or diffuse ML, lymphocytic, poorly differentiated, nodular or diffuse ML, mixed (lymphocytic-histiocytic), nodular or diffuse ML, histiocytic, nodular or diffuse
High-grade malignant lymphomas	
Centroblastic	⎰ ML, histiocytic, nodular or diffuse ⎱ ML, undifferentiated, nodular or diffuse
Lymphoblastic Burkitt type convoluted-cell type unclassified	ML, undifferentiated, diffuse ML, lymphocytic, poorly differentiated, diffuse
Immunoblastic	ML, histiocytic diffuse

ence between nodular and diffuse lymphomas was particularly emphasized. It soon became clear, however, that the Rappaport classification was not consistent with the results of modern immunology, i.e. with new concepts of the lymphoid system. Nevertheless, clinical oncologists and others in the United States insisted on further use of the Rappaport classification because of its simplicity and clinical relevance (clinical studies using the more modern classifications had not yet been done or were incomplete).

This did not solve the problem, however. Five other classifications had been proposed and were also defended emphatically by their proponents. A compromise agreement was not attained at the meeting at Airlie House in Warrenton, Virginia, USA (in 1975). In view of this situation, a large-scale study was designed, organized and supported financially by the National Cancer Institute (NCI) of the United States that would permit all authors of the new classifications of NHL, as well as selected pathologists who were not committed to any partic-

Table 9. Entities of the Working Formulation and their equivalents in the Kiel classification

Working Formulation	Kiel equivalent

Low grade

A. *Malignant lymphoma*
   Small lymphocytic
    consistent with CLL   ML lymphocytic, CLL
    plasmacytoid   ML lymphoplasmacytic/-cytoid

B. *Malignant lymphoma, follicular*
   Predominantly small cleaved cell
    diffuse areas
    sclerosis   ML centroblastic-centrocytic (small cell)
                                      follicular ± diffuse

C. *Malignant lymphoma, follicular*
   Mixed, small cleaved and large cell
    diffuse areas
    sclerosis

Intermediate grade

D. *Malignant lymphoma, follicular*
   Predominantly large cell   ML centroblastic-centrocytic (large cell),
    diffuse areas   follicular ± diffuse?
    sclerosis   ML centroblastic, follicular

E. *Malignant lymphoma, diffuse*
   Small cleaved cell   ML centrocytic, small cell?
    sclerosis

F. *Malignant lymphoma, diffuse*   ML centroblastic-centrocytic,
   Mixed, small and large cell   diffuse
    sclerosis   ML lymphoplasmacytic/-cytoid, polymorphic
    epithelioid cell component   T-zone lymphoma

G. *Malignant lymphoma, diffuse*
   Large cell
    cleaved cell   ML centrocytic, large cell?
    noncleaved cell   ML centroblastic, diffuse

High grade

H. *Malignant lymphoma*
   Large cell, immunoblastic   ML immunoblastic
    plasmacytoid
    clear cell
    polymorphous   Peripheral T-cell lymphomas
    epithelioid cell component   Lymphoepithelioid lymphoma

I. *Malignant lymphoma*
   Lymphoblastic   ML lymphoblastic
    convoluted cell
    nonconvoluted cell

J. *Malignant lymphoma*
   Small noncleaved cell   Burkitt's lymphoma
    Burkitt's
    follicular areas

Table 9. (continued)

Working Formulation	Kiel equivalent
Miscellaneous	
Composite	—
Mycosis fungoides	Mycosis fungoides
Histiocytic	—
Extramedullary plasmacytoma	ML plasmacytic
Unclassifiable	—
Other	—

ular classification, to review in a relatively short time a large number of previously untreated cases at different institutions. The clinical data on 1153 cases and all histopathological diagnoses according to the six available classifications were recorded at a central facility and subsequently collated for evaluation and discussion. The end result was the presentation of a "Working Formulation of Non-Hodgkin's Lymphoma for Clinical Usage" on 11 January 1980 in Palo Alto, California, USA.[59]

The Working Formulation (WF) is not a new classification of ML, but rather a terminological compromise for the definition of entities with different natural histories, prognoses and responses to therapy. The WF clearly incorporates concepts and terms that derive from the classifications proposed by LUKES and COLLINS, DORFMAN and the British National Lymphoma Investigation and, to a certain extent, the Rappaport classification. The WF also accepts the subdivision into "low grade", "intermediate grade" and "high grade", similar to the Kiel classification. The latter, however, speaks explicitly of morphologically defined grades of *malignancy*, whereas the WF avoids the term "malignancy" and makes only a prognostic subdivision. In the WF the three terms "low grade", "intermediate grade" and "high grade" are defined clinically, and not morphologically, which was justly pointed out by MUSSHOFF.[60] The WF includes ten different categories within the three grades. The term "follicular" was preferred to "nodular" to denote those ML showing a follicular growth pattern. The terms printed in italics applied to each category are mandatory for the diagnosis, whereas those not printed in italics are optional (Table 9). The categories of the WF were later given code numbers of the "International Classification of Diseases for Oncology" (ICD-O).[61]

One major difference between the Kiel classification and the WF is the subdivision of the latter into three "prognostic groups", whereas the Kiel classification comprises only two "grades of malignancy". The three groups of the WF were based exclusively upon survival curves. The two groups of the Kiel classification adhere to a morphological principle (which leads, none the less, to similar prognostic consequences). The low-grade malignant neoplasms are made up essential-

---

[59] The Non-Hodgkin's Lymphoma Pathologic Classification Project 1982.
[60] 1987.
[61] Percy et al. 1984; cf. the critical preliminary remarks by Robb-Smith 1982.

ly of "-cytes" with, in some instances, a minority population of "-blasts", whereas the high-grade malignant neoplasms consist mostly, or exclusively, of "-blasts". We should like to adhere to this principle for now, even though we have found certain differences in survival among the lymphomas in each of the two main groups. Our classification is based on morphology, and not on the results of clinical treatment. It defines biological entities. Nevertheless, it might be possible to subdivide the Kiel classification into three groups (low, intermediate, high), as suggested by SILVESTRINI et al.,[62] DIEHL et al.[63] and PILERI.[64] In our opinion, however, the time has not yet come to make changes in the concept used so far. At the time of the Palo Alto meeting, it was appreciated that the Kiel classification could not be dismantled and incorporated into such a formulation, and it was then agreed that the equivalent terms of the Kiel classification should stand next to each category of the WF. The users of the Kiel classification, and particularly those who wish to translate from the Kiel terminology into that of the WF (e.g. for institutional reasons or for the purpose of multicentre studies), will notice that there are problems and shortcomings in some areas, whereas other entities can be accommodated more easily. In our discussion of the individual entities later in this book we shall list the terms of the WF as synonyms wherever possible. This cannot be done with several entities that do not fit into the WF, e.g. LCAL and the AILD type of T-cell lymphoma. For comparison, the synonymous terms of the updated Lukes-Collins classification[65] (Table 10) are also listed for each entity.

Evaluation of the WF

Since the publication of the WF (in 1982) a number of commentaries have appeared, some of which have been positive, others critical. In most instances, the WF has been welcomed as an instrument for directly comparing various classifications and making clinicotherapeutic studies at least roughly comparable. According to the express will of the authors of the first publication (in 1982) and many others,[66] the *only function* of the WF should be that of a medium for translating different classifications into a sort of "lymphoma Esperanto".[67] Hence every pathologist and his clinical colleagues should agree to use the classification that the pathologist considers to be the best and with which he is most familiar. At the clinician's request, the pathologist may add the WF synonyms in brackets in his reports.

Although this principle was established at the Palo Alto meeting, it is often disregarded. Unfortunately, the WF was frequently considered to be *the* new classification and used for making diagnoses without one of the standard classifications. KRUEGER et al.[68] recommended the WF as a practical classification and

---

[62] 1977.
[63] 1979.
[64] 1985.
[65] R. J. Lukes, personal communication 1989; R. D. Collins, personal communication 1990.
[66] Moir 1983.
[67] Rilke and Lennert 1981; Robb-Smith 1982; Dorfman 1983; Lennert 1983; Leong 1983; Lukes 1983; Rosenberg 1983.
[68] 1983.

Table 10. Entities of the updated Kiel classification (1991) and their equivalents in the updated classification of LUKES and COLLINS[a]

Kiel classification	Lukes-Collins classification
Low-grade malignant B-cell lymphomas	
Lymphocytic	
CLL	Small lymphocyte B, B-CLL
PLL	Small lymphocyte B, PLL
HCL	Small lymphocyte B, HCL
Immunocytoma	Plasmacytic-lymphocytic
Plasmacytic	–
Centroblastic-centrocytic	Small cleaved FCC
Centrocytic	Small cleaved FCC
Monocytoid	Small lymphocyte B, monocytoid
Low-grade malignant T-cell lymphomas	
Lymphocytic	
CLL	Small lymphocyte T, knobby or cytopenic
PLL	Small lymphocyte T, prolymphocytic
Small cell, cerebriform (mycosis fungoides, Sézary's syndrome)	Cerebriform T
Lymphoepithelioid	Lymphoepithelioid
AILD (LgX) type	IBL-like T-cell lymphoma
T-zone lymphoma	T-immunoblastic sarcoma
Pleomorphic, small cell	T-immunoblastic sarcoma
High-grade malignant B-cell lymphomas	
Centroblastic	
Monomorphic	Large noncleaved FCC
Polymorphic	Large noncleaved FCC
Multilobated	Large cleaved FCC
Centrocytoid	Evolving FCC
Immunoblastic	B-immunoblastic sarcoma
Burkitt's lymphoma	Small noncleaved FCC, Burkitt and non-Burkitt variants
Large cell anaplastic	–
Lymphoblastic	–
High-grade malignant T-cell lymphomas	
Pleomorphic, medium-sized and large cell	T-immunoblastic sarcoma
Immunoblastic	T-immunoblastic sarcoma
Large cell anaplastic	T-immunoblastic sarcoma (anaplastic, Ki-1+)
Lymphoblastic	Convoluted T

[a] R. J. Lukes, personal communication 1989; R. D. Collins, personal communication 1990

considered it to be of limited value for translating the various classifications. These were not the only complaints. Numerous scientific investigations (e.g. cytogenetic studies) have also been carried out on the basis of the WF. This was supposed to be avoided since, according to the will of the authors of the WF, it was meant only for clinical usage. Even if that intention is ignored, there remain the repeatedly expressed serious doubts about the WF, which warn against considering this compromise formula to be a solid, scientifically founded system of lymphoma entities.[69]

In the meantime, NATHWANI,[70] an active proponent of the WF, has criticized the WF and suggested a revision in a lecture at a meeting of the American-Canadian Section of the International Academy of Pathology in New Orleans. He pointed out that categories are missing for immunocytoma, centrocytic lymphoma and peripheral T-cell lymphomas and that categories F ("mixed"), G ("large") and H ("large immunoblastic") are heterogeneous and should be subdivided. This would increase the number of categories in a revised WF to 22. In his criticism NATHWANI has appropriated many of our objections. We are not going to discuss them here. The problem will solve itself. We should like to stress, however, that it is not a matter of terms, as thought by MOIR[71] and many others. We think it is important to create a generally acceptable classification that defines biological *entities* by being based on subtle morphology and immunocytochemistry. All suggestions for improving the WF, of which there are already several,[72] will not reach this goal or will make the WF so complicated that it will no longer be teachable or learnable. Furthermore, only a classification of biologically defined lymphoma entities can be used as a basis for molecular genetic and epidemiological studies.

2.4 Cytological Basis

The scheme illustrated here (Fig. 4) is an attempt to demonstrate the most important cells of the lymphoid series, including their derivatives.[73] Our concept is based mainly on the experimental data of KEUNING's group (especially those of VELDMAN et al.[74]) and on our own morphological and kinetic studies of human lymphoid tissue.[75] We are aware that the scheme contains by no means all the functionally or morphologically definable cells. For example, the subtypes of T lymphocytes are missing, and the list of germinal centre cells is incomplete. The so-called plasmacytoid T cells, the monocytoid B cells of the sinus and marginal zone cells are also not included. We have consciously left out the MALT.

---

[69] E.g. Rilke and Lennert 1981; Lennert 1983; Lukes 1983; Diebold and Audouin 1985.
[70] 1987.
[71] 1983.
[72] Fifth International Workshop on Chromosomes in Leukemia-Lymphoma 1987; Nanba et al. 1987b; Nathwani 1987; Butler and Cleary 1988.
[73] Uckun 1990.
[74] 1978a,b; Veldman and Keuning 1978.
[75] Mitrou et al. 1969.

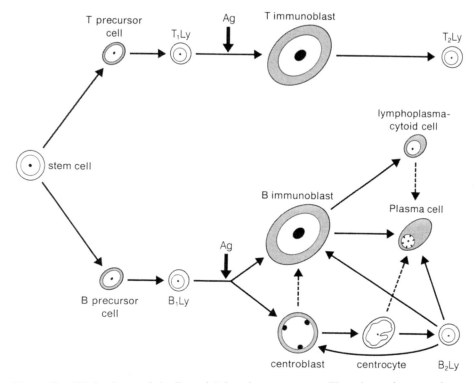

Fig. 4. Simplified scheme of the T- and B-lymphocyte systems. The scheme does not show marginal zone cells, monocytoid B cells or plasmacytoid T-zone cells, nor does it include the various functional subtypes of peripheral T cells. *Ag* = antigenic stimulation. *Ly* = lymphocyte

Precursor cells of the T-cell and B-cell series develop out of a haematopoietic stem cell.

2.4.1 T-Cell Series (see Fig. 5)

In the T-cell series maturation occurs partly in the bone marrow ("pre-thymical-ly") and partly in the thymus. CD7 is the earliest antigen that can be demonstrated constantly on pre-thymic and thymic T cells. In addition, terminal deoxynucle-otidyl transferase (TdT) is found in pre-thymic and thymic cells in various stages of maturation. Other T-cell antigens are expressed in a certain sequence during maturation. First there is the cytoplasmic expression of CD3, followed by expression of CD2 and CD5. At this level a rearrangement of the β chain of the T-cell receptor gene has already occurred, including a complete transcription. The expression of CD4 and CD8 largely coincides with the demonstration of thymic cortex antigen. The transition into a peripheral T cell is characterized by the exclusive expression of CD4 *or* CD8. In addition, in the blood there is a small T-cell population (approx. 3%) that expresses neither CD4 nor CD8 ("double negative"). These T cells show a rearrangement of TcR1, i.e. the γ- and δ-chain

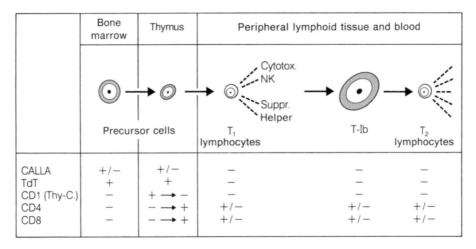

	Bone marrow	Thymus	Peripheral lymphoid tissue and blood		
	Precursor cells		T_1 lymphocytes	T-Ib	T_2 lymphocytes
CALLA	+/−	+/−	−	−	−
TdT	+	+	−	−	−
CD1 (Thy-C.)	−	+ → −	−	−	−
CD4	−	− → +	+/−	+/−	+/−
CD8	−	− → +	+/−	+/−	+/−

Fig. 5. Greatly simplified scheme of T-cell development. *Cytotox.* = cytotoxic cells. *NK* = natural killer cells. *Suppr.* = suppressor cells. *Helper* = helper cells. *T-Ib* = T immunoblast. *CALLA* = common ALL antigen (CD10). *TdT* = terminal deoxynucleotidyl transferase. *Thy-C.* = thymic cortex

genes. Functionally, they are largely cytotoxic T cells. Such cells can also be found in the epidermis and in the epithelium of the gastrointestinal tract. The CD4-positive or CD8-positive T lymphocytes show a rearrangement of TcR2, i.e. the α- and β-chain genes. They represent helper/inducer cells (CD4+) or suppressor cells (CD8+). When a T lymphocyte is stimulated by an antigen, it is transformed into a large basophilic blast cell (T immunoblast). This cell also shows the immunophenotype of mature peripheral T cells. T immunoblasts cannot as yet be morphologically distinguished from the cell of the B-cell series with the corresponding name (B immunoblast). T immunoblasts evidently give rise to T_2 lymphocytes; the latter function as "memory cells" that induce an accelerated and/or enhanced immune response to the same antigen. Most peripheral T cells have a characteristic antigen profile (CD2+, CD3+, CD5+ and CD4+ or CD8+).

Reactive lymph nodes contain groups of cells that we initially designated as clusters of lymphoblasts[76] but later interpreted as "plasmacytoid T cells" because they were CD4 positive.[77] Findings reported by HORNY et al.,[78] BEISKE et al.[79] and FACCHETTI et al.[80] indicated that these cells might not belong to the T-cell system. They express the monocytic antigen CD68 (Ki-M6[81]) and the T-cell-associated antigen CD4, which is also expressed by monocytes. Other myelomonocyt-

[76] Lennert 1961.
[77] Müller-Hermelink et al. 1983; Feller et al. 1983b.
[78] 1987.
[79] 1987.
[80] 1987.
[81] Horny et al. 1987.

ic antigens have been found as well.[82] The cells are also Ki-M1p positive. Hence the possibility that these cells have a myelomonocytic origin must be taken into serious consideration. The occurrence of tumour-like proliferations of "plasma-cytoid T cells" in chronic myelomonocytic leukaemia would be another argument favouring this possibility. On the other hand, "plasmacytoid T cells" occur preferably in T regions, even under neoplastic conditions, and are sometimes seen in low-grade malignant T-cell lymphomas (T-CLL, mycosis fungoides, T-zone lymphoma). In this uncertain situation, the term "plasmacytoid T-zone cell" proposed by BEISKE et al.[83] may be used until the origin of these cells has been fully elucidated.

2.4.2 B-Cell Series (see Figs. 4, 6–14)

In the bone marrow, stem cells give rise to pre-B cells, which initially contain CD19 and CD22 in their cytoplasm and then μ chains (without light chains) as well,[84] but do not exhibit complete sIg (IgM).[85] In contrast, the B_1 lymphocytes that develop out of pre-B cells are sIg positive. When B_1 lymphocytes encounter antigenic stimulation, they either transform directly into immunoblasts (this always happens in the primary immune response) or form germinal centres (this also happens in the primary immune response, but is particularly characteristic of the secondary immune response). These germinal centres produce not only precursor cells of immunoblasts and their derivatives, but also B_2 lymphocytes, which are the immunological memory cells of the B-lymphocyte series.

Germinal centres contain two main characteristic types of cells, viz. centro-blasts and centrocytes (Fig. 6). Centroblasts have scanty basophilic cytoplasm and a round nucleus with multiple, medium-sized, usually marginal nucleoli (these cells are called "non-cleaved FCC" by LUKES and COLLINS[86]). Centrocytes have about the same amount of cytoplasm, but it stains very weakly and is thus barely visible. The nucleus of the centrocyte is irregularly shaped and sometimes cleaved ("cleaved FCC"[87]), and it contains very small nucleoli and fine chromatin. In contrast to B_1 and B_2 lymphocytes, centroblasts and centrocytes show, at most, only very small amounts of sIg. A proportion of centroblasts and centrocytes appear to produce cIg of various classes.

Centroblasts are the precursor cells of centrocytes (and not vice versa). This definition contrasts with that of LUKES,[88] who maintained, even in a more recent publication, that centroblasts develop out of centrocytes.[89] A study of the development of germinal centres provides sufficient evidence supporting our view: At

---

[82] Beiske et al. 1987; Facchetti et al. 1987, 1988.
[83] Beiske et al. 1987.
[84] Cooper 1979.
[85] Uckun 1990.
[86] Lukes and Collins 1974a,b.
[87] Lukes and Collins 1974a,b.
[88] 1979.
[89] Lennert et al. 1983.

the beginning of their development, germinal centres consist exclusively of centroblasts; centrocytes do not appear until later.[90] An updated, convincing concept of germinal centre development has been presented by MACLENNAN.[91]

Besides the typical centroblasts and centrocytes, germinal centres contain several other cell types that are often easier to identify by electron microscopy than in immunohistochemically stained slides. New germinal centres and the dark zone of the later developmental phase show basophilic, medium-sized or large cells with multiple, central nucleoli. These probably represent the earliest transformation stages of lymphocytes and may therefore be interpreted as pre-centroblasts (Fig. 6). They correspond to the "B-cell blasts" that have been distinguished by MACLENNAN et al.[92] as different from centroblasts. They express sIg, whereas centroblasts do not.[91] In sections of resin-embedded tissue, some centrocytes may show pale (typical!) cytoplasm, while others have dark grey (protein-synthesizing, hence Ig positive?) cytoplasm (Fig. 7). Other investigators[92a] have described cIg-positive centrocytes. In addition, germinal centres always contain T cells (which are usually CD4 positive and CD26 negative) and natural killer (NK) cells (CD57+). The lymphoid cells are always interspersed with follicular dendritic cells (cf. p. 97), which have long, slim projections, an oval, often indented nucleus, and a solitary nucleolus (Figs. 7, 8). Binucleated cells are not uncommon.[93] The follicular dendritic cells can be identified best with specific monoclonal antibodies, even in paraffin sections (Ki-M4p and other antibodies), or by electron microscopy, but they are also recognizable by light microscopy in good sections. Depending on its developmental phase, the germinal centre also shows a small or large number of macrophages containing phagocytosed disintegrating cells ("tingible body macrophages", Fig. 8). In advanced phases of germinal centre development, marked plasmacytopoiesis (with immunoblasts, plasmablasts, proplasmacytes and plasma cells) may occur. Centroblasts and centrocytes occasionally show "multilobated" nuclei.[94]

Plasmacytopoiesis occurs mainly in the pulp, however. There B immunoblasts transform into plasma cells or lymphoplasmacytoid cells via plasmablasts and proplasmacytes (Fig. 9). The production of cIg increases markedly. The "plasma cell" shown in the scheme (Fig. 4) is the cell that has also been called the "Marschalkó type of plasma cell" or "reticular plasma cell". The lymphoplasmacytoid cell corresponds to the smaller "lymphatic plasma cell" of the literature. These two types of plasma cell secrete Ig. On electron microscopy, they contain rough endoplasmic reticulum; on light microscopy, they are basophilic (pyroninophilic). As a sign of Ig retention, they may contain intranuclear or intracytoplasmic PAS-positive inclusions (intranuclear inclusions are typical of plasma cells in lymphomas and are hardly ever seen in reactive plasma cells, except in the gastrointestinal mucosa!).

[90] Van Buchem 1962; Müller-Hermelink and Lennert 1978; Nieuwenhuis and Lennert 1980.
[91] 1991; Liu et al. 1992.
[92] 1989b.
[92a] Stein et al. 1982b; Close et al. 1990.
[93] Peters et al. 1984.
[94] Van der Putte et al. 1984

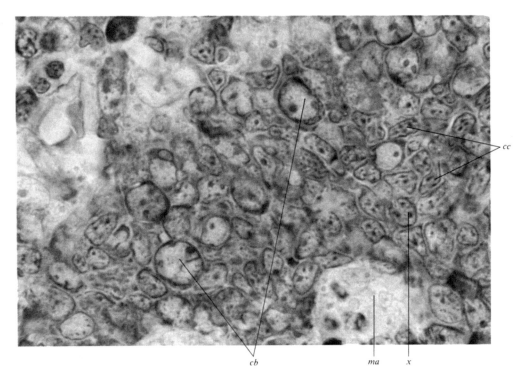

Fig. 6. Dark zone of a germinal centre containing several typical centroblasts (*cb*), one macrophage (*ma*) with tingible bodies ("starry-sky cell") and centrocytes (*cc*). Most of the cells are medium-sized and show scanty, basophilic cytoplasm and central nucleoli. They are probably cells in the process of transforming from lymphocytes into centroblasts ("pre-centroblasts", "B-cell blasts" of MacLennan et al.,[92] *x*). Giemsa. 1120:1

The relationship between germinal centres and the immunoblast–plasma cell system is probably of a manifold nature. We do not yet know enough about the transformation from non-secreting into Ig-secreting cells. For this reason, the arrows drawn in Fig. 4 should be conceived as possibilities only. One thing, however, appears to be certain, viz. that plasma cells can also develop directly ("metaplastically") out of small lymphocytes. Hence precursor cells are not always necessary for plasmacytopoiesis.

There are two other special types of B lymphocyte, which are relatively well characterized by their morphological and immunocytochemical features. Their derivation and function, however, are still largely obscure. These are the "monocytoid B cell" (also known as "sinusoidal B cell" or "parafollicular B lymphocyte") and the marginal zone cell.

The *monocytoid B cell* occurs, so to speak in pure culture, in a specific sinus reaction, which used to be known as immature sinus histiocytosis (Figs. 10, 11).[95] Now we know that it is actually a medium-sized B cell.[96] Monocytoid B cells are

---

[95] Lennert 1958, 1961.
[96] De Almeida et al. 1984; Stein et al. 1984; van den Oord et al. 1985; Piris et al. 1986.

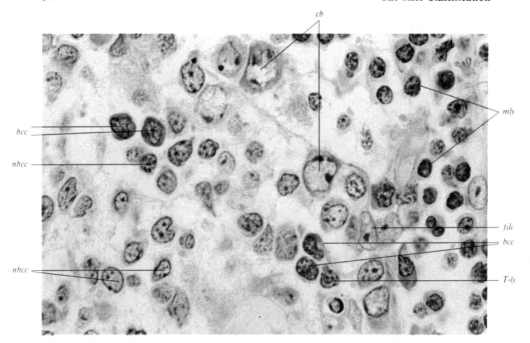

Fig. 7. Light zone of a germinal centre containing a moderate number of cells: centroblasts (*cb*), centrocytes with basophilic cytoplasm (*bcc*), centrocytes with pale cytoplasm (*nbcc*), follicular dendritic cell (*fdc*), T lymphocyte (*T-ly*), mantle zone lymphocytes (*mly*). Giemsa. 875:1

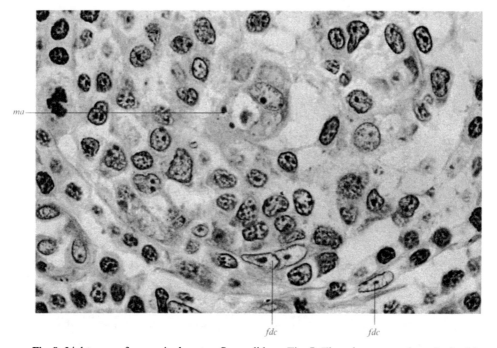

Fig. 8. Light zone of a germinal centre. Same slide as Fig. 7. There is a macrophage (*ma*) with "tingible bodies" (nuclear debris) above the *centre* of the picture. Binucleate and mononuclear follicular dendritic cells (*fdc*) are seen at the border of the mantle zone. Giemsa. 875:1

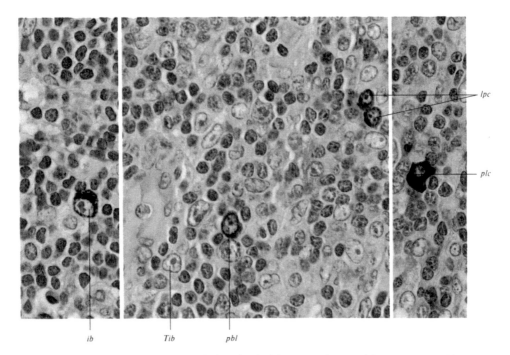

Fig. 9. Various forms of plasmacytopoiesis stained with PAP: B immunoblast (*ib*), plasmablast (*pbl*), lymphoplasmacytoid cell (*lpc*), plasma cell of Marschalkó type (*plc*). Several Ig-negative immunoblasts are present, mostly of T type (*Tib*). Piringer's lymphadenitis. Immunoperoxidase, *lambda* chains. 700:1

distinguishable from other B cells on the basis of their immunocytochemical properties. They are characterized for instance by the expression of CD22, CD35 and sIgM and by the absence of CD23 and CD5. A remarkable feature is the *granular* reaction seen in paraffin sections stained with the Ki-M1p antibody. The proliferation rate is usually low (2%–5% Ki-67-positive cells). In a freshly developed case of Piringer's lymphadenitis, however, we have seen 20%–30% Ki-67-positive cells. They may originate in the mantle zone of follicles (developing out of marginal zone cells?). This possibility was suggested by a montage of electron micrographs (cf. Fig. 40 in MORI and LENNERT[97]), which showed monocytoid B cells in perisinusoidal lymphoid tissue (follicular mantle) and some of them migrating through the sinus wall. The direction in which the lymphocytes migrated could be concluded from the position of the hand glass-shaped nuclei. They may also originate in the blood; we have observed emigration of monocytoid B cells out of an adjacent venule into the marginal sinus (Fig. 11). Monocytoid B cells are clearly larger than lymphocytes (the nuclear volume is twice that of lymphocyte nuclei[98]). They show a moderate amount of grey cytoplasm and

[97] 1969.
[98] Lennert and Remmele 1958.

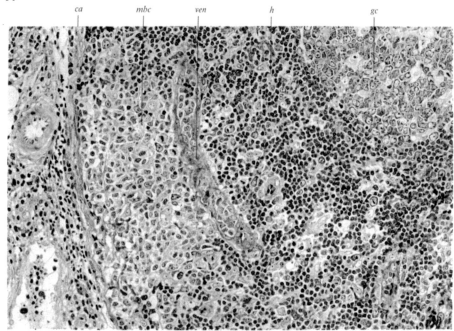

Fig. 10. Sinusoidal B-cell reaction (previously known as "immature sinus histiocytosis") in Piringer's lymphadenitis. The "monocytoid" B cells (*mbc*) are located under the capsule (*ca*) in the marginal sinus and near a venule (*ven*), in which monocytoid B cells are also recognizable. A germinal centre (*gc*) is seen in the top right corner. The tissue between the sinus and the germinal centre shows polymorphic hyperplasia (*h*). Giemsa. 220:1

plump oval or irregularly shaped nuclei with small nucleoli. Occasionally, there are also a few basophilic, relatively small blast cells (Fig. 11).

The *marginal zone cells* were found by KEUNING and his associates[99] in the spleen and lymph nodes. More recent studies have been focussed on these cells' immunological and functional characteristics.[100] In lymph nodes they are not as well defined as they are in the spleen, and are thus more difficult to find (Fig. 12).[101] They look somewhat larger than the mantle zone lymphocytes. They are IgD negative, Ki-B3 negative (Ki-B3 reacts with an antigen related to CD45), CD23 negative and alkaline phosphatase positive. Solitary marginal zone cells are hardly identifiable. They are usually interspersed in the follicular mantle. When they are hyperplastic, however, they are easily recognized because they form a dense band of somewhat enlarged lymphocytes. These are clearly distinguishable from the small lymphocytes of the mantle zone or T zones by their paler (more greyish blue) nuclei. They sometimes accumulate in the outer zone of the follicular mantle and thus cause widening of the corona, which completely surrounds the

---

[99] Keuning et al. 1963; Keuning and Bos 1967; Veldman et al. 1978a.
[100] Humphrey 1981; MacLennan et al. 1982, 1989; Van der Valk et al. 1984b; Timens and Poppema 1985; MacLennan and Gray 1986; Timens 1988.
[101] Veldman 1970; Kaiserling 1977, 1978; Stein et al. 1980; Van den Oord et al. 1986; Van Krieken et al. 1989.

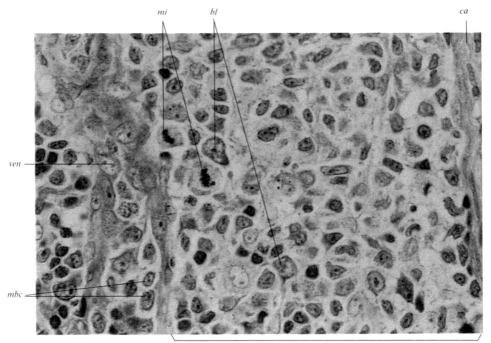

Marginal sinus showing predominance of monocytoid B cells

Fig. 11. Same area as Fig. 10 at a higher magnification. Among the monocytoid B cells in the marginal sinus one recognizes two medium-sized, basophilic blast cells (*bl*) and two mitotic figures (*mi*). The venule (*ven*) also contains monocytoid B cells (*mbc*). Evidently, they migrate from the venule into the marginal sinus. Lymph node capsule (*ca*). Giemsa. 695:1

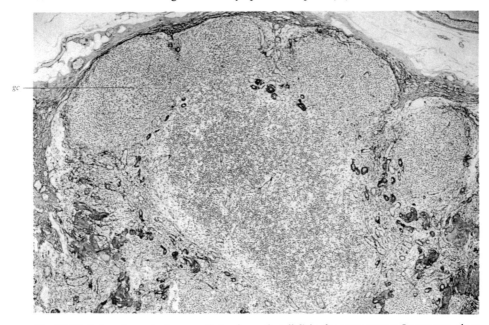

Fig. 12. Nodules of marginal zone cells (and mantle cells?) in the outer cortex. In one area there are remnants of a germinal centre (*gc*). Under this there is a large T nodule with epithelioid venules, most of which are located at the periphery. Gomori. 55:1

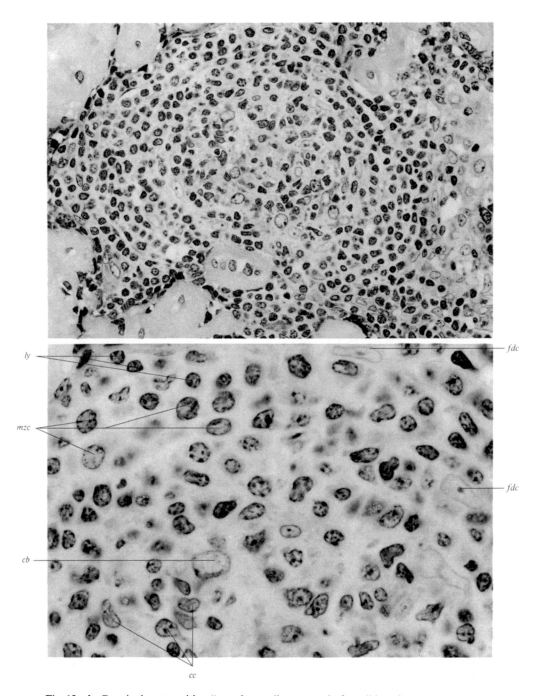

Fig. 13a, b. Germinal centre with a "mantle zone" composed of small lymphocytes (*ly*, IgD + , Ki-B3 +) and somewhat larger marginal zone cells (*mzc*, IgD − , Ki-B3 −). A few centroblasts (*cb*), centrocytes (*cc*) and follicular dendritic cells (*fdc*) are seen. Giemsa. **a** 440 : 1, **b** 1094 : 1

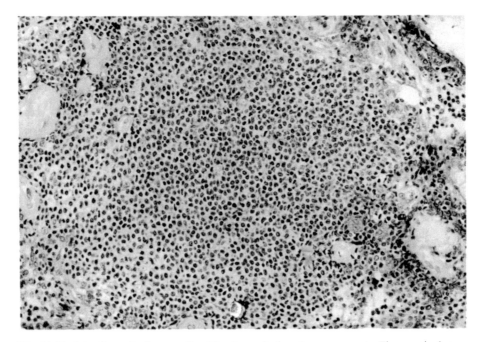

Fig. 14. Nodule of marginal zone cells without germinal centre components. The marginal zone cells are somewhat larger than lymphocytes. Same node as Fig. 13. Giemsa. 220 : 1

germinal centre (not just on one side! Fig. 13). This pattern is seen especially in mesenteric lymph nodes.[102] Peripheral lymph nodes may show another variant, viz. the solid marginal zone cell nodule (Fig. 14), which may also contain mantle cells. Such nodules should not be confused with the primary follicle (the latter consists of IgD-positive, Ki-B3-positive small lymphocytes!). The former may be associated with band-shaped accumulations right under the marginal sinuses. In all cases, there is an admixture of follicular dendritic cells.

Nota bene : The terms mantle zone ("corona") and marginal zone should not be used synonymously.[102a] It is easier to recognize the difference in the spleen. There the germinal centre is surrounded by a mantle composed of small IgD-positive lymphocytes. This mantle is then surrounded by the marginal zone, which contains somewhat larger, uniform cells with relatively abundant, pale cytoplasm and is therefore clearly distinct from the mantle zone lymphocytes. Marginal zone cells also differ from mantle zone lymphocytes because of their negative reactions for IgD, Ki-B3 and CD23.

---

[102] P. Isaacson, personal communication.
[102a] Keuning and Bos 1967.

2.5 Statistical Data

Frequency. The relative frequency of the various types of NHL in our collection is summarized in Table 11. The values reported for other countries or continents indicate that there are considerable differences, which are due not only to actual differences in incidence but also to variations in practice. In Germany, for example, biopsies are often performed in cases of acute and chronic lymphoid leukaemia, whereas in other countries such cases are frequently diagnosed on blood and bone marrow smears alone.

At the time of analysis (1983) our collection contained 78% B-cell lymphomas and 17% T-cell lymphomas. If all the unclassified cases were to be added to the T-cell lymphomas there would be 22%. Hence the actual frequency of T-cell lymphomas would be at most 20%. This is much higher than the percentage given in the table we published in 1981[103] (8.65% ± 6% unclear or null types). The reason for this was our inclusion of only the classifiable cases and exclusion of the unclassifiable cases (approx. 15%) at that time. In the United States LUKES et al.[104] found 21% T-cell lymphomas. In Japan[105] the proportion of HTLV-1-negative T-cell lymphomas is about one-third of all NHL. A look at the HTLV-1-positive T-cell lymphomas in Japan reveals that they make up 47% of all NHL in endemic regions and 8% of all NHL in non-endemic regions. If the virus-negative and virus-positive T-cell lymphomas are added together, then the endemic regions of Japan show 65% T-cell lymphomas and the non-endemic regions show 36%.

In our collection the ratio of low-grade ML to high-grade ML was 1.7:1. B-cell lymphomas showed a ratio of 2.3:1, T-cell lymphomas a ratio of 1.1:1. The most frequent types of lymphoma in our partially selected collection were centroblastic-centrocytic lymphoma (20.4%), centroblastic lymphoma (13.7%), immunocytoma (12.3%), and B-CLL (11.1%), all of which are B-cell lymphomas. The most frequent type of T-cell lymphoma was the AILD (LgX) type (3.6%).

The data listed in Table 11 differ somewhat from the frequency distribution we presented in 1981. There are several reasons for this: (a) Only nodal biopsies are included in the table presented here, because certain types of extranodal lymphoma follow their own laws and also show different morphologies. (b) As a result of our studies of high-grade malignant B-cell lymphomas after resin embedding, a considerably higher number of B-cell lymphomas, especially in the unclassified group, could be identified as centroblastic lymphomas.[106] (c) The lower percentage of immunoblastic lymphomas is a result of the somewhat refined definition of centroblastic and immunoblastic lymphomas.

The various new T-cell lymphoma entities are the fruit of world-wide efforts to classify these relatively rare tumours.[107] In particular, we have had to include

---

[103] Lennert 1981.
[104] 1978a,b.
[105] Suchi 1987.
[106] Hui et al. 1988.
[107] Suchi et al. 1987.

Table 11. Non-Hodgkin's lymphomas diagnosed on lymph node biopsies at the Lymph Node Registry in Kiel in 1983 (n = 1284). Repeated biopsies and extranodal lymphomas are not included

	B n	B [%]	T n	T [%]	Undefined[a] n	Undefined[a] [%]
Low-grade malignant lymphomas	**700**	**54.5**	**114**	**8.9**		
Lymphocytic						
CLL	141 } 143	11.1	7 } 10	0.8		
PLL	2 }		3 }			
HCL	0	–				
Small cell, cerebriform (mycosis fungoides and Sézary's syndrome)			12	0.9		
Immunocytoma	158	12.3				
Lymphoepithelioid (LeL)			18	1.4		
Plasmacytic	<7	<0.5				
AILD (LgX) type			46	3.6		
Centroblastic-centrocytic	262	20.4				
T-zone lymphoma			11	0.9		
Centrocytic	70	5.4				
Pleomorphic, small cell			17	1.3		
Monocytoid	6	0.5				
Borderline case	18 }					
Development into high-grade ML	17 } 54	4.2				
Unclassified	19 }					
High-grade malignant lymphomas	**300**	**23.4**	**106**	**8.2**	**64**	**5.0**
Centroblastic	176	13.7				
Pleomorphic, medium-sized and large cell			34	2.6		
Immunoblastic	55	4.3	14	1.1		
Burkitt's lymphoma	33	2.6				
Large cell, anaplastic	1	0.1	17	1.3	9	0.7
Lymphoblastic	11	0.9	41	3.2	27	2.1
Unclassified	24	1.9			28	2.2
	1000	**77.9**	**220**	**17.1**	**64**	**5.0**

[a] B-cell or T-cell-specific immunological markers were missing.

entities in our classification that previously were not, or were not definitely, recognized as T-cell lymphomas, viz. the AILD (LgX) type and lymphoepithelioid lymphoma (Lennert's lymphoma).

Age and Sex Distribution. The lymphomas of low-grade malignancy generally do not occur before the age of 20 years and show a peak incidence in the 7th decade. The only exception is centroblastic-centrocytic lymphoma, which shows a peak in the 6th decade (Fig. 15). For more details about the very rare low-grade ML in childhood see p. 43. Some types of high-grade ML (in the lymphoblastic category) are found more frequently in the first two decades of life than in adulthood (Fig. 16). Large cell anaplastic lymphoma is also observed more often in children and adolescents than in adults.

Almost all types of ML show a slight or moderate male predominance. Only centroblastic-centrocytic lymphoma exhibits a slight female predominance (male-to-female ratio of 1:1.2).

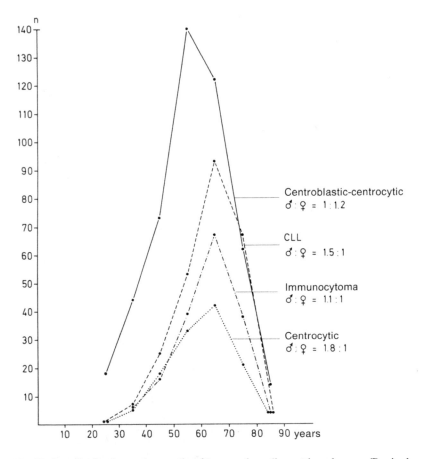

Fig. 15. Age distribution and sex ratio of low-grade malignant lymphomas. (Revised version of figure published by LENNERT et al. 1975)

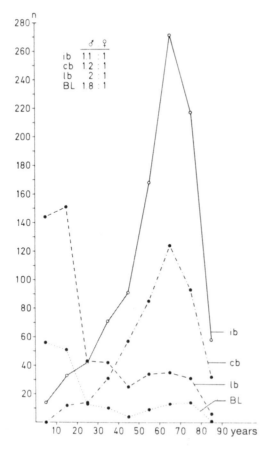

Fig. 16. Age distribution and sex ratio of high-grade malignant lymphomas. *ib* = immunoblastic lymphoma. *cb* = centroblastic lymphoma. *lb* = lymphoblastic lymphoma. *BL* = Burkitt's lymphoma. (Revised version of figure published by LENNERT et al. 1975)

2.5.1 Malignant Lymphomas of Childhood[108]

Between 1983 and 1987 we diagnosed a total of 448 ML in children under the age of 15 years; 56% of the cases were Hodgkin's lymphomas and 44% were NHL. The latter included only 6.6% low-grade ML (Table 12), most of which were of the pleomorphic, small cell T-cell type (5.1%). Only one case of immunocytoma and two cases of centroblastic-centrocytic lymphoma (making up a total of 1.5% low-grade malignant B-cell lymphomas) were found in children aged 13 and 14 years. Of the high-grade ML, the lymphoblastic type was diagnosed most frequently (45.9%), but these cases included a considerable number of ALL cases. The second most frequent type was Burkitt's lymphoma (24.5%), followed by

---

[108] Dura and Gladkowska-Dura 1981; Müller-Weihrich et al. 1984, 1985.

Table 12. Non-Hodgkin's lymphomas diagnosed on lymph node biopsies from children (0–14 years old) at the Lymph Node Registry in Kiel from 1983 through 1987

	n	[%]
Low-grade malignant lymphomas	13	6.6
Lymphoplasmacytic	1 ⎫	
Centroblastic-centrocytic, follicular	2 ⎬	1.5
Pleomorphic, small cell T-cell lymphoma	10	5.1
High-grade malignant lymphomas	171	87.2
Centroblastic	5 ⎫	
Immunoblastic	5 ⎬	5.1
Burkitt's lymphoma	48	24.5
Large cell, anaplastic (Ki-1 +)	24	12.2
Lymphoblastic (including ALL)	89	45.9
Unclassified	12	6.1
	196	

large cell anaplastic Ki-1-positive lymphoma (12.2%) and centroblastic lymphoma and immunoblastic lymphoma (totalling 5.1%). In 6.1% of the cases it was not possible to make a definitive diagnosis, usually for technical reasons. Since our data were partially based on a series of selected cases and hence do not allow conclusions about the actual incidence of the various lymphoma types, we are also displaying data that were obtained in two therapy trials in Germany (Table 13).[109] These series were quite different, however, because they included extranodal lymphomas and patients up to the age of 18 years. On the other hand, leukaemic lymphoblastic lymphomas (ALL) were excluded on the basis of strict criteria.

Table 13 reveals that Burkitt's lymphoma and centroblastic lymphoma were more frequent in the clinically investigated series than in our collection (40.4% versus 24.5% and 9.6% versus 2.5%, respectively), but that non-leukaemic lymphoblastic lymphoma accounted for only 38.3% of cases in the former series (versus 45.9% in our collection, which also contained leukaemic cases). The low percentage of large cell anaplastic lymphomas (3.7% versus 12.2% in our series) may have arisen because some cases in this category were not initially recognized as lymphomas and thus were not included in the study. On the other hand, the high percentage in our collection may be due to the consultative function of our Lymph Node Registry.

It is not possible to calculate the ratio of B-cell lymphomas to T-cell lymphomas in childhood on the basis of our data, because not all cases were examined immunohistochemically. An immunohistochemical analysis would be absolutely necessary in the cases of immunoblastic, lymphoblastic and large cell

---

[109] Bucsky et al. 1988; cf. Bucsky et al. 1989, 1990.

Table 13. Non-Hodgkin's lymphomas diagnosed on nodal and extranodal biopsies from children and adolescents (under the age of 18 years) during two clinical studies (NHL-BFM) in 1981 and 1983 (n = 262). Only the 188 biopsies that were diagnosed or examined at the Lymph Node Registry in Kiel are included in this list. The data were kindly provided by P. BUCSKY[a]

	n		[%]	
Low-grade malignant lymphomas	6		3.2	
Lymphoplasmacytic	1		0.5	
Centroblastic-centrocytic	1		0.5	
Pleomorphic, small cell T-cell lymphoma	4		2.1	
High-grade malignant lymphomas	179		95.2	
Centroblastic	18		9.6	
Immunoblastic, B	5		2.7	
Immunoblastic, T	1		0.5	
Burkitt's lymphoma	76		40.4	
Large cell, anaplastic (Ki-1 +)	7		3.7	
Lymphoblastic	72		38.3	
T		48		25.5
B		10		5.3
unclassified		14		7.5
Unclassified	3		1.6	
	188			

[a] BUCSKY et al. 1988.

Table 14. Relative frequency of T-cell lymphomas in childhood, approximated on the basis of the data listed in Table 12

	[%]
Pleomorphic, small cell T-cell lymphoma	5.1
$^2/_3$ of lymphoblastic lymphomas	≈ 30
$^4/_5$ of large cell, anaplastic lymphomas	≈ 10
$^1/_5$ of immunoblastic lymphomas	≈ 0.5
$^1/_2$ of unclassified lymphomas	≈ 3.0
	≈ 48.6

anaplastic lymphoma since they cannot be classified reliably as being of the B-cell or T-cell type by morphology alone. Hence we can make only a rough estimate by extrapolation on the basis of immunologically analysed cases of other series. We obtained the results listed in Table 14, showing that in childhood almost *half of the cases of NHL are of the T-cell type.* In adults the percentage of T-cell lymphomas is much lower (see p. 40).

2.6 Therapeutic Principles

by M. ENGELHARD and G. BRITTINGER

In a multicentre observation trial, 1127 patients with NHL diagnosed according to the Kiel classification (as published in 1975 and 1978) were recruited between 1975 and 1980[110] and observed for up to 10 years. The major results of this study[111] have added considerably to the understanding of the clinical characteristics of the various lymphoma entities. These observations have been supported by at least partially comparable experiences collected world-wide. A detailed analysis of the data disclosed the following general features of the biological behaviour of NHL.

Low-grade malignant NHL are characterized by a low rate of proliferation, as judged from the relatively favourable spontaneous clinical course, often lacking the need for treatment over a period of many years. These lymphomas are potentially curable by radiotherapy, at least in the localized stages of the disease. In cases of initially advanced disease requiring immediate therapy and in cases during the course of which therapeutic intervention is indicated (e.g. by development of B symptoms, anaemia and/or thrombocytopenia, or progression of the tumour mass), complete or partial remission in response to mild cytotoxic chemotherapy can be expected. The remissions are unstable, however, and, although a response can often be induced more than once, an inherent tendency to relapse will eventually lead to death.

High-grade malignant NHL show a high rate of proliferation, as evidenced by a clinically obvious tendency towards rapid generalization. Hence it is generally agreed that intensive therapy must be applied immediately. The induction of partial remission improves the prognosis only slightly, while the achievement of complete remission bears the chance of cure. In the strictly localized stage I/I_E (Ann Arbor classification) verified by invasive diagnostic procedures, radiotherapy of sufficient intensity is instrumental in inducing a cure in some entities, e.g. centroblastic lymphoma. In patients presenting with the advanced stage III or IV disease and in a majority of patients with stage II disease, a stable complete remission can be achieved only by applying intensive polychemotherapy. Relapses have to be expected, however, especially during the first 2 years after the end of induction therapy. The prognosis for the patients relapsing early and those who respond only insufficiently to induction therapy ("refractory cases") is still very poor.

These general observations are illustrated best by calculations of the overall probability of survival. As depicted in Fig. 17, advanced low-grade malignant NHL are characterized by continuously declining survival curves, whose slope corresponds to the persistent tendency to relapse that cannot be influenced significantly by treatment. In contrast to this pattern, the survival curves of patients with high-grade malignant NHL tend to form a plateau after a number of years, which indicates that there may be a group of potentially curable patients. Late

---

[110] Brittinger et al. 1984.
[111] Brittinger et al. 1986a, b.

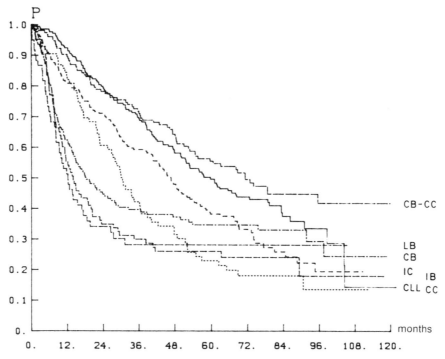

Fig. 17. Overall survival probability of patients with advanced non-Hodgkin's lymphoma (stage III/IV according to the Ann Arbor classification) diagnosed according to the Kiel classification. Results of a prospective observation trial carried out by the Kiel Lymphoma Study Group (1975–1980). The low plateau level of survival of patients with high-grade malignant lymphoma is due to the polychemotherapy of merely moderate intensity (predominantly COP ± methotrexate; C-MOPP) employed in this study, which started recruiting patients in 1975. *CB-CC* = centroblastic-centrocytic lymphoma (n = 113). *LB* = lymphoblastic lymphoma (n = 51). *CB* = centroblastic lymphoma (n = 89). *IC* = immunocytoma (n = 202). *IB* = immunoblastic lymphoma (n = 45). *CLL* = chronic lymphocytic leukaemia (n = 217). *CC* = centrocytic lymphoma (n = 76)

recurrences of disease are observed occasionally, however, which suggests that these tumours have inherent biological properties that are not yet fully understood. The decline of the curve of each histological entity depends considerably on the choice of therapeutic procedures. We should like to point out that the percentage of potentially curable patients with high-grade malignant NHL has been raised significantly in recent years by intensifying the induction chemotherapy protocols.

2.6.1 Requirements and Principles of Treatment

Besides an unequivocal histological and immunological diagnosis, supplemented in certain cases with molecular biological analyses, an extensive initial staging evaluation is the basic prerequisite for any therapeutic decision. The primary aim of the staging procedure is to define and separate a strictly localized disease from all cases of dissemination from the site of tumour origin, including those in their initial stages. In order to make a reliable distinction, it is necessary to perform roentgenological (standard X-ray and computed tomographic), ultrasound and, in some cases, scintigraphic examinations of the chest and abdomen, as well as cytological and histological analyses of the bone marrow (which may include molecular biological techniques to identify minimal tumour infiltration), a physical examination and all routine laboratory tests. The latter should include analyses of serum lactate dehydrogenase, albumin and β_2-microglobulin, since abnormal values are potential prognostic risk factors. A strictly localized stage I/I_E disease has to be substantiated by applying all modern imaging and endoscopic techniques, including lymphangiography, spinal fluid examination, liver biopsy and, in some cases, explorative (staging) laparotomy, at least if radiotherapy without additional chemotherapy is planned.

2.6.2 Treatment of Localized Disease

Under the assumption of a unifocal origin of most NHL, it may be expected that a strictly localized lymphoma manifestation, established preferably by pathological staging (as detailed below), can be controlled by local radiotherapeutic procedures, resulting in stable complete remissions. This would mean that such cases are potentially curable. This view is supported by numerous studies showing that 60%–90% of patients with low-grade malignant NHL in strictly localized stage I/I_E continue to be in complete remission 5 years after completion of involved or extended field radiotherapy.[112] Similar data have been obtained in cases of centroblastic lymphoma and immunoblastic lymphoma, with the remissions in the latter being slightly less stable than those of patients with centroblastic lymphoma.[112a] According to recent reports, a continuous relapse-free survival over many years in patients with stage I/I_E disease after radiotherapy alone can be expected only if the initial stage has been confirmed by pathological staging (PS) procedures, including staging laparotomy with splenectomy, liver biopsy, hepatic lobe excisions and multiple intra-abdominal lymph node biopsies. If stage I/I_E has been determined by less invasive diagnostic procedures (clinical staging, CS), relapses have to be expected in up to 50% of the patients within 2–5 years.[113] On the basis of these experiences, patients with incomplete verification of stage I/I_E have been submitted to intensive induction polychemotherapy in some centres, often followed by adjuvant radiotherapy.[114] Complete remission (90%–99%) and relapse-free survival rates (70%–100% after 2–5 years) achieved with this procedure correspond to the favourable results obtained by radiotherapy alone in patients with pathologically defined stage PS I/I_E.[115] In stage II/II_E disease or in the presence of B symptoms indicative of occult extension of the tumour, radiotherapy alone bears a high risk of relapse and can no

---

[112] Paryani et al. 1983.
[112a] Brittinger et al. 1986b.
[113] Bron and Stryckmans 1987; DeVita et al. 1988.
[114] Jones et al. 1989; Longo et al. 1989.
[115] DeVita et al. 1988.

longer be recommended. Only centroblastic-centrocytic lymphoma, which is characterized by a particularly high radiosensitivity, may be an exception to this rule, since tumour growth could be controlled by extensive radiotherapy in a number of patients even with advanced stage III disease. This procedure appears to be feasible, however, only in those cases of centroblastic-centrocytic lymphoma that show a low total tumour burden. The marked tendency of lymphoblastic lymphoma and Burkitt's lymphoma to early generalization, often with subsequent development of acute lymphoblastic leukaemia, and/or to involvement of the central nervous system precludes radiotherapy alone, even in apparently localized, initial stages of the disease. In the other types of high-grade malignant NHL it is not yet clear whether the efficacy of initial radiotherapy in stage I/I_E disease can be augmented by adjuvant polychemotherapy, or whether combined modality treatment, beginning with a limited number of chemotherapy courses followed by radiotherapy, would increase the chance of cure. These different approaches are currently being explored in clinical trials.

2.6.3 Treatment of Advanced Low-Grade Malignant NHL

Up until the early 1980s a "watch and wait" attitude was generally adopted in cases of advanced low-grade malignant NHL, moderately intensive chemotherapy only being administered when there were signs of progression, and then as a palliative measure.[116] With the aim of improving the prognosis of these cases and perhaps even achieving a cure, several new therapeutic approaches have been investigated recently.

In chronic lymphocytic leukaemia of B-cell type (B-CLL) chemotherapy of graded intensity, depending on the initial stage of disease, has been evaluated.[117] The staging classification applied was that of BINET, which defines stage A as the presence of less than three sites of lymph node involvement and stage B as the presence of three or more; erythrocytopoiesis and thrombocytopoiesis are virtually intact in both stages. The occurrence of anaemia and/or thrombocytopenia below a certain level characterizes stage C, irrespective of the nodal manifestation pattern. The administration of chlorambucil did not significantly improve the prognosis in stage A disease when compared with a control group that was not treated. The overall probability of survival for stage B patients treated with COP (cyclophosphamide, vincristine, prednisone) did not differ from that of patients exposed to chlorambucil alone. In the unfavourable stage C, however, a modified CHOP protocol (COP + adriamycin) proved to induce a prognostic advantage in comparison with the COP-treated control group; this was indicated by an increase in the 2- and 5-year survival rates. Whereas separate trials showed that remissions could be achieved with the CHOP protocol in symptomatic B-CLL, however, these studies did not demonstrate a favourable influence on survival in comparison with chlorambucil-prednisone therapy.[117a] As a novel approach, the

[116] Rosenberg 1985.
[117] French Cooperative Group on Chronic Lymphocytic Leukaemia 1986, 1991.
[117a] Hansen et al. 1991; Kimby and Mellstedt 1991.

introduction of fludarabine monophosphate or 2-chlorodeoxyadenosine (CDA) into the treatment of B-CLL may be promising, since first reports suggest that these are very active cytotoxic agents in low-grade malignant NHL.[118] The observed prognostic differences between B-CLL and immunocytoma[118a] remain to be validated in controlled treatment trials.

The unfavourable prognosis of centrocytic lymphoma was already evident during the multicentre observation trial mentioned above (Fig. 17).[119] The median survival of patients with centrocytic lymphoma (2.5 years) was considerably shorter than that observed in immunocytoma (4 years), B-CLL (5 years) and centroblastic-centrocytic lymphoma (5 years). In a subsequent prospective, randomized therapy trial in patients with advanced centrocytic lymphoma,[120] polychemotherapy was started immediately after completion of the staging procedures. Patients were randomly submitted to treatment with either the COP protocol or the more intensive CHOP protocol. A prognostic superiority of the latter could not be proven. These two groups were compared with the very similar group of centrocytic lymphoma patients who were observed in the first study with the "watch and wait" approach. It turned out that the immediate administration of polychemotherapy with the COP or CHOP regimen improved the prognosis slightly, as indicated by a prolongation of median overall survival by about 3 months, but the difference was not significant. In an independent study done elsewhere,[121] patients with centroblastic-centrocytic lymphoma, centrocytic lymphoma and immunocytoma who did not yet require treatment according to the conventional criteria listed above, were evaluated in a randomized trial. One group was merely observed and received palliative, low-intensity treatment only at signs of progression ("watch and wait"), while the second group was initially submitted to intensive induction polychemotherapy (ProMACE/MOPP protocol) with adjuvant low-dose total nodal irradiation. In the latter group 78% of the patients showed complete remission that proved to be stable for more than 4 years in 86%. Two-thirds of the patients in the control group ("watch and wait") required treatment during the study period, often repeatedly. With almost identical 5-year survival rates in both treatment groups (83% and 84%, respectively), intensive induction chemotherapy does not appear to have a prognostic advantage. This assumption may have to be revised, however, in view of the promising results obtained with ultra-intensive myeloablative therapy followed by autologous bone marrow or peripheral blood stem cell rescue.[121a] Nevertheless, in this group of slowly proliferating tumours, it is possible to detect significant differences between treatment approaches and to identify definitely cured patients only after longer observation periods.

---

[118] Cheson 1991; Keating et al. 1991.
[118a] Engelhard et al. 1991.
[119] Brittinger et al. 1984; 1986a.
[120] Meusers et al. 1989.
[121] Young et al. 1988.
[121a] Rohatiner and Lister 1991.

2.6.4 Treatment of Advanced High-Grade Malignant NHL

In contrast to the low-grade malignant NHL, the high-grade malignant entities definitely require immediate intensive polychemotherapy, since only the rapid achievement of complete remission offers the chance of cure. During the last 15 years, various polychemotherapy protocols have become available.[122] They show a few significant differences. Protocols employed up to the early 1980s were characterized by the cyclic application of a four- or five-component cytostatic drug combination (e.g. CHOP). In the subsequently investigated protocols, generally considered to be more intensive, six or more different components were combined (e.g. M-BACOD, COP-BLAM I, MACOP-B) and given to the patients according to various time schedules with the aim of decreasing the therapy-free intervals between drug exposures. Other concepts have required the response-adapted application of the fixed alternating or sequential administration of two drug combinations (e.g. ProMACE/MOPP, ProMACE/CytaBOM, LNH-80, COP-BLAM/IMVP-16). Initial results, e.g. complete remission rates of 60%–85% and a relapse-free survival of 40%–70% for at least 2 years, indicate that an increase in complete remission rates can be attained with various differentiated protocols. An evaluation of the remission stability and an estimation of the potential cure rate is still difficult, however, mainly because of differences in the follow-up periods. Another difficulty is the restricted comparability of the patient groups (e.g. homogeneity or heterogeneity of the lymphoma entities, age distribution, stage incidence, treatment at a single institution versus an oligocentre or multicentre trial).

The final percentage of patients cured is reduced not only by the 15%–40% of cases refractory to the induction chemotherapy, but also by those approx. 30% of patients who experience relapse after achieving complete remission. "Salvage" therapy approaches have included, for example, the administration of cytostatic drugs not employed in the induction regimen or of very intensive and/or highly toxic drug combinations. In patients who respond to this treatment it is feasible to add subsequent ultra-intensive therapy with bone marrow transplant rescue. It is still impossible, however, to make definite treatment recommendations that can significantly improve the generally unfavourable prognosis of these patients.

2.6.5 Prospects

A number of prospects for future therapeutic approaches can be deduced from the experiences gained internationally in the treatment of NHL. The conventional treatment strategies[123] can still be modified to improve the chance of curability. In the strictly localized stages, long-term disease-free survival rates after initial radiotherapy might be increased by adjuvant application of chemotherapy, if the prognostic relevance of this approach can be proven. As mentioned above, how-

---

[122] Recent reviews: Coleman et al. 1987; DeVita et al. 1988; Yi et al. 1990.
[123] Brittinger et al. 1986a.

ever, the positive results obtained with initial polychemotherapy, possibly followed by adjuvant radiotherapy,[124] may indicate that such an approach will become the appropriate strategy for centroblastic and immunoblastic lymphomas in stage I/I$_E$. In low-grade malignant NHL the identification of therapy-resistant and high-risk subgroups might contribute to a more precise set of indications for very intensive forms of treatment. In high-grade malignant NHL some modifications of the chemotherapy protocols[125] developed and used in recent years are still imaginable. It is also conceivable that adjuvant radiotherapy will occupy a firm position in the treatment approach, if current therapy trials provide proof that its use is indeed beneficial. The identification of high-risk subgroups may also prove to be of particular significance. A number of clinical and experimental observations already provide the basis for further meaningful modifications of conventional chemotherapy strategies. The consistent administration of the highest possible drug doses in a given combination, altering the dosage of certain components in a given combination, and changing the mode of administration appear to be prognostically relevant.[126] The objective of increasing the dosage of induction chemotherapy that derives from these observations necessarily requires a corresponding improvement in supportive care. The latter might include the administration of colony-stimulating factors that stimulate haematopoiesis, especially the formation of neutrophils.[127] In cases of refractory disease, ultra-intensive, bone marrow-ablative therapy with subsequent bone marrow transplantation rescue should be integrated early into the treatment plan in suitable patients. Moreover, the development of new strategies has to include a re-evaluation of both acknowledged prognostic factors (e.g. advanced age and tumour stage, reduced performance status, increased serum LDH activity and/or reduced serum albumin concentration) and newly identified ones for each lymphoma entity or patient subgroup. These new factors may include chromosomal aberrations, the proliferative activity of the NHL, the in vitro sensitivity to immune modulators and the early identification of multidrug resistance. The long-term clinical relevance of the aforementioned possibilities for developing more efficient therapeutic concepts can be determined only in prospective, randomized therapy trials.

---

[124] Jones et al. 1989; Longo et al. 1989.
[125] Coleman et al. 1987; DeVita et al. 1988; Yi et al. 1990.
[126] DeVita et al. 1988.
[127] Vadhan-Raj et al. 1988.

3 B-Cell Lymphomas

B-cell lymphomas are tumours of immunocompetent cells, whose function it is to produce Ig. Correspondingly, Ig can be demonstrated in most B-cell lymphomas, either on the surface of tumour cells (sIg) or in the cytoplasm (cIg). In principle, the demonstration of cIg is equivalent to Ig secretion. The latter can lead to monoclonal gammopathy when there is a sufficient number of cIg-positive cells. Mostly cIg is demonstrated when the PAP method used in our laboratory is applied to paraffin sections of formalin-fixed tissue. The positive cells show a dark brown, wide-rimmed reaction product. With the exception of IgM, sIg cannot be demonstrated with our PAP method after formalin fixation. The strept-avidin-biotin method is more sensitive and can be used to demonstrate sIg as well as cIg in properly fixed tissue. With this method the reaction product is seen as a narrow, light brown rim. The demonstration of only *one* light chain ("light chain restriction") is synonymous with clonality and thus an important criterion for determining malignancy of proliferating B cells. Approximately 30% of the cases of B-cell lymphoma, usually of high-grade malignancy, lack the expression of Ig. In such cases clonality can be determined only by demonstrating rearrangement of the Ig chain genes; this is necessary for a diagnosis in only a few cases, however.

We distinguish low-grade and high-grade malignant B-cell lymphomas. The high-grade ML are usually primary, but some of them develop secondarily from low-grade ML. Most B-cell lymphomas are derived from peripheral lymphoid tissue, most frequently from germinal centres. Lymphoblastic lymphomas are tumours of the precursor cells that develop in bone marrow. The origins of Burkitt's lymphoma and large cell anaplastic lymphoma have not yet been fully clarified.

3.1 Low-Grade Malignant Lymphomas of B-Cell Type

Low-grade ML are defined as lymphomas composed, in the main, of small, mostly non-basophilic cells. These are called "-cytes" to conform with haemato-logical usage. In some low-grade ML they are interspersed with larger, basophilic cells, which are correspondingly called "-blasts".

3.1.1 Lymphocytic Lymphomas

The term *lymphocytic lymphoma* is applied to all ML whose essential components are lymphocytes or certain lymphocytic variants (e.g. prolymphocytes, hairy cells). They usually belong to the B-lymphocyte series, less often to the T-lymphocyte series. As yet, we have never observed a lymphocytic lymphoma in a lymph node that could not be placed in one of the lymphocytic lymphoma categories. The Kiel classification differs in this respect from that of RAPPAPORT,[128] who separated lymphocytic lymphoma from CLL and macroglobulinaemia of Waldenström.

3.1.1.1 Chronic Lymphocytic Leukaemia of B-Cell Type (B-CLL)

WF: Malignant lymphoma, small lymphocytic, consistent with CLL (A)

Lukes-Collins: Small lymphocyte B, B-CLL

Definition and Origin. Chronic lymphocytic leukaemia of B-cell type (B-CLL) is a neoplasm of B lymphocytes whose normal counterpart might be a population of follicular mantle lymphocytes.[129] B-CLL does not show Ig-secreting cells in significant numbers. Hence involved lymph nodes do not contain lymphoplasmacytoid cells with CIg (light chains restricted to one type) or contain only a negligible number of them. Similarly, the neoplastic cells do not show any PAS-positive globular intranuclear inclusions. As a rule, the blood picture is leukaemic ($>4.0 \times 10^9$ lymphocytes/l). Bone marrow is always infiltrated by lymphocytes. Hypogammaglobulinaemia can often be demonstrated. Paraproteinaemia does not occur in B-CLL. Histologically, small lymphocytes predominate, but there are *always* at least a few large blast cells and some prolymphocytes.

Immunology. B-CLL lymphocytes bear sIg of the IgM type, often together with IgD, and Ig light chains of either the *kapppa* or the *lambda* type. Approximately 20% of the cases lack the expression of IgD, and occasional cases lack IgM as well. Cases that show IgG on the surface of tumour cells also reveal intracytoplasmic IgG. This finding is inconsistent with a diagnosis of B-CLL; such cases have to be diagnosed as immunocytoma (see p. 66). In paraffin sections monotypic cIg either is not seen or is found in only a few lymphoid cells. Paraimmunoblasts, however, may show moderate cIg reactivity (yellow reaction product with PAP staining), especially in the tumour-forming subtype (see Fig. 22b). B-CLL cells express the B-cell antigens CD22, CD23, and usually CD20. CD5 is another characteristic antigen of B-CLL cells. The proportion of proliferating cells (Ki-67+) is usually about 5%. Complement receptors (CD35) are not a constant finding. The T-cell content is low (<10%). Residual follicular dendritic cells are found only rarely, if at all.

Occurrence. At the present time, cases of B-CLL account for about 11% of the lymph node biopsy material among NHL encountered by pathologists in Germany. Outside Germany, lymph node biopsies are seldom performed in cases of CLL, because blood and marrow examinations are considered to be sufficient for a diagnosis.

---

[128] Pangalis et al. 1977.
[129] Gobbi et al. 1983.

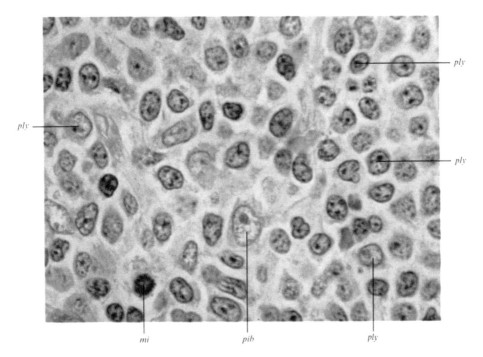

Fig. 18. B-CLL with Giemsa staining. Proliferation centre. Note one paraimmunoblast ("lymphoblast", *pib*), some prolymphocytes (*ply*) and one mitotic figure (*mi*). There are also a moderate number of small lymphocytes. Male, 70 years. Cervical node. 1550:1

B-CLL is usually a disease of late adult life and shows a peak occurrence in the 7th decade. B-CLL does not occur before the age of 20, and it is rare before the age of 30. The male-to-female ratio is approx. 1.5:1 (see Fig. 15).

Clinical Picture. See Definition.

Histology. The lymph node architecture is completely effaced, and sinuses cannot be recognized with standard stains. In sections stained for Ig, however, the sinuses can be identified because positively stained lymph marks the areas where numerous lymphocytes are migrating out of the node. The infiltration usually spreads into the tissue surrounding the node. When this happens, the fibres in the capsule usually remain intact, and only a small or moderate number of lymphocytes are found in the capsule, which is thus expanded. Residual lymphoid tissue is rarely seen; it is recognizable from the presence of lymphocytes that are smaller than the leukaemic lymphocytes and show a more intense nuclear staining. Remnants of germinal centres are also seldom. There are a small to moderate number of mostly fine reticulin fibres in a diffuse arrangement.

Cytologically, small lymphocytes with a usually round nucleus, coarse chromatin and scanty, pale-staining cytoplasm predominate (Fig. 18). Occasionally

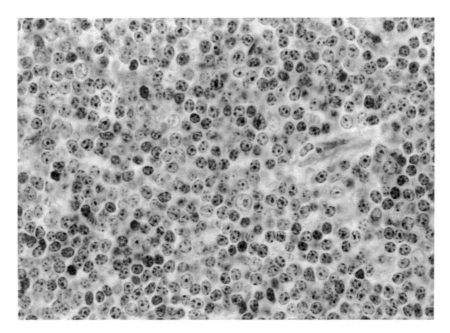

Fig. 19. B-CLL, diffuse subtype. Near the *centre*, one paraimmunoblast. There are no accumulations of prolymphocytes. Male, 61 years. Cervical node. Giemsa. 200 : 1

the nuclei are somewhat pleomorphic and hence suggestive of small centrocytes. Among the small lymphocytes are somewhat larger lymphocytoid cells ("prolymphocytes") with less dense chromatin and more abundant, pale-staining cytoplasm. Finally, one *always* finds at least a few large cells with a usually oval nucleus containing large, often solitary, central nucleoli. These cells have a moderate amount of cytoplasm that stains greyish blue with Giemsa, i.e. shows weaker staining than the cytoplasm of immunoblasts. Thus, we call these cells "paraimmunoblasts". Mitotic activity is low to moderate; mitotic figures are found only in paraimmunoblasts and prolymphocytes.

The histological impression of B-CLL varies with the number of prolymphocytes and paraimmunoblasts. (1) When there is only a small number of prolymphocytes and paraimmunoblasts, they cannot be recognized as such at a low magnification. Hence the growth pattern appears diffuse ("diffuse subtype", constituting about 7% of our cases; Fig. 19). (2) When there are moderate numbers of prolymphocytes and paraimmunoblasts, they are seen in clusters (proliferation centres), which are evident as light foci in Giemsa-stained slides at a low magnification ("pseudofollicular subtype", accounting for about 85% of our cases of B-CLL; Fig. 20). (3) Finally, prolymphocytes (and occasional or quite numerous paraimmunoblasts) may infiltrate large areas of the lymph node; these areas are clearly demarcated from the rest of the CLL infiltration ("tumour-forming subtype", constituting about 8% of our biopsy cases; Figs. 21, 22).

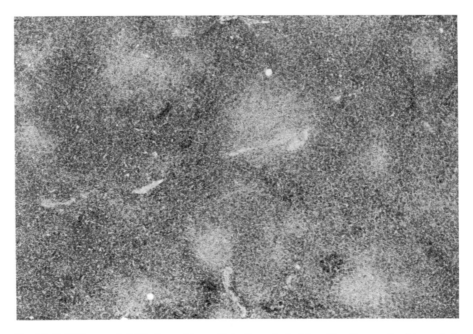

Fig. 20. B-CLL, pseudofollicular subtype. Note the pale foci (proliferation centres) irregularly distributed throughout the section. These should not be confused with neoplastic germinal centres. Male, 41 years. Axillary node. Giemsa. 56:1

Only a small number of macrophages and "reticulum cells"[130] are seen. There is no significant increase in mast cells, and eosinophils are absent. In occasional cases, there are a few typical plasma cells, sometimes with plasmablasts; they are found especially near vessels, the capsule or trabeculae. Immunohistochemical staining reveals that the light chains in the plasma cells are not restricted to one type ("polyclonal pattern", i.e. *kapppa* and *lambda* positive); hence the cells can be interpreted as reactive plasma cells and not as components of CLL. Giant cells of the Sternberg-Reed type are seldom seen.

---

[130] We have used the term "reticulum cell" for the non-lymphoid cells forming the framework of lymph nodes. Reticulum cells have an oval, round or irregularly shaped nucleus with fine chromatin and small or medium-sized nucleoli. They show relatively abundant, non-basophilic cytoplasm. On the basis of cytochemical and ultrastructural features, reticulum cells could be divided into four subtypes: the dendritic reticulum cell (B-zone specific; now called follicular dendritic cell), the interdigitating reticulum cell (T-zone specific; now called interdigitating cell), the histiocytic reticulum cell (also called histiocyte or macrophage) and the fibrogenic reticulum cell (also called myofibroblast). It is not always possible to make this distinction on paraffin sections, i.e. with ordinary light microscopic techniques. Hence one may continue to use the old term "reticulum cell", which originally meant nothing more than the large cells forming the framework between lymphoid cells (production of fibres was not recognized until later). In order to avoid confusion, however, we are using the generally accepted names in this edition.

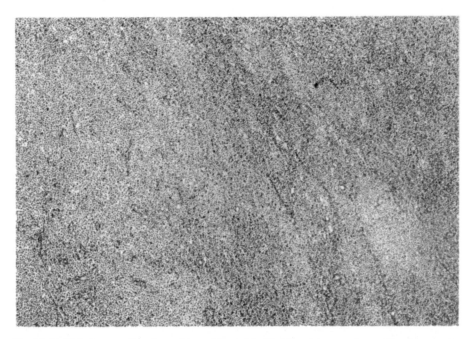

Fig. 21. B-CLL, tumour-forming subtype. The *left half* of the picture and a smaller focus at the *lower right* show cells that are paler and larger than those in the rest of the field. Male, 51 years. Cervical node. PAS. 56:1

Cytochemistry. Cytochemical analysis does not provide any diagnostically important information.

Differential Diagnosis

1. Immunocytoma. This type of lymphoma shows cIg in at least one cell per microscopic field with a 40 × objective or in large groups of cells. The light chains are restricted to one type ("monoclonal" pattern). There are often PAS-positive globular inclusions in the nuclei of neoplastic cells.

2. Centrocytic lymphoma. There are no blast cells. The reticulin fibres are thick.

3. Chronic lymphocytic leukaemia of T-cell type. T regions are infiltrated, and there is a marked increase in the number of epithelioid venules. A pseudofollicular pattern is not seen. T immunoblasts are extremely rare.

4. Sézary's syndrome. T regions are infiltrated, and a marked increase in the number of epithelioid venules is seen. Nuclei of lymphocytes are pleomorphic. Interdigitating cells are increased in number. There may be giant cells of the mycosis fungoides type.

5. Hairy cell leukaemia. B regions and connective tissue (trabeculae, capsule) are infiltrated. The lymph node is usually only partially involved. Nuclei are often reniform. Blast cells are absent, and mitotic figures are very rare.

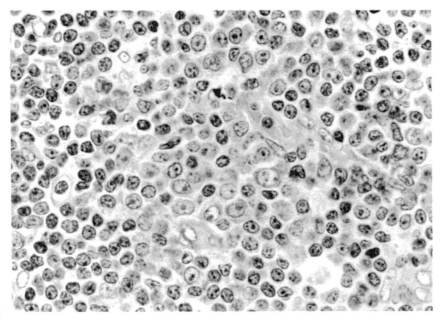

a

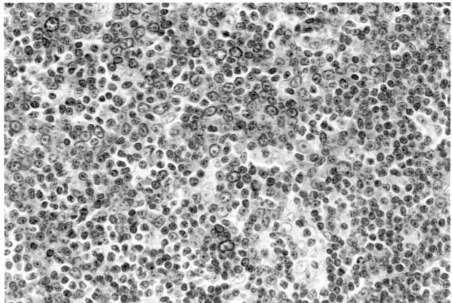

b

Fig. 22a, b. B-CLL, tumour-forming subtype. **a** Numerous paraimmunoblasts and pro-lymphocytes in a pale zone. **b** Corresponding area with staining for IgM. Numerous paraimmunoblasts and prolymphocytes contain a yellow reaction product. Female, 51 years. Cervical node. **a** Giemsa. 650:1. **b** PAP. 440:1

6. Hodgkin's lymphoma with lymphocytic predominance. This type of lymphoma contains Sternberg-Reed cells of the L & H type. It often shows infiltration by clusters of epithelioid cells. The growth pattern is frequently nodular ("nodular paragranuloma"); silver impregnation is the best staining for recognizing this.

7. Diffuse lymphoid hyperplasia. The sinuses are clearly demarcated, often dilated and filled with lymphoid cells.

Development into a Lymphoma of Higher-Grade Malignancy. About 16 % of cases of B-CLL terminally develop a tumour-like macroscopic appearance. Histologically, this corresponds in about 12 % of cases to the "tumour-forming subtype", which can often be recognized in the blood from an increase in the number of prolymphocytes. Such cases have been described as "transition into prolymphocytic leukaemia"[131], but this must not be confused with the primary prolymphocytic leukaemia of GALTON[132] (see below). Some cases of the tumour-forming subtype with a high content of prolymphocytes also contain numerous paraimmunoblasts; such cases correspond to the paraimmunoblastic variant described by PUGH et al.[133] Approximately 4 % of the B-CLL cases with a terminal tumour-like appearance show a large cell lymphoma, viz. immunoblastic or centroblastic lymphoma (so-called Richter syndrome; Fig. 23a). In contrast, a terminal lymphoblastic phase is evidently rare in CLL. Figure 23b shows a case that was interpreted as the blastic phase of B-CLL. The "blasts" contained a large amount of cytoplasmic IgM and were CD23 negative. They looked more like prolymphocytes than immunoblasts.

Prognosis. The duration of survival of patients with B-CLL is relatively long, but depends on the stage of the disease at the time of diagnosis. According to RAI et al.[134] and BINET[135] the stage of the disease is determined by other criteria than those used for other types of NHL. We assumed that it would be possible to make a more specific prognostic prediction from the histological subtype, even though the results of a study by DICK and MACA[136] do not appear to support this assumption. The pseudofollicular subtype shows the most favourable prognosis, while the prognosis for patients with the other two subtypes is significantly worse.[137]

Addendum: Prolymphocytic Leukaemia of B-Cell Type (B-PLL)

GALTON et al.[138] separated a special type of leukaemia from typical B-CLL: the lymphocytes are larger and have a large, prominent nucleolus (Fig. 24). The patients have marked splenomegaly. Initially, the lymph nodes are only slightly

---

[131] York et al. 1984; Stark et al. 1986.
[132] Galton et al. 1974.
[133] 1988.
[134] 1975.
[135] French Cooperative Group on Chronic Lymphocytic Leukaemia 1986.
[136] 1978.
[137] Brittinger et al. 1984.
[138] 1974.

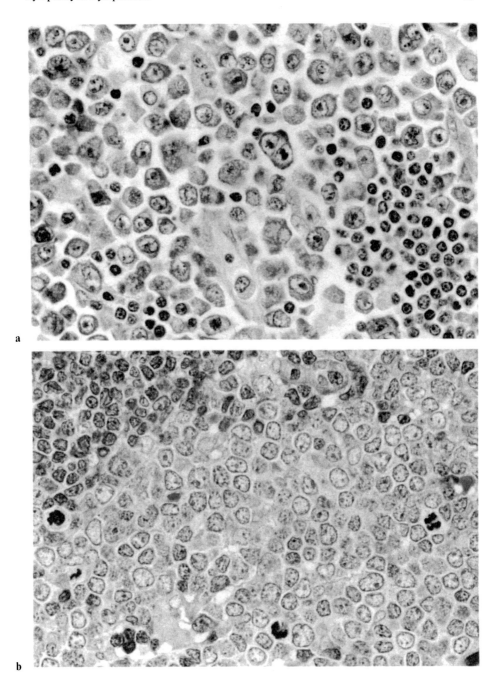

Fig. 23. a Immunoblastic lymphoma that developed terminally in a patient with CLL ("Richter's syndrome"). Only δ chains could be demonstrated with immunohistochemical staining. Post-mortem tissue specimen. **b** Blast crisis in B-CLL. The cells show small or medium-sized nucleoli and scanty, weakly basophilic cytoplasm. There are numerous mitotic figures. Biopsy. Male, 76 years. Giemsa. 695:1

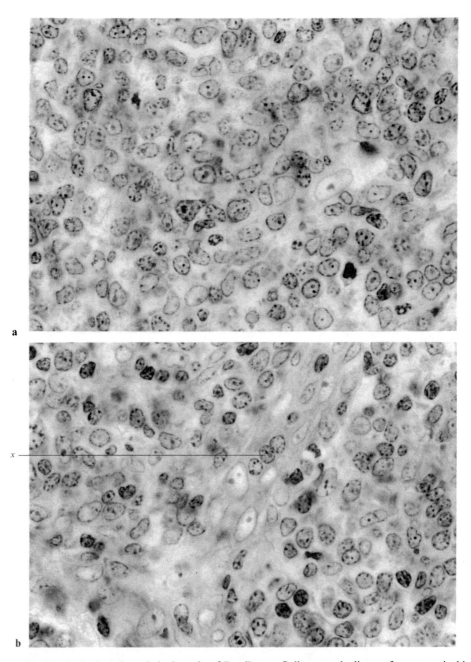

Fig. 24a, b. Prolymphocytic leukaemia of B-cell type. Solitary nucleoli are often recognizable next to the coarse nuclear chromatin. In **b** there is a venule with three prolymphocytes (*x*) located in the lumen. The walls of the vein are not effaced (cf. prolymphocytic leukaemia of T-cell type, Fig. 95). Giemsa. 875 : 1

infiltrated, but later they may be massively infiltrated by prolymphocytes. The prolymphocytes are quite monotonous looking. They are much larger than B-CLL lymphocytes and show more abundant, weakly basophilic cytoplasm. There are no proliferation centres. The large paraimmunoblasts seen in B-CLL do not occur in this type of leukaemia, but occasionally one finds a somewhat larger, basophilic cell with a larger nucleolus. The lymphoma types to be considered in a differential diagnosis are centrocytic lymphoma and lymphoblastic lymphoma.

Immunology. B-PLL shows more sIg than does B-CLL. Stainings for the light Ig chains reveal *lambda* more often than *kapppa*. The antigen profile is almost identical with that of B-CLL except that CD23 is not expressed. The number of cells expressing the proliferation-associated antigen (Ki-67 +) is larger than in B-CLL.

3.1.1.2 Hairy Cell Leukaemia (HCL)

WF: Not listed

Lukes-Collins: Small lymphocyte B, hairy-cell leukemia

Definition. Hairy cell leukaemia (HCL) is a neoplasm of small lymphoid cells that often reveal hair-like surface projections in blood smears (especially in unfixed slides)—thus the term "hairy cells". They are a special type of B lymphocyte, but an equivalent cell has not yet been found in normal or reactive lymphoid tissue. Hairy cells are characterized by tartrate-resistant acid phosphatase activity, although this is not specific to HCL.

Immunology.[139] Hairy cells always express sIg. Stainings for heavy chains reveal the expression of only *one* type (usually γ) about as often as that of two types (usually μ and δ). Our relatively large haematological collection shows a slight predominance of Ig light chains of *kapppa* type. Hairy cells also express the B-cell antigens CD22, CD20 and CD19.[140] They are CD5 and CD23 negative, but a few partially CD23-positive cases have been observed. Ninety percent of hairy cells show TAC reactivity (IL-2 receptor α chain). A special feature of hairy cells is their expression of the myelomonocytic antigen CD11c (Ki-M1 +) in frozen sections. There is also an intensely positive reaction with the monoclonal antibody Ki-M1p, which is not fully identical with Ki-M1 but can be applied to paraffin sections. Moreover, hairy cells can be stained with HML-1 antibody, which also recognizes intraepithelial intestinal T cells,[141] and the equivalent antibodies B-ly7[141a] and Ber-ACT8.[141b] The number of Ki-67-positive cells is smaller (< 5%) than in all other types of ML.

---

[139] The immunological analyses were done with the assistance of S. Bödewadt-Radzun.
[140] Cf. Schwarting et al. 1985.
[141] Moldenhauer et al. 1990; Möller et al. 1990.
[141a] Visser et al. 1989.
[141b] Schwarting et al. 1990; Kruschwitz et al. 1991.

Occurrence. HCL occurs in patients between the ages of 20 and 80. The age curve shows a peak in the 6th decade. There is a slight male predominance (male-to-female ratio 1.4:1).

Clinical Picture. HCL is a markedly chronic disease. The paramount signs are splenomegaly and pancytopenia. Lymphadenopathy does not appear until late in the course of the disease and is not pronounced. In the bone marrow there is a massive increase in the number of fibres and infiltration by small lymphoid cells; the latter eventually replace the whole of the normal marrow. Substantial enlargement of mediastinal and retroperitoneal lymph nodes has been reported.[142] The peripheral blood contains a small or moderate number of hairy cells. There is a relatively high incidence of infections with *M. kansasii*[143] and of secondary malignant tumours[144] in cases of HCL.

Histology. Lymph nodes show infiltration by monomorphic lymphocytoid cells that are somewhat larger than lymphocytes (Fig. 25). The nuclei of the tumour cells are somewhat irregular and often reniform; they lie farther apart from each other than do the nuclei of CLL cells because the cytoplasm is more abundant. Blast cells are not found in HCL. Mitotic figures are seen only rarely. The hairy cells are usually interspersed with some polyclonal plasma cells and some mast cells. The infiltration begins in B regions and connective tissue.

Cytology and Cytochemistry. In imprints the hair-like processes of "hairy cells" can be recognized most easily with acid phosphatase staining. Hairy cells show a granular acid phosphatase reaction, which is tartrate resistant in a variable number of cells in almost all cases. The acid non-specific esterase reaction is strongly positive and granular.[145]

3.1.2 Lymphoplasmacytic/Lymphoplasmacytoid Lymphoma (Immunocytoma)

WF: Malignant lymphoma, small lymphocytic, plasmacytoid (A)

Lukes-Collins: Plasmacytic-lymphocytic

Definition. Immunocytoma is a monoclonal neoplasm of B lymphocytes and is thus similar to B-CLL. In addition to lymphocytes, however, immunocytoma always contains some lymphoplasmacytoid cells or plasma cells that express the same type of Ig. The lymphocytes show sIg, while the lymphoplasmacytoid cells or plasma cells (including precursor cells) contain cIg of the same type.

We distinguish two subtypes of immunocytoma,[146] viz. the lymphoplasmacytoid type and the lymphoplasmacytic type. In the past, we have also included a third subtype known as the polymorphic type, but we have since found that this

---

[142] Vardiman and Golomb 1984; Malik et al. 1989.
[143] Rice et al. 1982.
[144] Jacobs et al. 1985.
[145] Tolksdorf and Stein 1979.
[146] Lennert et al. 1991.

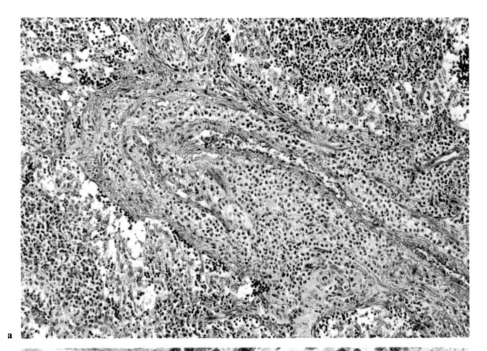

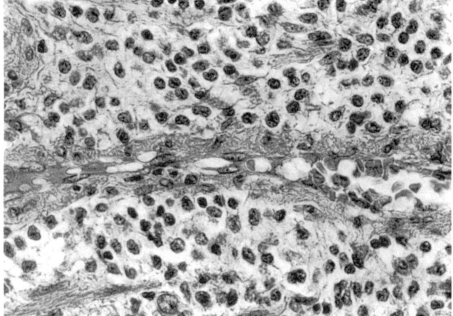

Fig. 25a, b. Hairy cell leukaemia. Perivascular leukaemic infiltration of a trabecula. The nuclei of the "hairy cells" are fairly far apart in comparison with those in the surrounding lymphoid tissue at *upper right* and *lower left* in **a**. Note the pleomorphic, sometimes reniform, nuclei in **b**. Male, 61 years. Axillary node. H & E. **a** 140:1, **b** 560:1

category is merely confusing. The lymphoplasmacytoid subtype is usually CD5 positive; it is more often leukaemic and less often paraproteinaemic. In contrast, the lymphoplasmacytic subtype is always CD5 negative; it is less often leukaemic and more often paraproteinaemic. The lymphoplasmacytoid subtype occurs about three times more often than does the lymphoplasmacytic subtype. The paraproteinaemia is frequently of the IgM type ("macroglobulinaemia"), but there may also be monoclonal IgG or, rarely, IgA synthesis. Histologically, intranuclear PAS-positive inclusions are found in about one-quarter of the cases of immunocytoma.

Remarks on the Definition Underlying Other Classifications. Although some classifications recognize a "lympho-plasmacytic" category of ML, cases of immunocytoma are often simply classified as "ML lymphocytic". The reasons for this are mainly technical: In H & E-stained slides, plasmacytoid differentiation can be recognized only when it is pronounced; hence it is often necessary to apply special stains or immunological analysis to make the correct diagnosis.

Immunology.[147] The tumour cells express monoclonal sIg. In contrast to B-CLL cells, some plasma cells, plasmacytoid cells and immunoblasts also contain cIg of the same isotype as the sIg when examined on paraffin sections (Figs. 33, 34). The most frequent heavy chain class is μ. Approximately 70% of the cases show both IgM and IgD. IgG can be demonstrated in about 10% of cases. IgA and IgE are rarely found. The tumour cells express CD22, CD19 and CD20. At least 80% of the cases of the lymphoplasmacytoid subtype express CD5 and CD23, whereas the lymphoplasmacytic subtype is always CD5 negative and shows CD23 expression in only half the cases.[147a] The proportion of proliferating cells (Ki-67 +) is, on the average, somewhat larger in immunocytoma than in B-CLL. In about 40% of cases the tumour cells express C3b receptors (CD35 +). A diffuse admixture of T cells (both CD4 positive and CD8 positive) is a regular finding in immunocytoma. Remnants of follicular dendritic cells are found with or without germinal centre cells in about 50% of the cases of lymphoplasmacytic immunocytoma, whereas they are hardly ever seen in the lymphoplasmacytoid subtype (similar to B-CLL).[147a] The presence of follicular dendritic cells and complete, polytypic germinal centres is reminiscent of findings in low-grade malignant B-cell lymphomas of MALT type.

Occurrence. When lymph node biopsies are often performed in cases of B-CLL, as is true in Germany, the number of cases of immunocytoma is also higher than it is in other countries. We diagnosed 12.4% of our cases of NHL as immunocytoma. In the United States immunocytoma appears to be less common (approx. 5% of the NHL), but this may be due to differences in the definition.

The age distribution of immunocytoma is approximately the same as that of B-CLL, except for the occasional case of immunocytoma in childhood. Our youngest patient was 13 years old. The male-to-female ratio is about 1.1 : 1 (see Fig. 15).

[147] Cf. Harris and Bhan 1985b; Hall et al. 1987.
[147a] Lennert et al. 1991.

Immunocytoma often develops in patients with autoimmune diseases, especially Sjögren's syndrome.[148]

Clinical Picture. In most patients, lymphadenopathy develops slowly and affects many regions. In some cases, however, an excessively enlarged spleen is the first sign of disease.[149] The so-called splenomegalic type, in which there is gross splenomegaly but no enlargement of peripheral lymph nodes, is not infrequent.[150] Immunocytoma may develop primarily at an extranodal site and occasionally does not involve lymph nodes at all. The blood serum of at least 36% of patients shows monoclonal gammopathy, usually IgM, sometimes IgG, rarely IgA or IgE. A few cases exhibit light chains or heavy chains alone. About 60% of patients have lymphocytosis ($>4 \times 10^9$ lymphocytes/l), which looks very much like B-CLL, but is sometimes striking owing to the presence of basophilic lymphoplasmacytoid cells. Coombs-positive haemolytic anaemia was reported in 13.5% of patients,[151] whereas it is rarely, if at all, seen in patients with B-CLL.

Histology. As in B-CLL, small lymphocytes predominate markedly in immunocytoma. They always make up more than 50%, and usually more than 90% of the tumour cells. In contrast to B-CLL, however, there is also a number of lymphoplasmacytoid cells or plasma cells, i.e. cells with more abundant, basophilic cytoplasm. These cells rarely amount to more than 10% of the tumour cells. In addition, there are always a few immunoblasts. Some cases show a larger number of immunoblasts, and there may be very large proliferation centres, as in tumour-forming B-CLL. Nevertheless, lymphocytes are still the predominant cells. In the past, we have classified such cases as the *polymorphic subtype* of immunocytoma (Fig. 28). Now we consider this category to be superfluous. When we diagnose a case of immunocytoma of the lymphoplasmacytoid or lymphoplasmacytic subtype we can say whether there is a large number of immunoblasts, which is a sign of a higher proliferation rate. By making a diagnosis of this sort one can avoid the danger of overdiagnosing immunocytoma of the polymorphic subtype. Over the years, the immunocytoma category has become a collection box for many different lesions with a high content of plasma cells and immunoblasts, e.g. immunoblastic lymphoma with plasmacytic differentiation, immunocytoma transforming into immunoblastic lymphoma, T-cell lymphomas with a high content of plasma cells, Hodgkin's lymphoma and infectious mononucleosis. By avoiding the term "polymorphic immunocytoma" it is possible to place a case of immunocytoma with a high content of blast cells in either the lymphoplasmacytoid category or the lymphoplasmacytic category, which are evidently different in nature.

Histologically, the *lymphoplasmacytic subtype* fully corresponds to Waldenström's macroglobulinaemia as described in the earlier literature (Figs. 26, 29). Classic plasma cells of the Marschalkó type and immunoblasts are interspersed

---

[148] Lennert et al. 1979.
[149] Heinz et al. 1979.
[150] Theml et al. 1977; Audouin et al. 1988.
[151] Heinz et al. 1979.

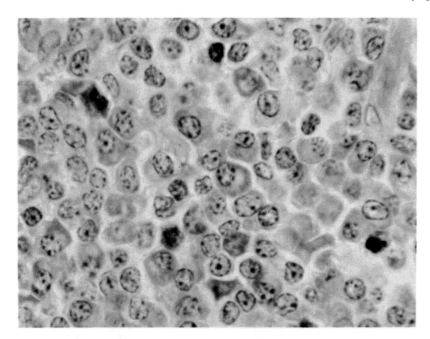

Fig. 26. Immunocytoma, lymphoplasmacytic subtype, with Giemsa staining. Most of the cells are lymphocytes. They are interspersed with typical Marschalkó plasma cells ("reticular" plasma cells). Male, 66 years. Cervical node. 1550:1

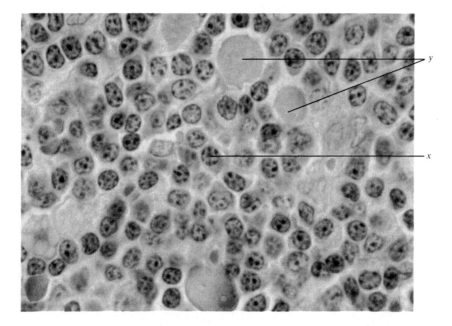

Fig. 27. Immunocytoma, lymphoplasmacytoid subtype, with Giemsa staining. The predominant lymphocytes are interspersed with some lymphoplasmacytoid cells (*x*) and a few large Russell bodies (*y*). Male, 69 years. Axillary node. 1550:1

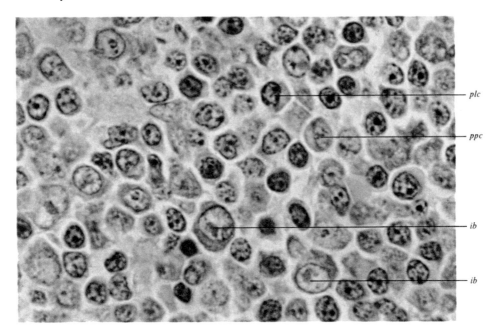

Fig. 28. Immunocytoma with a moderate content of blast cells (previously called the polymorphic subtype), with Giemsa staining. Small lymphocytes predominate. There are also large cells (immunoblasts, *ib*), medium-sized cells (proplasmacytes, *ppc*) and plasma cells (*plc*). Female, 80 years. Supraclavicular node. 1550 : 1

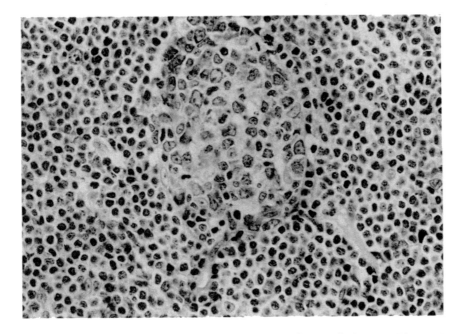

Fig. 29. Immunocytoma, lymphoplasmacytic subtype. Active germinal centre. Giemsa. 440 : 1

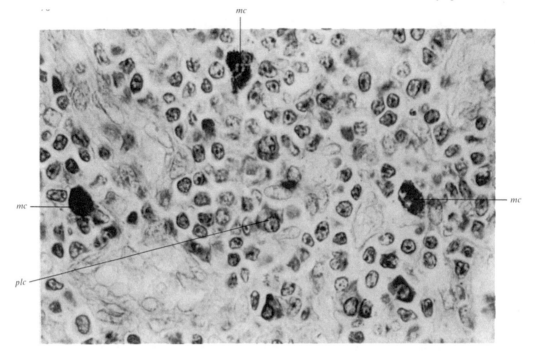

Fig. 30. High content of mast cells (*mc*) in immunocytoma, lymphoplasmacytic subtype. Numerous lymphocytes and some Marschalkó plasma cells (*plc*). Male, 73 years. Inguinal node. Giemsa. 880 : 1

among the predominant lymphocytes. The numbers of immunoblasts and mitotic figures are low. Proliferation centres like those seen in the pseudofollicular subtype of B-CLL are rarely found in the lymphoplasmacytic subtype of immunocytoma. An increase in the number of mast cells is observed in about two thirds of the cases (Fig. 30). The lymph node sinuses are usually dilated; occasionally they show cavernous dilatation, which is not seen in any other type of lymphoma. Haemosiderosis is often evident, especially in the sinuses.

The *lymphoplasmacytoid subtype* (Figs. 27, 32) is more like B-CLL: Lymphoplasmacytoid cells are seen instead of plasma cells. Lymphoplasmacytoid cells do not have prominent Golgi bodies. Their cytoplasm is less basophilic and less abundant than that of the plasma cells in the lymphoplasmacytic subtype. We are often surprised to find a large number of lymphoplasmacytoid cells with immunostainings, since these cells may be overlooked in sections stained with Giemsa. A significant increase in the number of mast cells is found in one-third of the cases. Sinuses are seldom recognizable in sections stained with Giemsa, but they can be identified with stainings for Ig (as in B-CLL, cf. p. 55). There is sometimes a pseudofollicular pattern. Haemosiderosis is not seen.

In the diagnosis of immunocytoma the most valuable histological feature is the presence of globular PAS-positive inclusions ("Dutcher bodies") in the *nucleus* of lymphoplasmacytoid cells or plasma cells (Figs. 31, 32). PAS-positive inclusions in the cytoplasm are not as significant, because they also occur in B-CLL. Intranuclear PAS-positive inclusions are found in only one-quarter of the cases.

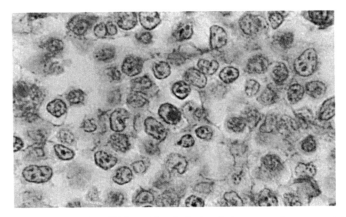

Fig. 31. Intranuclear PAS-positive inclusion in immunocytoma associated with μ-chain disease. Male, 43 years. Cervical node. PAS. 1000:1

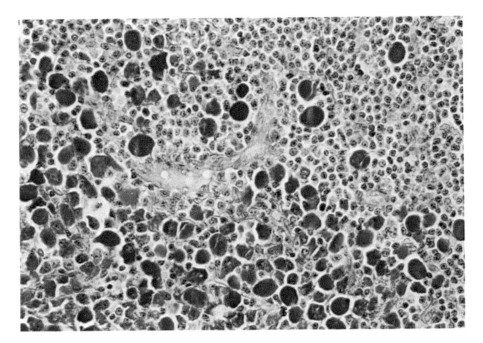

Fig. 32. PAS-positive globules in immunocytoma, lymphoplasmacytoid subtype. Female, 74 years. Inguinal node. Marked increase in IgM in tissue homogenate. PAS. 350:1

If we find them, however, we may be quite sure that the neoplasm is an immuno-cytoma and not B-CLL. With Goldner or Ladewig staining one can determine whether the PAS-positive globules represent IgM or another Ig class: IgM stains green or greyish blue, and the other Ig classes stain red. Besides globular inclusions, crystalline deposits are rarely seen in plasma cells, whereas diffuse PAS positivity is found more often. Paraproteins are rarely seen in the form of amorphous masses between the tumour cells. In such cases one sometimes finds foreign-body giant cells attempting to remove the deposits. The paraproteins seldom induce amyloidosis of the AL type[152] (usually *lambda* subtype). Some cases show groups of epithelioid cells. These may be so numerous as to simulate lymphoepithelioid T-cell lymphoma (Lennert's lymphoma). Such cases often show myoepithelial sialadenitis (sometimes with the clinical picture of Sjögren's syndrome) as well. This special type of immunocytoma is described on pp. 192 ff. Giant cells of the Sternberg-Reed type are found in occasional cases, especially when there is a high content of epithelioid cells.

Cytology and Cytochemistry. Imprints reveal the degree of basophilia better than do sections. For this reason it is easier to identify lymphoplasmacytoid cells in imprints. Cytochemical analysis does not provide any diagnostically helpful information.

Diagnosis. The diagnosis is based on the demonstration of lymphoplasmacytoid cells or plasma cells among the *predominating* small lymphocytes. It is seldom possible to recognize the lymphoplasmacytoid cells with H & E staining—one needs Giemsa staining to recognize them as basophilic cells or MGP staining to recognize them as pyroninophilic cells. The most reliable way to identify them is an immunohistochemical analysis, which makes it possible not only to determine the number of lymphoplasmacytoid cells and plasma cells, but also to demonstrate that the proliferation is monoclonal (light chains of only *one* type). In all doubtful cases (e.g. PAS-negative cases), the demonstration of monoclonality is essential. The presence of typical plasma cells and plasma cell precursors may be merely due to reactive changes; in such cases, the CIg in these cells is not restricted to one light chain type.

Differential Diagnosis. The most frequent problem is the distinction between immunocytoma and *B-CLL*. In one-quarter of such cases it is possible to make this distinction by looking at the PAS reaction: PAS-positive nuclear inclusions in the lymphoplasmacytoid cells or plasma cells are an indication of immunocytoma. In the remainder we have to do an immunohistochemical analysis to determine whether the lymphoplasmacytoid cells or plasma cells contain monotypic CIg; if they do, the neoplasm is definitely immunocytoma (Figs. 33, 34). Other histological or cytological criteria are of limited value and should be supplemented with one of the two reliable criteria.

Other diseases to be considered in the differential diagnosis of immunocytoma have been described in the section on B-CLL (see p. 58).

---

[152] Newland et al. 1986.

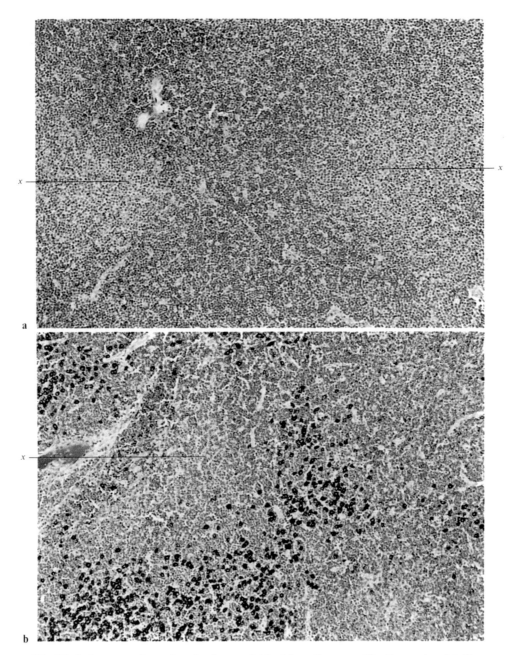

Fig. 33a, b. Immunocytoma, lymphoplasmacytoid subtype. Large proliferation centres (*x*). The surrounding tissue contains *kapppa*-negative (**a**), *lambda*-positive lymphoplasmacytoid cells (**b**). PAP. 100:1

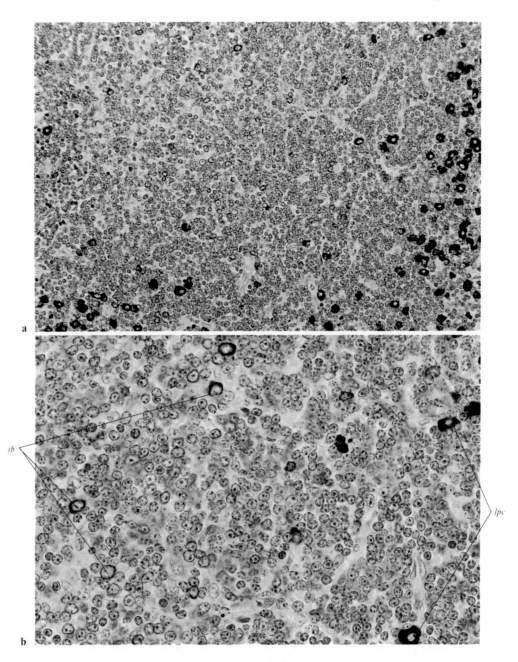

Fig. 34a, b. Immunocytoma, lymphoplasmacytoid subtype. Same case as Fig. 33. **a** IgM-positive lymphoplasmacytoid cells at the edge of a proliferation centre. **b** Immunoblasts (*ib*) in the proliferation centre. Only a few lymphoplasmacytoid cells (*lpc*). PAP. **a** 205:1, **b** 450:1

Borderline Cases. The borderline between immunocytoma and *B-CLL* is not sharp. In a systematic study using immunohistochemical methods,[153] we found a small group of "borderline cases" between B-CLL and immunocytoma. These cases looked like B-CLL, but contained a few lymphoplasmacytoid cells with cIg whose light chains were restricted to one type ("monoclonal" pattern). Since we may assume that the defect in the development of Ig-secreting cells in CLL does not have to affect all of the cells, we can draw only an arbitrary line between CLL and immunocytoma. We shall have to check whether this line is really of clinical significance. For immunocytoma we drew the line at one lymphoplasmacytoid cell or plasma cell per microscopic field at a magnification of 500 × – these cells had to show a monotypic light-chain staining pattern. Cases with less than one lymphoplasmacytoid cell or plasma cell per field were classified as B-CLL or as borderline cases between B-CLL and immunocytoma.

The borderline between immunocytoma and *immunoblastic lymphoma* is not sharp when the number of immunoblasts is high. When may one speak of an immunoblastic lymphoma, and when is the neoplasm still immunocytoma? The presence of *large accumulations* of immunoblasts is an indication of immunoblastic lymphoma. A high content of lymphocytes evenly spread about the section is inconsistent with a diagnosis of secondary immunoblastic lymphoma.

Development into a High-Grade Malignant Lymphoma. About 4% of cases of immunocytoma show transformation into immunoblastic lymphoma. In some instances, this may already be evident in the first biopsy, but immunoblastic lymphoma can also appear after immunocytoma has existed for a variable period of time. When immunoblastic lymphoma has developed, one finds a "pure" proliferation of immunoblasts, replacing part, or all, of the immunocytoma. An immunoblastic lymphoma that develops from an immunocytoma is often derived from the same cell clone,[154] but the immunoblastic lymphoma cells are often no longer capable of Ig secretion. The process may also be leukaemic. Secondary development of centroblastic lymphoma is rarely observed.

Prognosis. On the whole, the overall survival rate is somewhat lower than that of B-CLL (see Fig. 17). A study done by the Kiel Lymphoma Study Group[155] did not reveal any significant differences between the two subtypes. According to KIMBY and MELLSTEDT[156] the prognosis for immunocytoma patients with a leukaemic blood picture is more favourable than the prognosis for those with aleukaemic immunocytoma.

Addendum: Heavy Chain Diseases

In rare cases of paraproteinaemia the blood serum shows an elevated level of heavy chains of one class. In "γ-chain disease" and "μ-chain disease", immunocy-

---

[153] Papadimitriou et al. 1979.
[154] Brouet et al. 1976; Habeshaw et al. 1979.
[155] Heinz et al. 1979.
[156] 1991.

toma is the underlying disorder. The disorder known as "α-chain disease" is a subtype of immunoproliferative small intestinal disease (IPSID), which eventually develops into so-called Mediterranean lymphoma. In α-chain disease there is at first heavy infiltration of the small intestinal mucosa by monoclonal (α_1-positive) plasma cells, which can be controlled with antibiotics. In a later phase, low-grade malignant MALT lymphoma[157] develops, and this may finally transform into a high-grade malignant B-cell lymphoma (centroblastic or immunoblastic lymphoma).

3.1.3 Plasmacytic Lymphoma (Plasmacytoma)

WF: Extramedullary plasmacytoma

Lukes-Collins: Not listed, but the term "plasmacytoma" would be used.[158]

Definition. In this group we include only the "extramedullary" plasmacytomas that develop primarily in lymphoid tissue (lymph nodes and tonsils). The reasons for excluding plasmacytic myeloma are mainly practical ones. We certainly do not intend to imply that myeloma is completely different from lymph node plasmacytoma. "Extramedullary" plasmacytomas have also been found outside lymphoid tissue, e.g. in the upper respiratory tract, where they are of the same appearance as lymph node plasmacytoma.[159]

Immunology. The tumour cells contain cIg, usually of IgA type, less often of IgG type, rarely of IgM type.[160] A characteristic feature of this B-cell lymphoma category is the absence of the B-cell antigen CD22. Some cases, however, show expression of CD45R (Ki-B3 +). The tumour cells do not express the B-cell antigens CD19 and CD20. The reactions for PCA1 and CD38 antibodies are positive.

Occurrence. Primary lymph node plasmacytoma is a rare disease (<0.6% of the NHL in our collection). Most patients are between the ages of 30 and 70 years. The male-to-female ratio is about 2.6:1.

Clinical Picture. Involved lymph nodes are mostly cervical; axillary lymph nodes are also involved quite often, whereas lymph nodes in other regions are rarely affected. In general, paraproteinaemia is not found in early stages (because of the low tumour cell mass). The possibility of myeloma has to be excluded by bone marrow examination and skeletal x-rays.

---

[157] Isaacson 1979.
[158] R. D. Collins, personal communication.
[159] Wiltshaw 1971.
[160] Papadimitriou and Schwarze 1983.

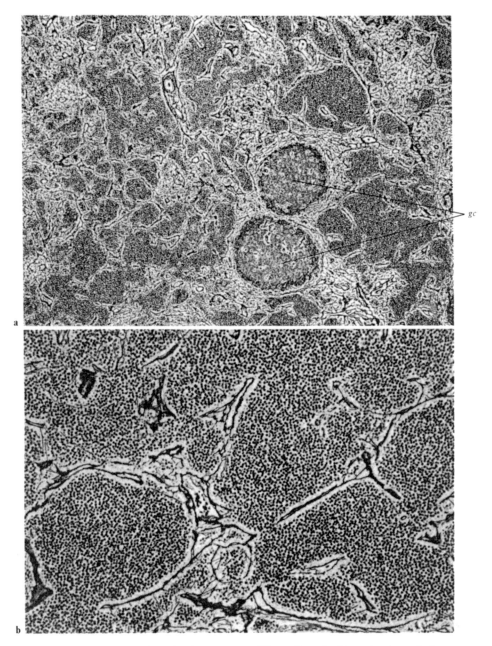

gc

Fig. 35a, b. Primary lymph node plasmacytoma. The uniform-looking, closely packed tumour cells form large clusters and masses surrounded by thick fibres and vessels producing an alveolar pattern. Residual germinal centres (*gc*) in **a**. Male, 70 years. Cervical node. Gomori. **a** 56:1, **b** 140:1

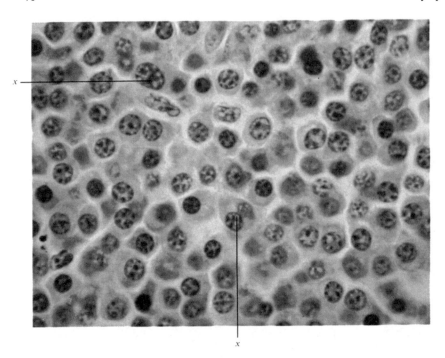

Fig. 36. Primary lymph node plasmacytoma with Giemsa staining. Somewhat polymorphic plasma cells. Two binucleate plasma cells (*x*). Same node as Fig. 35. 1550:1

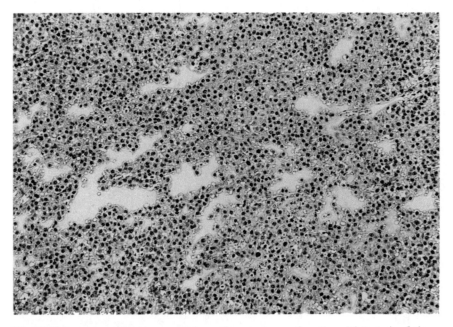

Fig. 37. Plasmacytoma showing a pseudo-angiomatous growth pattern. Metastasis of plasmacytoma in the nasopharynx 15 years after removal of the primary tumour. Male, 66 years. Cervical node. Van Gieson. 140:1

Histology. The tumour consists exclusively of typical ("reticular") plasma cells (Figs. 35, 36). Immunoblasts, plasmablasts and lymphocytes are not found. The reticulin fibres are thick and produce an alveolar pattern (Fig. 35). Occasionally, amyloid deposits can be demonstrated in the tumour tissue or vessel walls. Pseudo-angiomatous structures are occasionally evident (Fig. 37). In such cases bleeding into the tumour causes the formation of vessel-like lacunae that are not lined with endothelial cells.

Diagnosis and Differential Diagnosis. The main characteristics of lymph node plasmacytoma are the "monotony" and predominance of small cells. Although the plasma cells may show a certain degree of pleomorphism, with giant or multinucleate forms, there are no large basophilic cells with large nucleoli. The nuclear structure of the giant cells is the same as that of the mature plasma cells. This uniformity distinguishes plasmacytoma from most cases of *reactive plasmacytosis*, in which one can recognize all maturational stages of plasmacytopoiesis (immunoblasts, plasmablasts, proplasmacytes and plasma cells).

In comparison with lymph node metastasis of *myeloma*, primary lymph node plasmacytoma usually consists of smaller cells and shows a higher degree of differentiation. One of the reasons for this difference is probably that myeloma usually spreads to lymph nodes late in the course of the disease and after the cells have become anaplastic.

In contrast, *plasma cell leukaemia* shows a small-cell picture like that of lymph node plasmacytoma,[161] but there is a greater tendency to infiltration of the capsule and surrounding tissue in plasma cell leukaemia. It should not be difficult to diagnose plasma cell leukaemia, however, because of the obvious changes in the blood picture.

In contrast to *immunocytoma*, plasmacytoma does not contain lymphocytes. When we find lymphocytes (of B type) in a tumour otherwise composed of plasma cells, we diagnose immunocytoma, even if the lymphocytes are confined to small areas or are relatively sparse.

Prognosis. Lymph node plasmacytoma shows a much more favourable prognosis than does myeloma, because it is generally recognized at an earlier stage and the tumour can often be completely removed by surgery.

Addendum: Angiofollicular Hyperplasia (Castleman's Disease) with a High Content of Plasma Cells

Castleman's disease with a high content of plasma cells may simulate plasmacytoma, especially when the plasma cells are monotypic. Such plasma cells were found in seven of 18 biopsies in our collection.[162] IgG was detected more often than IgA (five vs. two cases, respectively). The light chains were of the *lambda* type in our cases and in almost all cases reported in the literature. Two of our cases showed monoclonal gammopathy. Histologically, the follicles exhibited regres-

---

[161] Isobe et al. 1979.
[162] Radaszkiewicz et al. 1989.

sive changes, with perivascular hyaline deposits and small germinal centres containing fewer cells; these are not features of plasmacytoma. Only two of the cases in our collection showed generalized lymphadenopathy ("multicentric angiofollicular lymph node hyperplasia"[163]).

A similar histological picture can be seen in a clinicopathological syndrome that has been described in the literature under various names, viz. osteosclerotic myeloma, Takatsuki's disease and POEMS (i.e. polyneuropathy, organomegaly, endocrinopathy, M proteins, skin changes) syndrome.[164] This syndrome is characterized by polyneuropathic and endocrinological symptoms and a usually monoclonal increase in plasma cells in lymph nodes and bone marrow.

HANSON et al.[165] found clonal rearrangements of Ig and TcR genes in three of four cases of systemic Castleman's disease, but not in four localized cases. ISAACSON[166] was motivated by that investigation and those of RADASZKIEWICZ et al.[167] and HALL et al.[168] to speculate on the topic of prelymphomas and early lymphomas.

3.1.4 Centroblastic-Centrocytic Lymphoma

*WF:*Malignant lymphoma, follicular, predominantly small cleaved cell (B)
Malignant lymphoma, follicular, mixed, small cleaved and large cell (C)
Malignant lymphoma, follicular, large cell (D)?
Malignant lymphoma, diffuse, small cleaved cell (E)?
Malignant lymphoma, diffuse, mixed, small and large cell (F)
Malignant lymphoma, diffuse, large cell, cleaved cell (G)?

Lukes-Collins: Small cleaved FCC

Definition. Centroblastic-centrocytic lymphoma is a neoplasm of germinal centres and thus consists of all their elements, viz. centroblasts, centrocytes, follicular dendritic cells and macrophages. Centrocytes always predominate. The tumour may show a follicular, a follicular and diffuse, or (rarely) a diffuse growth pattern. Tumours with a follicular or follicular and diffuse growth pattern are also known as follicular lymphoma (once called Brill-Symmers' disease). Between the neoplastic follicles there are variable-sized T regions containing T lymphocytes and epithelioid venules. Even in cases with a diffuse growth pattern, T lymphocytes can always be recognized among the germinal centre cells. About 30% of cases show sclerosis as well. Translocation of t(14;18) and rearrangement of *bcl*-2 on the molecular level are characteristic features of centroblastic-centrocytic lymphoma that are not found in other types of low-grade malignant B-cell lymphoma.

---

[163] Leibetseder and Thurner 1973; Diebold et al. 1980; Frizzera et al. 1983; Weisenburger et al. 1985b.
[164] Takatsuki et al. 1976b; Gaba et al. 1978; Kojima et al. 1983; Takatsuki and Sanada 1983.
[165] 1988.
[166] 1989.
[167] 1989.
[168] 1989.

Immunology[169] **and Cytogenetics.** The tumour cells bear sIg, mostly IgM and IgD; at least 30% of cases show IgG. Paraffin sections prepared from formalin-fixed tissue usually reveal cIg whose heavy chains are of the same classes as the sIg and whose light chains are restricted to one type. A few cases of centroblastic-centrocytic lymphoma showing biclonal cell proliferation have been reported.[170] Such proliferation may have resulted, however, from the development of sub-clones.[171]

Centroblastic-centrocytic lymphoma is characterized by the constant expression of CD22, CD19, CD20 and common ALL antigen (CD10). The expression of CD10 is more pronounced in neoplastic follicles than in reactive follicles. Interfollicular areas contain CD22-positive B cells that belong to the same cell clone as do those in the follicles. In the follicular structures there is generally a network of follicular dendritic cells, which appears to be less dense than that seen in reactive follicles. In a majority of cases of centroblastic-centrocytic lymphoma, stainings with monoclonal antibodies against bcl-2 protein show a positive reaction confined to neoplastic germinal centres, whereas reactive germinal centres are negative.[172] When the growth pattern becomes more diffuse, common ALL antigen may disappear and be replaced by the expression of CD23. The network of follicular dendritic cells is also much thinner in areas with a diffuse growth pattern and in the diffuse subtype. Rare cases of the diffuse subtype show no such network at all. The number of T cells may be high, reaching as much as 40%, even within the follicular structures. CD4-positive lymphocytes usually predominate. The number of Ki-67-positive cells varies from case to case (range: 4%–55%; mean: approx. 25%).

Both chromosomal analyses and molecular genetics have shown the frequent occurrence of t(14;18) chromosomal translocation involving the bcl-2 gene. Application of monoclonal antibodies directed against the bcl-2 oncogene protein has revealed that bcl-2 protein expression is not specific to t(14;18) translocation. Nevertheless, it is helpful in the distinction between neoplastic and reactive follicles.[173]

Occurrence. Centroblastic-centrocytic lymphoma accounts for about one-fifth of all cases of NHL in our collection. In the United States more than half and in Italy (Milan) only about 13% of all cases of NHL are of this type.

Centroblastic-centrocytic lymphoma shows a peak in the 6th decade of life. Our youngest patient was 13 years old and the oldest was 88. Hence centroblastic-centrocytic lymphoma does occur (very rarely) in childhood[174]; this was not evident in our previous investigations. A diagnosis of centroblastic-centrocytic lymphoma in a child must be substantiated, however, by the immunohistochem-

---

[169] Harris et al. 1984; Swerdlow et al. 1985.
[170] Sklar et al. 1984; Swerdlow et al. 1985.
[171] De Jong et al. 1989.
[172] Pezzella et al. 1990a, b; H. Griesser, personal communication.
[173] Weiss et al. 1987; Ngan et al. 1989; Pezzella et al. 1990; Wotherspoon et al. 1990; Ott et al. 1991.
[174] Frizzera and Murphy 1979; Winberg et al. 1979.

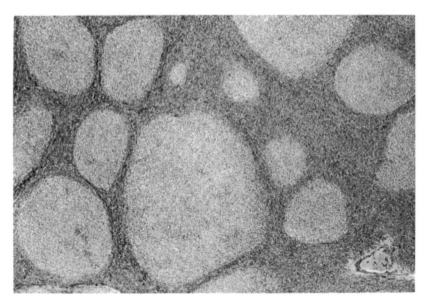

Fig. 38. Follicular centroblastic-centrocytic lymphoma. Female, 51 years. Axillary node. Giemsa. 31 : 1

Fig. 39a–c. Centroblastic-centrocytic lymphoma, follicular and diffuse. **a** On the *left* diffuse, on ▶ the *right* follicular growth pattern. **b** Follicular area. **c** Diffuse area. There is no significant cytological difference between the follicular and diffuse areas. Female, 57 years. Inguinal node. Giemsa. **a** 31 : 1, **b,c** 1000 : 1

ical demonstration of light chain restriction. Centroblastic-centrocytic lymphoma is the only type of ML that shows a slight female preponderance (the male-to-female ratio is about 1 : 1.18; see Fig. 15).

Clinical Picture.[175] The disease begins insidiously and is therefore often in an advanced stage when the patient seeks medical care. About 67% of patients are in stage III or IV at the time of diagnosis. B symptoms are noted by only 17% of patients. Cervical and inguinal lymph nodes are involved most frequently, but even lymph nodes in unusual sites (e.g. epitrochlear) may be affected. Mediastinal lymph nodes are often bypassed and do not appear to be a site of primary involvement.[176] The sclerotic type develops relatively frequently in the abdomen and groin. There are no changes in blood protein levels for a long period of time; paraproteinaemia (usually IgM) is seldom observed (about 1% of cases[177]). About 33% of patients show a leukaemic blood picture, usually with only a slight increase in the number of centrocytes, at some time during the course of the disease.

---

[175] Jones et al. 1973; Spiro et al. 1975; Brittinger et al. 1976; Bartels et al. 1979; König et al. 1979a,b.
[176] Bartels 1980.
[177] Bartels 1980.

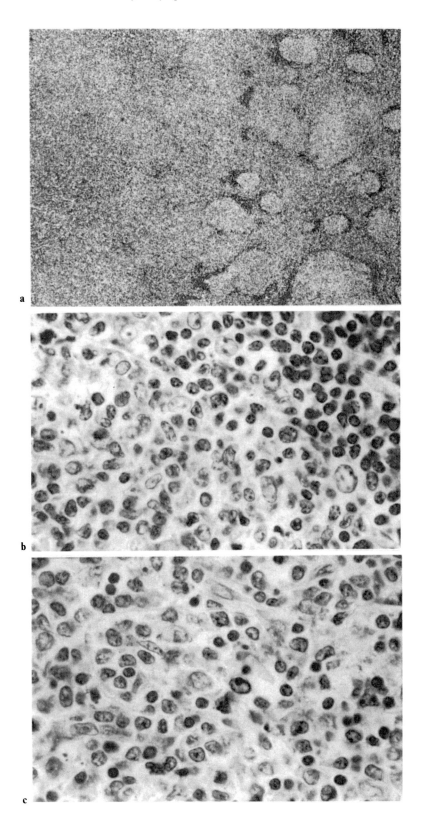

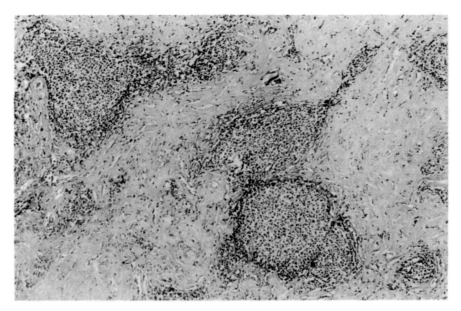

Fig. 40. Centroblastic-centrocytic lymphoma, follicular, with sclerosis. Sclerotic areas are hyalinized. Female, 69 years. Inguinal node. H & E. 96 : 1

A very small number of patients have centrocyte counts of up to 1×10^{11} cells/l. The centrocytes can be recognized from their "notched"[178] or "cleaved" nuclei. In our collection a significant primary extranodal localization was the *spleen*.[179] In 70% of those cases the spleen was the only infiltrated organ. Some of the patients recovered after splenectomy, while others later showed recurrence elsewhere. DIEBOLD et al.[180] also described a splenomegalic type of centroblastic-centrocytic lymphoma showing a relatively favourable prognosis.

Histology. On the basis of the growth pattern, centroblastic-centrocytic lymphoma can be divided into three subtypes, viz. follicular, follicular and diffuse, and diffuse. The purely follicular type (Fig. 38) is the most frequent (50%–70%), followed by the follicular and diffuse variant (25%–40%; Fig. 39) and, finally, the rare diffuse variant (5% or even less;[181] cf. Fig. 2b). Besides the growth pattern, we always indicate whether there is sclerosis (Fig. 40). Sclerosis is seen least often in the purely follicular variant (approx. 17%) and most often in the diffuse variant (100%); the follicular and diffuse variant shows an intermediate frequency of sclerosis (approx. 67%). This means that a diffuse growth pattern and a tendency to sclerosis go hand in hand.

---

[178] Galton 1964.
[179] Bartels 1980.
[180] 1987.
[181] Molenaar et al. 1984.

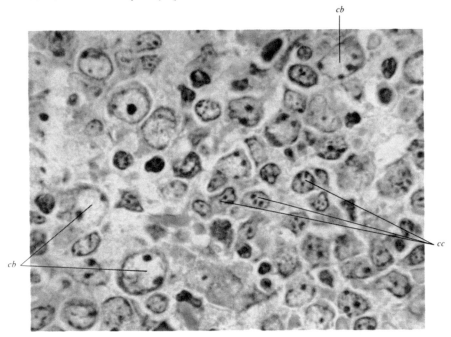

Fig. 41. Centroblastic-centrocytic lymphoma with Giemsa staining. Centrocytes (*cc*) and a relatively large number of centroblasts (*cb*) are present. Female, 71 years. Cervical node. 1550 : 1

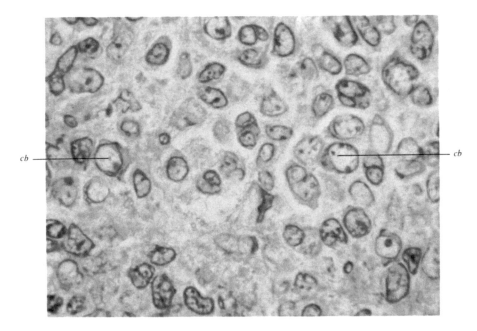

Fig. 42. Another case of centroblastic-centrocytic lymphoma with Giemsa staining. Only a few centroblasts (*cb*). Numerous, relatively large, pleomorphic centrocytes. Some "multilobated" cells. Female, 26 years. 1550 : 1

In follicular centroblastic-centrocytic lymphoma, formation of follicles is seen in the lymph node cortex and medulla. The lymph node architecture thus appears to be effaced. Between the neoplastic follicles, however, there are variable-sized T regions containing small lymphocytes, epithelioid venules and some reticulin fibres. These regions occasionally show a large number of plasma cells that are of the same immunophenotype as the neoplastic germinal centre cells. Paraproteinaemia is often seen in such cases.[182] The follicles contain only a small number of fibres; often they are almost completely devoid of fibres.

The neoplastic follicles consist chiefly of small or medium-sized centrocytes, but they always contain centroblasts, follicular dendritic cells and macrophages as well (Fig. 41). The centroblasts are medium sized or large and have scanty, basophilic cytoplasm and a round or oval nucleus with multiple, medium-sized, often marginal nucleoli. In some instances, centroblasts are evident in only some of the follicles, and these centroblasts may be present only in very small numbers. Occasionally, the follicles also show immunoblasts. Van der Putte et al.[183] pointed out the presence of germinal centre cells with lobated nuclei (see Fig. 42). The neoplastic follicles differ from reactive follicles in the uniform, dense arrangement of the cells and the absence of starry-sky cells (see p. 89). Neoplastic follicles may contain some or only one or two large, atypical lymphoid cells, and basophilic giant cells of an uncharacteristic appearance are seen in rare instances. Kjeldsberg and Kim[184] described polykaryocytes resembling Warthin-Finkeldey giant cells. These cells, or at least most of them, probably represent multinucleate follicular dendritic cells. Occasionally, one finds epithelioid cell granulomas ("tubercles") without evidence of tuberculosis or sarcoidosis.[185] Clusters of epithelioid cells are rarely seen.

In both the neoplastic follicles and the interfollicular tissue there are occasionally deposits of a PAS-positive substance in centrocyte-like or plasma cell-like cells. The PAS-positive deposits are often globular and may lead to a signet-ring cell-like deformation of the cells. The term "signet-ring cell lymphoma" has been applied to cases showing substantial numbers of such cells (see pp. 91 f.). Sometimes the PAS-positive substance is stored outside the cells in clumps and larger, amorphous aggregates in the neoplastic germinal centres (Fig. 43).[186] The deposits are sometimes phagocytosed by macrophages. They probably represent Ig, specifically IgM.

A diagnostically important, although infrequent, lesion in centroblastic-centrocytic lymphoma is total necrosis of infiltrated lymph nodes. It is found almost exclusively in this type of ML. In such cases it is easy to diagnose the lymphoma on sections stained by silver impregnation.

When purely follicular centroblastic-centrocytic lymphoma starts to show a diffuse growth pattern, the neoplastic follicles appear to be split into pieces and permeated with numerous reticulin fibres and lymphocytes. The diffuse areas consist chiefly of a mixture of centrocytes, lymphocytes and a few centroblasts.

---

[182] Cf. Alberti and Neiman 1984; Mann 1985; Frizzera et al. 1986.
[183] 1984.
[184] 1981.
[185] Kim and Dorfman 1974.
[186] Chittal et al. 1987.

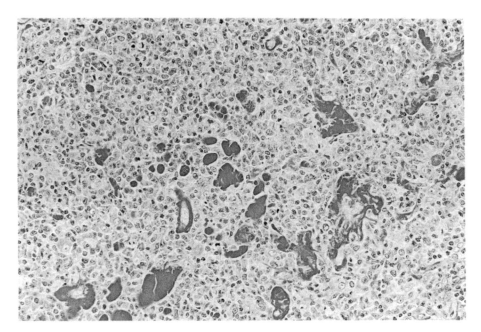

Fig. 43. Follicular centroblastic-centrocytic lymphoma. PAS-positive deposits in a neoplastic germinal centre. The deposits were produced by neoplastic germinal centre cells. Some of the deposits have been ingested by macrophages. Female, 33 years. Cubital node. PAS. 220:1

One must make a clear distinction between this picture and the development of diffuse centro*blastic* lymphoma from centroblastic-centrocytic lymphoma.

Sclerosis, which often affects only one side of the lymph node, appears to begin near the capsule and sometimes within it, and to spread first into the outer lymph node regions and surrounding tissue. Eventually, one finds large bundles of fibres, and these show a pronounced tendency to hyalinization. If the sclerosis progresses, then large areas of the lymph node may be replaced by hyaline fibrous tissue (this has been called "nodular sclerotic lymphosarcoma" by BENNETT and MILLETT[187]). In such cases the tumour develops a certain similarity to the nodular sclerosis type of Hodgkin's lymphoma.

Various other classifications distinguish several types of follicular lymphoma. The way we understand these types, they correspond to the following three morphological variants of centroblastic-centrocytic lymphoma:

1. With small centrocytes and only a few centroblasts (*WF:* B)
2. With small centrocytes and a large number of centroblasts (*WF:* C)
3. With large centrocytes and a large number of centroblasts (*WF:* D?)

Making these distinctions is supposed to allow certain prognostic predictions. This hypothesis has been tested on our own collection of cases by MOLENAAR et al.[188] (see p. 90).

---

[187] 1969.
[188] 1984.

Table 15. Differential diagnosis of follicular centroblastic-centrocytic lymphoma and follicular lymphoid hyperplasia

Histological features	Follicular centroblastic–centrocytic lymphoma	Follicular lymphoid hyperplasia
Lymph node architecture	Effaced	Largely preserved
Sinus catarrh	–	Sometimes +
Germinal centres		
Outline	Ill-defined	Distinct
Size and shape	Relatively uniform	Variable
Lymphocyte mantle	Absent or narrow	Usually well developed
Zonal architecture	Never	Often
In perinodal tissue	Often	Very rarely
Mitotic figures	Often only a few	Often very many
Protein precipitates	Almost never found	Frequently found
Cytology of follicles		
Centrocytes	Large number	Relatively small number
Centroblasts	Often small number	Often very large number
Starry-sky cells	None	Often abundant
Follicular dendritic cells	Relatively large number	Relatively small number
Interfollicular tissue	Monotonous; small cells	Sometimes polymorphic
Cytology of the interfollicular tissue (besides lymphocytes)		
Plasma cells	Sometimes (monotypic)	Often (polytypic)
Immunoblasts	–	Sometimes
Neutrophil granulocytes	–	Occasionally
Eosinophils	Occasionally	Occasionally
Mast cells	Occasionally	Occasionally

Cytology and Cytochemistry. Cytological or cytochemical analysis does not provide any diagnostically helpful information.

Differential Diagnosis. It is most important, and sometimes difficult, to distinguish *follicular* centroblastic-centrocytic lymphoma from *follicular lymphoid hyperplasia* (e.g. that associated with rheumatoid arthritis). It is usually possible to make a distinction on the basis of the criteria given in Table 15.[189] Important information is already provided by a low-power view (see MANN[190] for some very informative illustrations). Follicular centroblastic-centrocytic lymphoma shows relatively poorly defined germinal centres without, or with a merely narrow lymphocyte mantle and without a zonal arrangement. In contrast, the germinal centres in follicular hyperplasia are more clearly defined and often have a broad lymphocyte mantle; they also frequently show a zonal arrangement, with a lower dense zone containing numerous blast cells (basophilic!) and an upper, less dense zone containing numerous centrocytes (non-basophilic!). Cytologically, neoplastic germinal centres as a rule contain many more centrocytes than do reactive

---

[189] Reviews: Rappaport et al. 1956; Nathwani et al. 1981; Mann 1985.
[190] 1985, see the same publication for more literature.

germinal centres. In addition, mitotic activity is generally much lower in neoplastic germinal centres than in reactive ones. Starry-sky cells (macrophages with "tingible bodies") are not seen in centroblastic-centrocytic lymphoma unless the tumour is transforming into centroblastic lymphoma, whereas such cells are often found in reactive germinal centres.

Of the criteria listed in Table 15, the following are particularly important. An admixture of other types of "inflammatory" cells (especially large groups of well-differentiated, polyclonal plasma cells) and sinus reactions occur only in follicular lymphoid hyperplasia. *Very* large germinal centres containing numerous centroblasts and starry-sky cells are also typical of lymphoid hyperplasia, especially in children and in early stages of HIV infection. Since centroblastic-centrocytic lymphoma very rarely occurs in patients younger than 20 years of age, the patient's age is another important criterion.

A histological and cytological analysis can now be supplemented with immunohistochemical stainings. An immunohistochemical analysis is the most reliable way to distinguish between reactive and neoplastic germinal centres in paraffin sections from ambiguous cases. Reactive germinal centres contain *kapppa* and *lambda* chains, whereas neoplastic germinal centres contain light chains of only *one* type. Although rare cases of biclonal follicular lymphoma have been described,[191] light chain restriction is the most reliable criterion for substantiating a diagnosis of follicular centroblastic-centrocytic lymphoma. When light chain staining does not allow a clear distinction between centroblastic-centrocytic lymphoma and follicular hyperplasia, the use of anti-*bcl*-2 antibodies may be helpful.

Diffuse centroblastic-centrocytic lymphoma is diagnosed much too often.[192] At a workshop of the European Lymphoma Club, 80% of cases that had been interpreted as diffuse centroblastic-centrocytic lymphoma proved to be immunocytoma, centrocytic lymphoma or centrocytoid centroblastic lymphoma. Immunocytoma consists predominantly of lymphocytes, which can be misinterpreted as centrocytes on poorly prepared slides (!) and contains CIg-positive plasma cells or lymphoplasmacytoid cells. The larger blast cells do not correspond to centroblasts, but rather to immunoblasts or plasmablasts. Centrocytic lymphoma does not contain blast cells, with the exception of polyclonal plasma cell precursors or residual germinal centre cells. Centrocytoid centroblastic lymphoma shows a monotonous-looking proliferation of cells with a morphological appearance between that of centrocytes and that of centroblasts. Typical centroblasts are found in merely small numbers or not at all; immunoblasts do not occur. Mitotic activity is higher in centrocytoid centroblastic lymphoma than in centroblastic-centrocytic lymphoma.

Development into a High-Grade Malignant Lymphoma. Centroblastic-centrocytic lymphoma evolves into a high-grade ML (viz. secondary centroblastic lymphoma) more often than does any other type of B-cell lymphoma of low-grade malignancy. In our autopsy collection we found such a development in 40% of

---

[191] Sklar et al. 1984.
[192] E.g. Lieberman et al. 1986.

the cases of centroblastic-centrocytic lymphoma; in the other 60% the centrob-lastic-centrocytic lymphoma diagnosed on a lymph node biopsy was still evident at autopsy. An analysis of 424 cases in our biopsy collection revealed only 18 (4.2%) with development into centroblastic lymphoma.[193] The transformed tu-mour is made up of medium-sized or large cells of only *one* type and shows a *diffuse* growth pattern. In the literature there have been reports of sporadic cases of centroblastic-centrocytic lymphoma showing secondary development of dif-fuse peripheral T-cell lymphoma.[194]

Borderline Cases between Centroblastic-Centrocytic Lymphoma and Centroblastic Lymphoma. We do not draw the line between centroblastic-centrocytic lymphoma and centroblastic lymphoma simply on the basis of the number of centroblasts. We diagnose transformation into centroblastic lymphoma only when circum-scribed areas of the lymph node have been replaced by centroblasts (cf. p. 126).

Prognosis. Of all lymphomas of low-grade malignancy, centroblastic-centrocytic lymphoma shows the most favourable prognosis (see Fig. 17). Long-term survival is relatively high when the disease is diagnosed in stages I or II.[195] The growth pattern has hardly any influence on survival so long as at least part of the lymphoma exhibits a follicular pattern. The purely diffuse variant apparently has a significantly poorer prognosis than do other types.[196] The available data on the prognostic significance of sclerosis are contradictory, but we presume that sclero-sis does not have any significant influence on ultimate survival.

The size of the centrocytes and the number of centroblasts also have a merely limited effect on survival: large centrocytes and numerous centroblasts seem to indicate a somewhat poorer prognosis.[197] There was no statistically significant difference in survival between the small cleaved cell type and the mixed, small cleaved and large cell type of follicular ML as defined by the WF.[198] Different results were obtained in earlier investigations and in a study by LIEBERMAN et al.[199] These differences may be a matter of definition: the large cell type as defined in those studies may have corresponded to centroblastic lymphoma with a follicular growth pattern instead of centroblastic-centrocytic lymphoma.

The survival rate is somewhat higher when the primary localization of the tumour is extranodal and when the patients are women. When centroblastic-cen-trocytic lymphoma develops into centroblastic lymphoma, the survival rate drops considerably (see p. 126).

---

[193] Molenaar et al. 1984.
[194] Jennette et al. 1982; York II et al. 1983.
[195] Brittinger et al. 1978, 1984; Kuse et al. 1983.
[196] Meugé et al. 1978; The Non-Hodgkin's Lymphoma Pathologic Classification Project 1982.
[197] Rappaport et al. 1956; Jones et al. 1973; van Unnik et al. 1975; Molenaar et al. 1984.
[198] Molenaar et al. 1984.
[199] 1986.

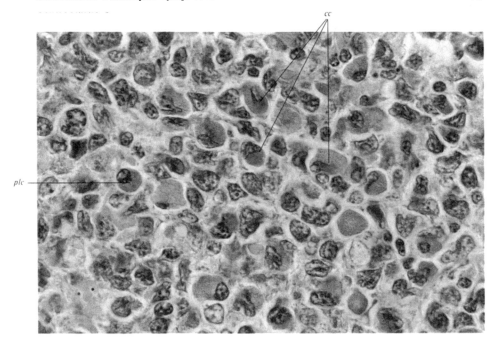

Fig. 44. "Signet-ring cell lymphoma". Follicular centroblastic-centrocytic lymphoma. PAS-positive, IgG/*kapppa*-positive deposits that stain red with Giemsa in the cytoplasm of centrocytes (*cc*) and plasma cells (*plc*) in a neoplastic germinal centre. Female, 67 years. Cervical node. Giemsa. 440:1

Addendum: Cytological Variants of Centroblastic-Centrocytic Lymphoma

1. Signet-Ring Cell Lymphoma.[200] A few cases of centroblastic-centrocytic lymphoma show globular or diffuse, PAS-positive deposits in numerous centrocytes, lymphoplasmacytoid cells and plasma cells (Fig. 44). These deposits represent IgM. Occasionally, they cause displacement and indentation of the nuclei;[201] this gives the vague impression of signet-ring cells. Hence such tumours have been called signet-ring cell lymphoma.[202]

The term "signet-ring cell lymphoma" is also applied to another morphological picture, in which vacuoles of various sizes fill the cytoplasm and push the nucleus to the periphery (Fig. 45).[203] The picture is otherwise that of centroblastic-centrocytic lymphoma with a follicular or follicular and diffuse growth pattern. In our cases the vacuoles were PAS negative or showed, at most, a very weak PAS reaction. In most cases the tumours were IgG-positive lymphomas.[204] The large vacuoles have been interpreted as giant multivesicular bodies, although they are lysozyme negative.[205]

---

[200] See Weiss et al. 1985a for review of English literature.
[201] Lennert and Mohri 1978; van den Tweel et al. 1978.
[202] Kim et al. 1978a.
[203] Kim et al. 1978a; see Weiss et al. 1985a for review of English literature.
[204] Weiss et al. 1985a.
[205] Harris et al. 1981.

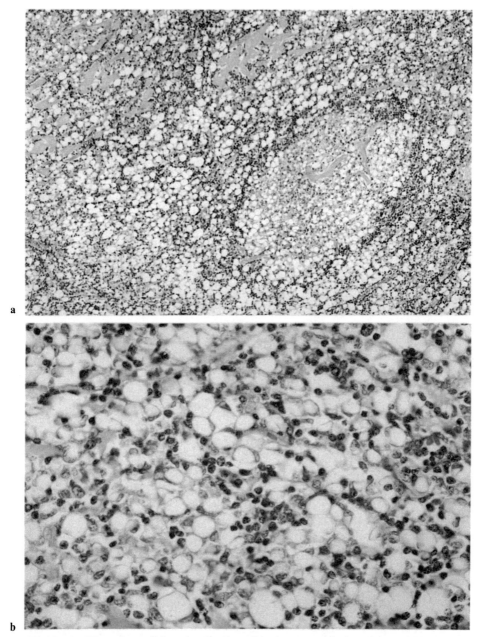

Fig. 45a, b. Signet-ring cell lymphoma. Centroblastic-centrocytic lymphoma, follicular and diffuse. **a** Neoplastic germinal centre embedded in an accumulation of diffusely infiltrating signet-ring cells. **b** Signet-ring cells in a diffuse area. Giemsa. **a** 110:1, **b** 440:1

We agree with STANSFELD[206] that the term "signet-ring cell lymphoma" should be used only for the second type of tumour with large cytoplasmic vacuoles, because only this type is confined to *one* cytologically defined entity, viz. centroblastic-centrocytic lymphoma. In contrast, PAS-positive Ig deposits occur in cytologically different lymphoma types, e.g. immunocytoma and centroblastic-centrocytic lymphoma. The term "signet-ring cell lymphoma" is superfluous, and even confusing, in such cases. Signet-ring cell lymphoma of T-cell type[207] is discussed on p. 260.

2. Centroblastic-Centrocytic Lymphoma with a High Content of Cells Containing Lobated Nuclei (Fig. 42). VAN DER PUTTE et al.[208] described two cases of follicular centroblastic-centrocytic lymphoma and one case of follicular and diffuse centroblastic-centrocytic lymphoma in which numerous germinal centre cells showed "multilobated" nuclei. The nuclear lobation was seen in centroblasts, centrocytes and lymphoplasmacytoid cells in the neoplastic germinal centres. Subsequently, the investigators looked in reactive germinal centres for cells with multilobated nuclei and actually found them in 5 of 40 cases.

3. Follicular Plasmacytoma. SCHMID et al.[209] described a case of follicular lymphoma in which the neoplastic follicles consisted predominantly of typical plasma cells. Some of the follicles, however, contained centroblasts and centrocytes. Hence the tumour was considered to be a special variant of centroblastic-centrocytic lymphoma.

3.1.5 Centrocytic Lymphoma (Mantle Cell Lymphoma)[209a]

WF: Not listed; categories E and G show similarities

Lukes-Collins: Small cleaved FCC

Other synonyms: Mantle zone lymphoma; intermediate lymphocytic lymphoma

Definition. Until now we have defined centrocytic lymphoma as a tumour derived from the centrocytes of germinal centres. It consists exclusively of the cells that we have designated as "centrocytes" and contains no centroblasts. In this definition the Kiel classification differs from that of LUKES and COLLINS,[210] who apply the term "cleaved FCC lymphoma" to all lymphomas that consist of cleaved cells (centrocytes), irrespective of whether there is an admixture of non-cleaved cells (centroblasts). Our investigations[211] shed doubt on their definition. Now there is a new, weighty argument in favour of separating centrocytic lymphoma from

---

[206] 1985.
[207] Weiss et al. 1985a.
[208] 1984.
[209] 1985.
[209a] Banks et al. 1992.
[210] 1974a,b, 1975a,b.
[211] Cf. Lennert and Mohri 1978.

centroblastic-centrocytic lymphoma, viz. the immunophenotype of centrocytes of centrocytic lymphoma differs from that of centrocytes of centroblastic-centrocytic lymphoma.[212] This confirmed our long-time morphological impression, viz. that the centrocytes of centrocytic lymphoma differ from those of centroblastic-centrocytic lymphoma. But what is the origin of the tumour cells of centrocytic lymphoma? At present there are four possible answers to this question:

1. The tumour cell is a special variant of centrocytes ("centrocyte II" according to STEIN et al.[213]). HARRIS and BHAN[214] and PILERI et al.[215] supported this assumption.
2. Centrocytic lymphoma is a tumour of follicular mantle lymphocytes, which compose the primary follicles (without germinal centres). Correspondingly, one could use the term "mantle zone lymphoma". This is now preferred by JAFFE et al.[216] to the term "intermediate lymphocytic lymphoma" used in the past.[217] WEISENBURGER et al.,[218] however, still make a distinction between mantle zone lymphoma and intermediate lymphocytic lymphoma.
3. FALINI et al.[219] proposed that the tumour cells of centrocytic lymphoma "might represent cells in transition from one compartment to the other but blocked in their development, or be derived from a minor cell population, such as that described by BOFILL et al.[220] in primary follicles around the 18th to 20th gestational week."
4. WEISENBURGER[221] has said that the cells of centrocytic lymphoma are derived from precursor cells of the normal germinal centre reaction and do not represent follicular or postfollicular cells.

It is now obvious to us that the tumour cells are not derived from the centrocytes of germinal centres, but rather from a small, CD5-positive subpopulation of cells in the mantle zone. Hence we can accept the proposal made by BANKS et al.[222] by calling centrocytic lymphoma "mantle *cell* lymphoma". We avoid the term "mantle *zone* lymphoma", however, because there are other cells (mostly CD5 −) in the follicular mantle and there are other types of lymphoma that show a mantle zone growth pattern.

It is conceivable that centrocytic lymphoma is the malignant equivalent of the nodular and band-shaped proliferation of cells that we have interpreted tentatively as marginal or mantle zone cells (see pp. 36 ff.).

We agree with SWERDLOW and MURRAY[223] that cases showing proliferation centres or blast cells of the same clone should not be included in the centrocytic

---

[212] Swerdlow et al. 1983; Stein et al. 1984a.
[213] 1984a.
[214] 1985a.
[215] 1985.
[216] 1987.
[217] Berard and Dorfman 1974; Berard 1975; Weisenburger et al. 1981.
[218] 1987b, 1991.
[219] 1989.
[220] 1985.
[221] 1990.
[222] 1992.
[223] 1988.

lymphoma category. WEISENBURGER et al.[224] now accept this view and have reported that cases with proliferation centres have a much more favourable prognosis than do those without.

It is possible to distinguish centrocytic lymphoma from centroblastic-centrocytic lymphoma because of a characteristic molecular genetic feature. Centrocytic lymphoma shows the translocation t(11;14)(q13;q32), which involves rearrangement of the *bcl*-1 locus.[224a] In contrast, centroblastic-centrocytic lymphoma often shows the translocation t(14;18), which corresponds to rearrangement of the *bcl*-2 locus.

Immunology.[225] The tumour cells show marked surface expression of Ig, chiefly of IgM/*kapppa* or *lambda* type with a slight predominance of the latter. In 60% of cases the cells simultaneously express IgD. In addition, the B-cell antigens CD22, CD19 and CD20 are found. Centrocytic lymphoma is CD5 positive and CD23 negative; this constellation distinguishes it from other low-grade malignant B-cell lymphomas. In 90% of cases stained for complement receptors (CD35) or with Ki-M4, either loose networks of follicular dendritic cells or small groups of follicular dendritic cells, i.e. remnants of germinal centres, can be identified. The T-cell content (a mixture of CD4-positive and CD8-positive cells) amounts to 5%–10% and is thus usually much lower than that of centroblastic-centrocytic lymphoma. The number of Ki-67-positive cells lies between 5% and 50%, with a mean of approximately 20%. In a few cases the centrocytes on paraffin sections show strongly stained monoclonal Ig in their scanty cytoplasm, without exhibiting a plasmacytoid morphology (Fig. 46).

Occurrence. In our collection centrocytic lymphoma accounts for 5.4% of the cases of NHL. The age curve shows a peak in the 7th decade (see Fig. 15). Our youngest patient was 16 years old and the oldest was 86. There is a clear preponderance of males, with a male-to-female ratio of 2.7 : 1.

Clinical Picture.[226] Most patients show generalized lymphoma (stage III or IV) at the time of diagnosis. Approximately 50% of patients present with B symptoms.[227] A small number of centrocytes are usually found in the blood, but the count is higher than 4×10^9/l in only about 25% of patients.

Histology. Even at a low magnification, it is possible to make a tentative diagnosis of centrocytic lymphoma on Giemsa-stained slides: there is a monotonous-looking proliferation of small to, at most, medium-sized cells whose nuclei show

---

[224] 1991.

[224a] Weisenburger et al. 1987b; Medeiros et al. 1990; Vandenberghe et al. 1991.

[225] Cf. Weisenburger et al. 1987b for comparison with immunohistochemical findings in intermediate lymphocytic lymphoma; also Strickler et al. 1988; Close and Lauder 1990; Weisenburger et al. 1991.

[226] Clinicopathological correlations have been studied by: Swerdlow et al. 1983; Engelhard et al. 1989; Meusers et al. 1989.

[227] Meusers et al. 1989.

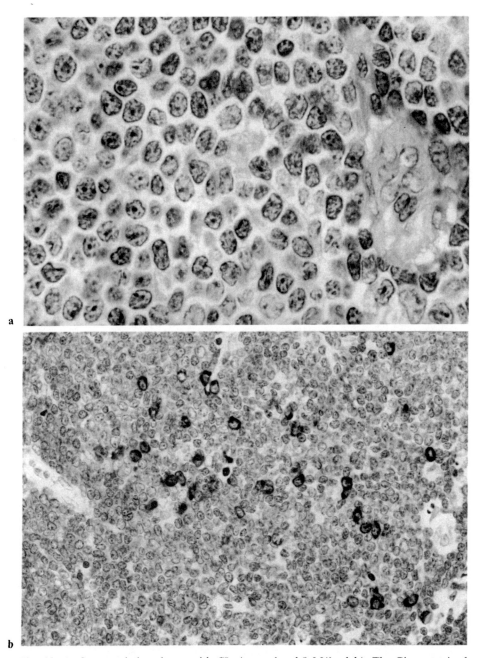

Fig. 46a, b. Centrocytic lymphoma with CIg (monoclonal IgM/*lambda*). The Giemsa-stained section (**a**) does not reveal any lymphoplasmacytoid cells. **a** Giemsa. 1094:1. **b** PAP, *lambda*. 440:1

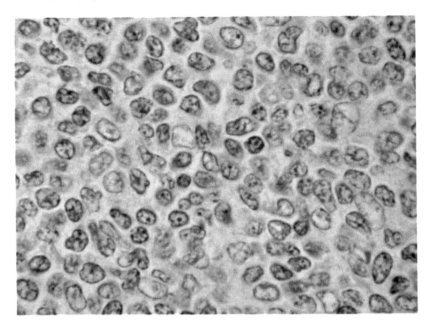

Fig. 47. Centrocytic lymphoma, small cell type, with Giemsa staining. The overall impression suggests uniformity, but the individual nuclei vary considerably in shape. Some cells contain cleaved nuclei. The chromatin pattern is fine, the nucleoli are small. Cytoplasm cannot be identified. Male, 53 years. Axillary node. 1550:1

weaker (greyer) staining than do those of CLL or immunocytoma (Figs. 47, 48). The nuclei are usually irregularly shaped and occasionally cleaved. The cytoplasm of the tumour cells shows practically no staining with Giemsa. There are no monotypic blast cells (basophilic cells) of any type (centroblasts, immunoblasts). Polytypic blast cells (centroblasts, immunoblasts), however, may be found as remnants of germinal centres. Plasmablasts, i.e. precursors of polytypic (reactive) plasma cells, are sometimes scattered among the tumour cells. The number of mitotic figures varies from case to case. The tumour cells are interspersed with macrophages. There is a loose network of follicular dendritic cells, which usually show relatively large, round nuclei and solitary, medium-sized nucleoli. These cells sometimes contain two or more nuclei and may finally turn into multinucleate giant cells, which KJELDSBERG and KIM[228] reported to be similar to Warthin-Finkeldey giant cells. Such giant cells also occur in other types of neoplasms of the follicles (centroblastic-centrocytic lymphoma, nodular paragranuloma) and in low-grade malignant B-cell lymphomas of MALT type. They are often Ki-M4p positive.

Hyaline deposits are frequently found around small blood vessels (capillaries, not epithelioid venules; Fig. 48a); this finding is highly characteristic of centrocytic lymphoma. The reticulin fibres are usually thick and form a coarse alveolar network, which surrounds large, solid groups of tumour cells (Fig. 49). Band-forming sclerosis or a diffuse increase in fibres is also occasionally found.

---

[228] 1981.

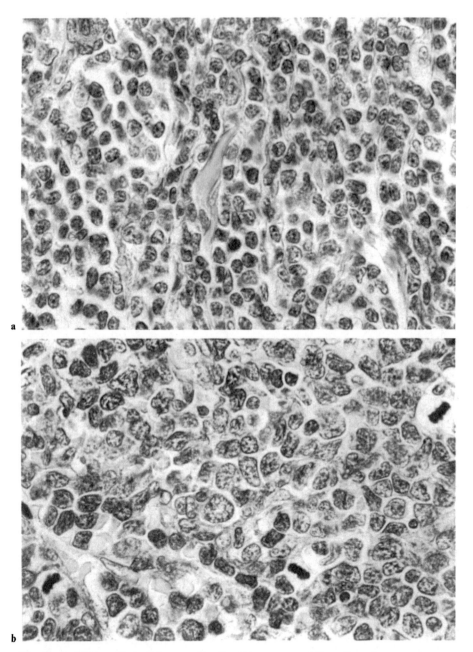

Fig. 48a, b. Centrocytic lymphoma. **a** Small cell tumour consisting of small centrocytes, sometimes with cleaved nuclei. In the *centre*, there is a hyaline deposit in tissue surrounding a small vessel. No mitotic activity. Male, 42 years. Inguinal node. **b** Large cell ("anaplastic") variant, 2 years after the first diagnosis of centrocytic lymphoma, small cell type, was made. The tumour is more pleomorphic. Three mitotic figures. Male, 63 years. Inguinal node. **a, b** PAS. 875:1

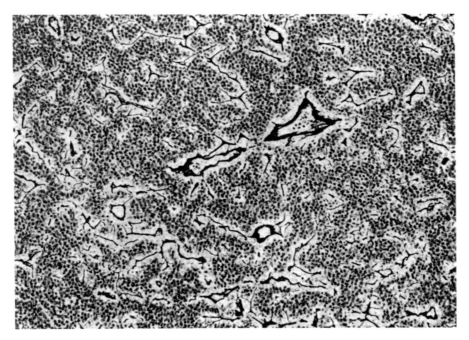

Fig. 49. Centrocytic lymphoma with silver impregnation. The tumour cells form tightly packed masses without any follicular arrangement. The fibres are thick and very sparse; they are usually located around small vessels. Same node as Fig. 47. Gomori. 140:1

The growth pattern is either diffuse or nodular or both, as is readily appreciated with silver impregnation. In early stages there may be a band-shaped infiltrate in the outer cortex of the node (Fig. 50). In a recent investigation[229] we found nodularity in 46% of cases. In 17% it affected the whole lymph node section; in 28% it was merely partial. In the same study, we also looked for a mantle zone pattern, i.e. the band-like growth of "centrocytes" around reactive (polyclonal) or residual germinal centres. Of our cases, 43% showed this growth pattern, but it was usually recognizable in only part of the lymph node. A mantle zone growth pattern and nodularity were usually demonstrable in the same node. Diffuse centrocytic lymphomas showed a partially developed mantle zone growth pattern in only about 20% of cases. It is conceivable that the proliferation of centrocytic lymphoma initially develops in the areas surrounding reactive germinal centres (mantle zone pattern; Fig. 51). Then the germinal centres might disappear, which would result in a nodular pattern. Finally, the tumour cells grow diffusely.

It might be helpful to distinguish a small cell and a large cell ("anaplastic") type of centrocytic lymphoma, although the borderline between the two types would not be sharp. The large cell centrocytic lymphoma described by STANS-FELD[230] corresponds to the centrocytoid centroblastic lymphoma recently identi-

---

[229] Plank et al. 1991.
[230] 1985.

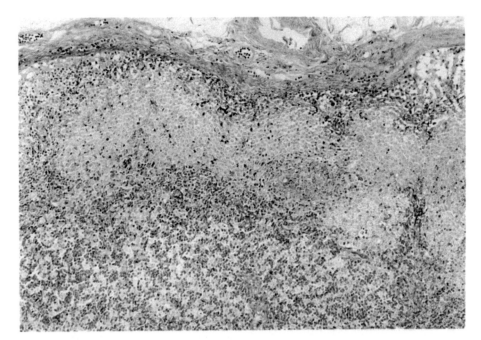

Fig. 50. Centrocytic lymphoma. Early stage of infiltration. There is a band-shaped infiltrate under the marginal sinus. A T nodule is located beneath the infiltrate. Cf. Fig. 12. Male, 57 years. Axillary node. Giemsa. 110:1

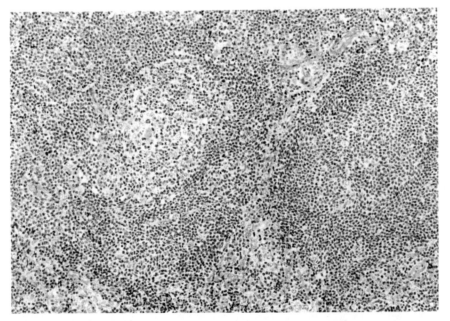

Fig. 51. Centrocytic lymphoma. Early stage of infiltration. On the *left* a germinal centre surrounded by a "mantle of centrocytes" (mantle zone pattern). On the *right* the remains of a follicle with a germinal centre that has been completely infiltrated and obliterated by "centrocytes". Male, 60 years. Nuchal node. Giemsa. 140:1

fied by our research group (see p. 122), i.e. it must be classified as a high-grade
ML.[231]

Cytology and Cytochemistry. It is easier to distinguish centrocytes from
lymphoblasts in imprints than in sections, because the cytoplasm of lymphoblasts
is more basophilic than that of centrocytes. The usual cytochemical reactions are
negative, or merely weakly positive, and thus of no help in characterizing the cells.
In 1977, NANBA et al. described a type of ML that was characterized by a
positive alkaline phosphatase reaction. The neoplasm was interpreted as ML of
follicular mantle lymphocytes and thus roughly corresponds to centrocytic
lymphoma. A positive alkaline phosphatase reaction has also been described,
however, in other types of B-cell lymphoma (B-CLL, immunocytoma, centroblastic-centrocytic lymphoma, centroblastic lymphoma and immunoblastic
lymphoma).[232]

Diagnosis and Differential Diagnosis. The diagnosis is based on the monotony of
the cell picture and the absence of markedly basophilic blast cells belonging to the
same clone as the centrocytes. A similarly monotonous picture is found in
lymphoblastic lymphomas, including acute lymphoblastic leukaemia (ALL). In
lymphoblastic lymphoma the nuclei are rounder than those of centrocytes, but
they occasionally show protrusions. In centrocytic lymphoma the nuclei are generally more elongate or irregular, but sometimes round. The cytoplasm of
lymphoblastic lymphoma cells is clearly basophilic, but very scanty and thus
hardly visible in sections. Lymphoblastic lymphoma shows, on the average, a
larger number of mitotic figures than does centrocytic lymphoma. Imprints are
helpful in the differential diagnosis, especially when focal acid phosphatase reactivity is seen (this is characteristic of T-lymphoblastic lymphoma). In lymphoblastic lymphoma the reticulin fibre pattern is finer, and the age curve shows a much
earlier peak.
Monocytic and *myelomonocytic leukaemia* may also be confused with centrocytic lymphoma because of the polymorphic nuclei in the former neoplasms.
Consideration of the following criteria should prevent misinterpretations. In
monocytic leukaemia the nuclei are occasionally reniform, deeply indented or
folded and usually contain a larger nucleolus than do centrocytic nuclei. With
Giemsa staining the cytoplasm of monocytic leukaemia cells is grey or greyish red
and more abundant than that of centrocytes. Among these leukaemic cells there
are almost always a few, or even numerous, chloroacetate esterase-positive myelocytes and promyelocytes. Reticulin fibres and capillaries are increased in number. In imprints monocytes show a diffuse reaction for non-specific esterase.
In a few cases the morphological borderline between centrocytic lymphoma
and *centroblastic-centrocytic lymphoma* is not sharp. The presence of a few
(markedly basophilic) centroblasts is required for a diagnosis of centroblastic-
centrocytic lymphoma. One often has to search for them carefully. They should

---

[231] A. G. Stansfeld, personal communication 1988.
[232] Lennert et al. 1961; Berard et al. 1978; Poppema et al. 1978; Schwarze 1979, 1986; Abe et
al. 1988.

not be confused with centroblasts or immunoblasts (residual germinal centre cells) or with plasmablasts (precursors of reactive plasma cells). In such cases an immunohistochemical analysis easily reveals the polyclonality of the blast cells and plasma cells.

Very rare cases of *small cell pleomorphic T-cell lymphoma* may be very similar to centrocytic lymphoma. The application of pan-B-cell or pan-T-cell antibodies is the only available aid in making a differential diagnostic decision. In almost all cases, however, small cell T-cell lymphoma shows more pleomorphic nuclei and never a nodular or "mantle zone" growth pattern (see p. 218).

The distinction between centrocytic lymphoma and *centrocytoid centroblastic lymphoma* is discussed on p. 125.

Development into a Lymphoma of High-Grade Malignancy. Occasionally, biopsies obtained some time after the diagnosis of centrocytic lymphoma disclose larger cells with more pronounced nuclear polymorphism and higher mitotic activity (Fig. 51). We consider these to be signs of advancing anaplasia and thus indications of an unfavourable prognosis.

Our collection contains only one case in which a B-immunoblastic lymphoma with PAS-positive inclusions evolved out of a centrocytic lymphoma. We have never observed transformation of centrocytic lymphoma into centroblastic lymphoma.

Prognosis. Centrocytic lymphoma shows a much poorer prognosis than do B-CLL, immunocytoma and centroblastic-centrocytic lymphoma (see Fig. 17). The median survival time was 32 or 37 months, depending on the method of treatment.[233] Less than 10% of patients survived 5 years. The prognosis is less favourable in cases with high mitotic activity (or marked Ki-67 positivity) than in cases with a small number of mitotic figures.[234]

3.1.6 Monocytoid B-Cell Lymphoma (Including Marginal Zone Cell Lymphoma)[235]

WF: Not listed

Lukes-Collins: Small lymphocyte B, monocytoid B

History and Definition. The lesion formerly known as immature sinus histiocytosis or monocytoid sinus reaction has been identified as a special B-cell reaction and may be referred to as monocytoid B-cell reaction (see p. 33). We have observed "monocytoid B cells" in myoepithelial sialadenitis and especially in the immunocytoma that may subsequently develop in the salivary gland.[236] SHEIBANI

---

[233] Engelhard et al. 1989; Meusers et al. 1989.
[234] Swerdlow et al. 1983; Plank et al. 1991.
[235] This section was written in collaboration with C. von Schilling, S. B. Cogliatti and J. Paulsen.
[236] Schmid et al. 1982.

et al.,[237] COUSAR et al.,[238] PIRIS et al.[239] and NG and CHAN[240] have described a number of cases of lymphoma that they considered to be derived from monocytoid B cells.

Since 1982 we have diagnosed 28 cases of B-cell lymphoma in lymph nodes in which a considerable portion of the lymphoma was composed of large collections of small and medium-sized "monocytoid B cells".[241] Nine of the patients also showed an extranodal lymphoma of similar histology that was diagnosed as low-grade malignant B-cell lymphoma of MALT type; the tumours were located in the stomach (four cases), salivary gland (two cases), thyroid gland (one case), nasopharynx (one case) and hypopharynx (one case). In all these cases the lymph node lesions were of the small cell type (marginal zone cell type? cf. p. 109).

According to the general principles of the Kiel classification, monocytoid B-cell lymphoma (and the lymphoma of MALT type) should be classified as a low-grade ML (composed of "-cytes" and blasts).

Immunology. cIg can be demonstrated in about half the cases of monocytoid B-cell lymphoma. The tumour cells are interspersed with plasma cells that belong to the same cell clone. IgM is found in approx. 80% of the cases, IgG in approx. 20%. A varying number (20%–60%) of the monocytoid B cells show monoclonal Ig on their surface, chiefly IgM. The antigens CD19, CD20, CD22 and Ki-B3 (antigen related to CD45) are expressed constantly and CDw75 (LN1) weakly or not at all. The C3b receptor (CD35) is usually demonstrable on only a small number (10%–20%) of the infiltrating cells. Recently, the new macrophage antibody Ki-M1p[242] has proved to be quite useful. It can be applied to paraffin sections for identifying both macrophages (strong, diffuse reaction) and monocytoid B cells (granular reactivity). Ki-M1p is positive in all cases, but a reaction with this antibody is also found in marginal zone cells and in other types of low-grade malignant B-cell lymphoma.

Clinical Picture.[243] Monocytoid B-cell lymphoma of the lymph node chiefly occurs in cervical regions. Occasionally, however, axillary or inguinal nodes are primarily involved. Most patients present in stage IA. According to the clinical reports, only a small percentage of the patients show B symptoms. In one case there was a leukaemic blood picture (Fig. 52).[244] This patient's blood showed not only monocytoid B cells but also some lymphoplasmacytoid forms. In another case monoclonal gammopathy (IgG/*kapppa*) was documented clinically.

---

[237] 1986, 1988.

[238] 1987.

[239] 1988.

[240] 1987.

[241] Von Schilling et al. 1987; Cogliatti et al. 1990; Nizze et al. 1991.

[242] Wacker et al. 1990; Radzun et al. 1991.

[243] Cogliatti et al. 1990.

[244] Other leukaemic cases have been described by Carbone et al. 1989; Traweek et al. 1989.

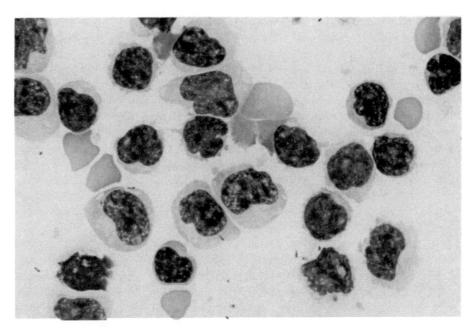

Fig. 52. Monocytoid B-cell lymphoma, leukaemic. Leucocyte concentrate of peripheral blood. Note the pleomorphic cells, some of which are somewhat similar to monocytes. Pappenheim. 1094:1

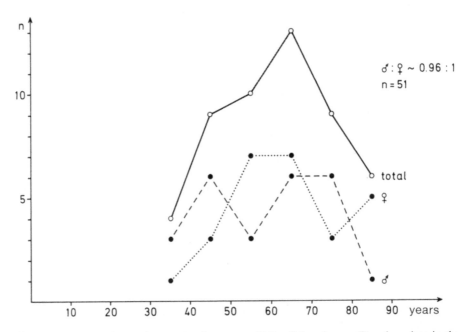

Fig. 53. Age distribution and sex ratio of monocytoid B-cell lymphoma. (Based on data in the literature and those of COGLIATTI et al. 1990)

Occurrence. Monocytoid B-cell lymphoma is rare. It probably accounts for about 0.2%–0.3% of the NHL. The age curve shows a peak in the 7th decade of life (Fig. 53). The youngest patient was 30 years old, the oldest was 87. Neither sex appears to predominate.

Histology. In most cases, monocytoid B-cell lymphoma can be suspected at a low magnification (Figs. 54, 55). One sees compact, sharply demarcated plaques or less sharply delineated, peritrabecular and subcapsular collections of medium-sized cells that look relatively pale. These cells stand out clearly against the other lymph node structures, whose cells have darker nuclei. The nuclei of the pale cells lie relatively far apart from one another, which indicates that the cytoplasm is relatively abundant. The infiltrations are located in the sinuses, chiefly the intermediate and marginal ones. The monocytoid B cells have medium-sized, round or somewhat indented or cleaved nuclei with moderately coarse chromatin and small, usually solitary nucleoli. The cytoplasm is moderately abundant and stains grey with Giemsa (Figs. 56, 57). With L26 (CD20-like) or Ki-B3 (CD45-related) staining it looks cohesive. In some of the cases typical large (cIg +) immunoblasts are interspersed among the monocytoid B cells. Small numbers of neutrophil granulocytes are often found. Mitotic figures are quite numerous.

At first glance, the rest of the lymphoid tissue stands out because of its large germinal centres. They show a typical, mixed cytology and polytypic Ig, and they are always surrounded by follicular mantle lymphocytes. Remnants of lymphoid tissue (pulp) are not always recognizable between the follicles and the collections of monocytoid B cells. Large areas are often infiltrated by somewhat larger (B) lymphocytes and a variable number of plasma cells. In one case there were so many plasma cells that we were tempted to diagnose plasmacytoma. In the other cases there were usually areas that corresponded in appearance to immunocytoma. Some of these areas were circumscribed, others were extensive.

In many cases that we had diagnosed as the subtype of immunocytoma with a high content of epithelioid cells we later saw some foci of monocytoid B cells as well (Fig. 58). These were sometimes surrounded by a ring of epithelioid cells (Fig. 59). At times the monocytoid B cells appeared to lie in thin-walled vessels of an indeterminable type. At other times the cells were arranged in large clusters enclosed by a wall of collagenous fibres. In all of these cases of immunocytoma with a high content of epithelioid cells and monocytoid B-cell clusters there was involvement of the parotid gland by myoepithelial sialadenitis or merely sicca syndrome.

With silver impregnation, either the monocytoid B-cell foci are sharply bounded by a dense network of fibres, or only a few fibres occur with about equal frequency in the monocytoid B-cell clusters and surrounding pulp. A remarkable, and still incomprehensible, finding is the increase in typical epithelioid venules (Fig. 57) often seen within large, poorly demarcated monocytoid B-cell clusters.

Besides the typical lesion consisting of medium-sized cells that primarily infiltrate the sinuses, we have observed a second variant. Initially, we placed it in the monocytoid B-cell lymphoma category, but it might be necessary to place it in another category. We have described the second variant as the "small cell

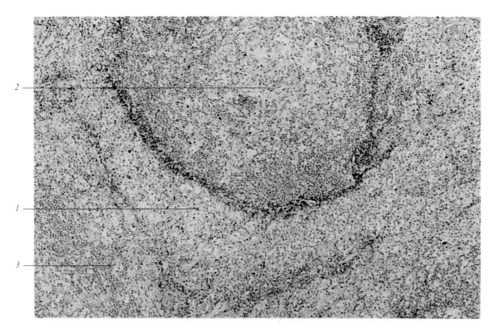

Fig. 54. Monocytoid B-cell lymphoma. Band-shaped intrasinusoidal infiltrate (*1*). Hyperplastic, poorly demarcated germinal centre (*2*). Diffuse infiltration of the pulp ("immunocytoma", *3*). Female, 55 years. Nuchal node. Giemsa. 110 : 1

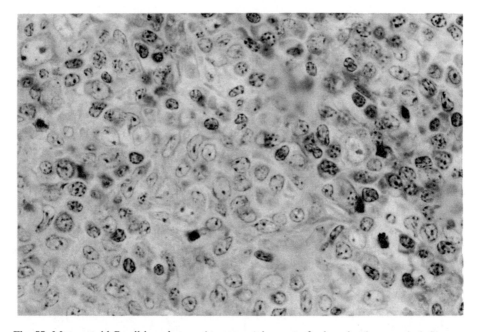

Fig. 55. Monocytoid B-cell lymphoma. At *upper right*, part of a lymphoplasmacytic infiltrate ("immunocytoma"). Female, 68 years. Giemsa. 700 : 1

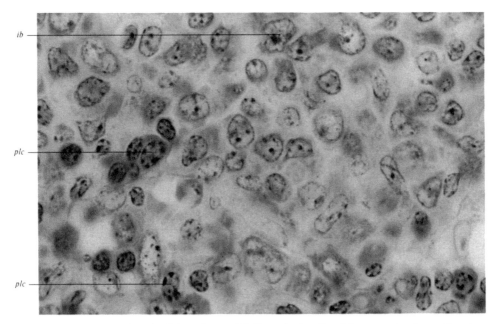

Fig. 56. Monocytoid B-cell lymphoma. Medium-sized cells with grey cytoplasm. One immunoblast (*ib*). A few plasma cells (*plc*) and lymphocytes. Components of the "immunocytoma" that developed in surrounding tissue. Same case as Fig. 55. Giemsa. 1100:1

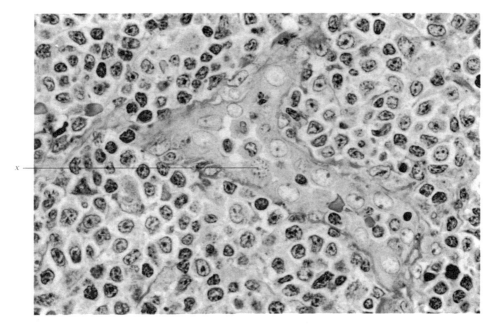

Fig. 57. Monocytoid B-cell lymphoma. Relatively pleomorphic nuclei. Some immunoblasts. The infiltrate surrounds an epithelioid venule showing typical vesicular nuclei and one mitotic figure (prophase, *x*). Female, 55 years. Nuchal node. Giemsa. 700:1

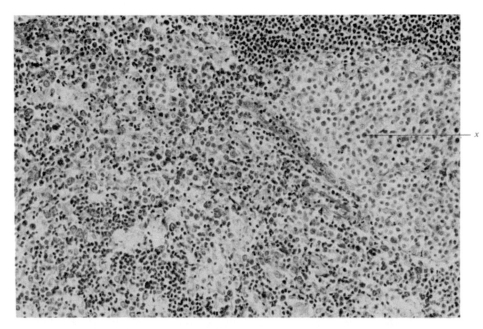

Fig. 58. Immunocytoma with a high content of epithelioid cells and a cluster of monocytoid B cells (*x*). Clinically, the patient showed IgA/*kapppa* paraproteinaemia and sicca syndrome of the eyes. Sjögren's syndrome was suspected. Female, 54 years. Giemsa. 220:1

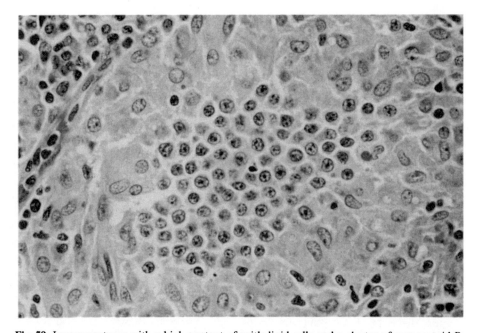

Fig. 59. Immunocytoma with a high content of epithelioid cells and a cluster of monocytoid B cells, which is enclosed by epithelioid cells. Female, young adult. Cervical node. H & E. 256:1

variant of monocytoid B-cell lymphoma".[245] It consists of smaller cells that usually show round nuclei. The cytoplasm is less abundant and also non-basophilic (cf. Fig. 2c in NIZZE et al.[246]). The cells are frequently located in the marginal zone, from where they invade and massively infiltrate the lymphoid tissue (cf. Fig. 1b in NIZZE et al.[247]). A plasmacytic component has not been found. The reaction for Ki-B3 (CD45-related) was negative.

Clinically, cases of the small cell type were combined with a low-grade ML of MALT type. This may lead one to suspect that such cases correspond to the lymphoma that ISAACSON calls "centrocytoid" and says may be derived from marginal zone cells[248] (see p. 111).

Since we have observed a case that contained both a medium-sized and a small cell component, we are not presently in a position to make a sharp distinction between the two variants.

Cytology and cytochemistry. The monocytoid B cells can be readily recognized in imprints (cf. Fig. 52). They are medium-sized, and their (bean-shaped) nuclei resemble those of monocytes in shape more often than they do in sections. The chromatin is darker than that of monocytes. Nucleoli usually cannot be recognized. The cytoplasm is a rich greyish blue, and in one of our cases it was highly vacuolated (on electron microscopy the vacuoles proved to be fat). The PAS reaction is often finely or coarsely granular; sometimes it is diffusely positive (glycogen). With non-specific esterase or acid phosphatase staining one finds a few unevenly distributed positive granules. The alkaline phosphatase reaction is negative.

Development into a High-Grade Malignant Non-Hodgkin's Lymphoma. In two cases out of 28 we observed transformation into a high-grade ML of the B-cell series (polymorphic centroblastic lymphoma in one case, unclassified in the other).

Diagnosis. The pathologist can often decide in favour of a monocytoid B-cell lymphoma when examining a slide at a low magnification, which reveals that the sinuses are infiltrated by medium-sized cells. These infiltrates stand out clearly against the rest of the lymph node, which shows follicular hyperplasia (with follicular mantles) and sometimes infiltration of the pulp resembling immunocytoma. With immunohistochemical methods one can determine that the monocytoid B cells, plasma cells and immunoblasts all belong to the same clone (frequently IgM/*kapppa*+), whereas the germinal centres usually show polytypic Ig. Staining with Ki-M1p reveals granular reactivity (Fig. 60). The reaction to L26 (CD20-like) is strong, and the tumour cells look cohesive with this stain.

If the monocytoid B-cell foci are sparse, and if the predominant picture is that of immunocytoma, one may at least pose the fundamental question whether it

---

[245] Nizze et al. 1991.
[246] 1991.
[247] 1991.
[248] Spencer et al. 1985.

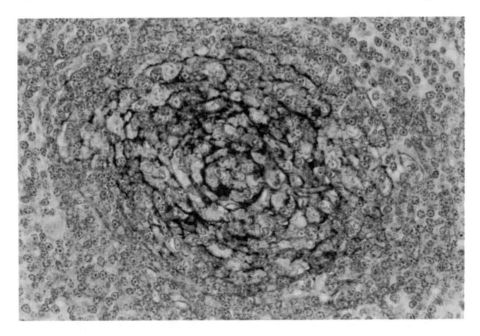

Fig. 60. Monocytoid B-cell lymphoma with Ki-M4p staining. APAAP method. 1094:1

would not be better to speak of an immunocytoma. One would have to point out that such a picture, especially when it is connected with a focal epithelioid cell reaction, is typical of lymphomas of the salivary gland (immunocytoma) associated with myoepithelial sialadenitis.

Differential diagnosis. Monocytoid B-cell lymphoma is usually distinguishable from *inflammatory lesions* showing a pronounced monocytoid B-cell reaction combined with marked follicular hyperplasia (toxoplasmosis, infectious mononucleosis, AIDS, purulent inflammation of tissue drained by a node). In such cases immunohistochemistry quickly substantiates the diagnosis, depending on the monoclonality or polyclonality of the sinusoidal B cells.

The types of ML that occasionally cause difficulty in a diagnosis include centroblastic-centrocytic lymphoma and centrocytic lymphoma. *Centroblastic-centrocytic lymphoma* usually shows a follicular growth pattern. In contrast, there is interfollicular growth in monocytoid B-cell lymphoma. In centroblastic-centrocytic lymphoma the neoplastic germinal centre cells are monotypic and mostly Ki-M1p negative.

Centrocytic lymphoma sometimes shows a nodular growth pattern and completely replaces the follicular mantle, whereas monocytoid B-cell lymphoma always reveals remnants of the follicular mantle. Moreover, centrocytic lymphoma does not contain blast cells or plasma cells of the same clone. With Ki-M1p staining, about two-thirds of the cases show circumscribed, focal reactivity (and not a granular, disseminated reaction product!).

Finally, cases of *B-CLL* or *immunocytoma* may show some similarity with monocytoid B-cell lymphoma, but they do not exhibit marked Ki-B3 expression. With Ki-M1p staining, however, B-CLL and immunocytoma may reveal granular reactivity.

Prognosis. We were able to evaluate the clinical course of 18 of the cases of monocytoid B-cell lymphoma in our collection.[249] Patients in early stages (I and II) were treated mainly with radiotherapy (involved/extended field radiation), patients in later stages (III and IV) mostly with chemotherapy (COP, CHOP, ABVD, Knospe, COP-BLAM). Cases of extranodal primary lymphoma were usually subjected to local postoperative irradiation following resection. Complete remission, lasting from 1–78 months (mean: 28 months), was achieved in 15 patients. Over an average observation period of 34 months (the maximum was more than 6½ years) six patients remained free of disease. In more than half the cases there was a relapse after a mean remission period of 20 months (range: 1–55 months). Five patients (28%) died after 3–54 months (mean: 24 months), in each case from causes related to the lymphoma.

Addendum: Low-Grade Malignant B-Cell Lymphoma of MALT Type

Since the first publication of ISAACSON and WRIGHT[250] in 1984, pathologists have become aware of low-grade malignant B-cell lymphomas of MALT type. It has proved to be a common tumour that can be distinguished clearly from most nodal ML and whose clinical behaviour also clearly differs from that of nodal lymphomas.

The tumour is distinguishable by the following criteria:

1. The lymphoma arises in the stomach immediately underneath the mucosal epithelium. It invades and effaces adjacent columnar epithelium. This leads to development of the so-called *lymphoepithelial lesions*, which are highly characteristic of low-grade malignant B-cell lymphomas of MALT type (Fig. 61).

2. The lymphoma cells usually show a certain similarity to centrocytes, i.e. they are somewhat larger than lymphocytes and sometimes have irregularly shaped nuclei. Hence they were called "centrocyte-like cells" by ISAACSON and WRIGHT. In the meantime, there has been growing evidence that the cells are neoplastic marginal zone cells.[251] According to an agreement that we reached with ISAACSON in 1991, we also include in this category cases in which the majority of cells are small lymphocytes or medium-sized monocytoid B cells. This means that we include lymphoplasmacytic immunocytoma and a very small number of cases of monocytoid B-cell lymphoma in the group of low-grade malignant B-cell lymphomas of MALT type.

3. In contrast to centrocytic lymphoma, the centrocytoid cells are, as a rule, interspersed with large, basophilic blast cells, usually of the immunoblast type.

---

[249] Cogliatti et al. 1990.
[250] 1984; cf. Isaacson and Spencer 1987; Myhre and Isaacson 1987.
[251] Spencer et al. 1985, 1990.

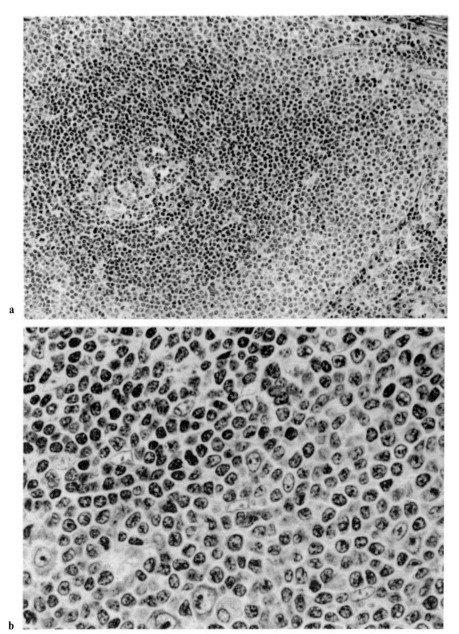

Fig. 61a, b. Nodal metastasis of low-grade malignant B-cell lymphoma of MALT type. The primary tumour was located in the stomach. A germinal centre (*gc*), follicular mantle (*fm*) and marginal zone (*mgz*) are recognizable. The marginal zone cells are somewhat larger than the follicular mantle lymphocytes and include some large blast cells. They are Ki-B3 negative (not shown). Paragastric lymph node. Giemsa. **a** 220:1, **b** 700:1

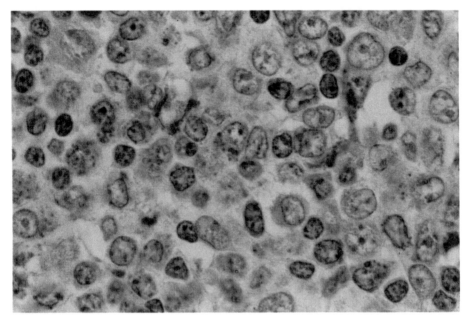

Fig. 62. Low-grade malignant B-cell lymphoma of MALT type (immunocytoma, lymphoplasma-cytic subtype). Lymph node infiltration, arising after involvement of skin, orbits and fallopian tubes. One germinal centre, which is recognizable from the red-stained follicular dendritic cells and is colonized by neoplastic lymphocytes. Ki-M1p staining, APAAP method. 440:1

These blast cells exhibit CIg of the same type as the SIg of the centrocytoid cells or of the lymphocytes and monocytoid cells.

4. One usually finds polytypic germinal centres. According to ISAACSON, these can be colonized by "centrocytoid" cells or lymphocytes and may then look like monotypic germinal centres. The germinal centres eventually lose all centroblasts and centrocytes and are finally recognizable only from the network of follicular dendritic cells (Fig. 62). There are also networks of follicular dendritic cells, however, that contain no other germinal centre cells and may never have done so previously. Such networks are seen especially in the outermost ramifications of the tumour.

5. The tumour always contains monotypic plasma cells. In areas near the mucous membrane these cells often cannot be distinguished from the numerous reactive, polytypic plasma cells. In deeper layers, however, it is easy to identify the mono-typic nature of the plasma cells. Here they are often accumulated in groups or sheets.

Low-grade malignant B-cell lymphomas of MALT type occur in numerous or-gans, including some that do not contain mucous membranes. On the other hand, one always finds columnar epithelium at sites involved by lymphomas of this type. The various sites at which low-grade ML of MALT type have been found are listed in Table 16. The most common localization is undoubtedly the stomach.

Table 16. Sites of development of low-grade malignant B-cell lymphomas of MALT type

Conjunctiva, including the orbit	Lung	Uterus?
Salivary glands	Stomach	Prostate gland
Waldeyer's ring	Thymus	Skin
Thyroid gland	Small and large intestines	(Lymph node)[a]
Breast	Rectum	
Larynx	Fallopian tube	

[a] Apparently, lymph nodes are never primarily involved.

Table 17. Types of non-Hodgkin's lymphoma (NHL) that can develop primarily in the gastrointestinal tract

B-cell types

Lymphomas of mucosa-associated lymphoid tissue (MALT)
   Low-grade malignant B-cell lymphomas of MALT type
      Immunocytoma, lymphoplasmacytic subtype
      Centrocyte-like (derived from marginal zone cells?)
      Monocytoid
   High-grade malignant B-cell lymphomas of MALT type with a low-grade malignant component
   Immunoproliferative small intestinal disease (IPSID), low-grade, high-grade, or both
Centrocytic lymphoma (lymphomatous polyposis)
Burkitt's lymphoma or Burkitt's lymphoma-like lymphoma
Other types of low-grade or high-grade ML corresponding to nodal NHL

T-cell types

Enteropathy-associated T-cell lymphoma (EATL)
Other types of ML not associated with enteropathy

Other important sites are the intestine, lungs, orbit and salivary gland. Common features of all the lymphomas are the development of lymphoepithelial lesions and the occurrence of polytypic germinal centres, monotypic plasma cells that are of the same clone as the majority of the tumour cells, lymphocytes, centrocyte-like cells (marginal zone cells) and monocytoid B cells. All low-grade malignant B-cell lymphomas of MALT type show a relatively favourable prognosis, as demonstrated, for example, in our studies of lymphomas of the lungs[252] and stomach.[253] Patients with lymphomas of the orbit or salivary gland are also known to have a relatively high survival rate.

It is notable that low-grade malignant B-cell lymphomas of MALT type can develop one after another in various organs showing columnar epithelium or glands. It is plain from this that the lymphomas belong to one particular system.

Table 17 is a scheme worked out by P. ISAACSON and ourselves showing where low-grade malignant B-cell lymphomas of MALT type belong in a classification of gastrointestinal lymphomas.

[252] Li et al. 1990.
[253] Cogliatti et al. 1991.

3.2 High-Grade Malignant Lymphomas of B-Cell Type

All B-cell lymphomas of high-grade malignancy are composed, at least in the main, of blast cells, which are medium-sized or large cells with moderately to intensely basophilic cytoplasm. Such lymphomas may be primary, i.e. of high-grade malignancy from the beginning, but some of them develop secondarily from low-grade ML.

3.2.1 Centroblastic Lymphoma

WF:
Subtype I = malignant lymphoma, diffuse, large cell, non-cleaved cell (G)
Subtype II = malignant lymphoma, large cell, immunoblastic (H)
Subtype III: not listed
Subtype IV: not listed

Lukes-Collins:
Subtypes I and II = large non-cleaved FCC
Subtype III = large cleaved FCC
Subtype IV = evolving FCC

Definition. So far, we have applied the term "centroblastic" to all high-grade ML whose blast cells are exclusively or partially centroblasts. In the first instance, the tumour was called "pure-cellular" or "monomorphic", and in the second instance, "mixed-cellular" or "polymorphic". In addition to centroblasts, the latter type contains immunoblasts; the borderline between this type and B-immunoblastic lymphoma is not sharp and has to be drawn arbitrarily (centroblastic lymphoma contains, at most, 90% immunoblasts, i.e. at least 10% centroblasts).[254]

By re-embedding tissue specimens in synthetics it has become possible to classify a number of previously unclassified high-grade malignant B-cell lymphomas and to define the various morphological variants more clearly.[255] We now distinguish four subtypes of centroblastic lymphoma, viz. the monomorphic (I) and polymorphic (II) types mentioned above, a multilobated type (III) and a centrocytoid type (IV).

Morphologically, the multilobated subtype of centroblastic lymphoma largely corresponds to the "multilobated type" of PINKUS,[256] which was originally described as a special type of T-cell lymphoma (see p. 252). It soon became obvious, however, that a large number of "multilobated" lymphomas are derived from B cells.[257] Electron microscopic studies by the research group of VAN UNNIK[258] revealed cells with lobated nuclei in normal germinal centres. Those inves-

---

[254] Cf. Lukes and Collins 1975a,b.
[255] Hui et al. 1987.
[256] Pinkus et al. 1979; Weinberg and Pinkus 1981.
[257] Weinberg and Pinkus 1981; Pileri et al. 1982; Cerezo 1983; Van der Putte et al. 1984; R. L. Weiss et al. 1985; Chan et al. 1986; Baroni et al. 1987.
[258] Van der Putte et al. 1984.

tigators logically concluded that the "multilobated" B-cell tumour is derived from germinal centre cells. Based on our own experience and that of van Un-nik,[259] we maintain that more than 90% of the lymphomas of "multilobated type" are germinal centre cell lymphomas. In contrast to van Unnik, however, we consider them to be centro*blastic* lymphomas, because they show medium-sized, often marginal nucleoli, slightly basophilic but clearly recognizable cyto-plasm, numerous mitotic figures and a large number of Ki-67-positive cells.

Centrocytoid centroblastic lymphoma is described on pp. 122 and 125f.

Centroblastic lymphoma may be either primary or secondary. A secondary centroblastic lymphoma may develop out of centroblastic-centrocytic lymphoma or, in rare cases, out of immunocytoma.

3.2.1.1 Primary Centroblastic Lymphoma

Immunology. sIg, chiefly of IgM type, can be demonstrated in 60%–70% of cases of centroblastic lymphoma. A small number of cases show expression of IgG. The other cases are sIg negative. The light chains are usually of *kapppa* type. In a small number of cases, cIg can also be demonstrated. The B-cell-associated antigens CD19, CD20 and CD22 are found in all cases. The expression of CD23 is an exception. CD5 is detectable in approximately 10% of cases. Follicular dendritic cells (usually in small residual foci) are seen in about one-third of cases that do not have a follicular growth pattern. Approximately 25% of cases show common ALL antigen (CD10). The number of cells expressing Ki-67 lies between 25% and 80% (mean: 50%).

Occurrence.[261] Because of the addition of new subtypes and the redefinition of polymorphic centroblastic lymphoma (requiring at least 10% centroblasts in-stead of more than 50%), centroblastic lymphoma has become the most frequent type of high-grade ML in our collection. In 1983, 13.7% of cases were classified as centroblastic lymphoma. The various morphological subtypes showed the frequency distribution presented in Table 18. The polymorphic subtype account-ed for almost half the cases of centroblastic lymphoma; the multilobated subtype showed the lowest frequency, while the other two subtypes were somewhat more frequent.

Primary centroblastic lymphoma (all subtypes) occurs in all age groups, but there is a peak incidence in the 7th decade. Our youngest patient was 1 year old, the oldest 97. The four subtypes do not show any significant differences in age distribution. The male-to-female ratio is about 1.2:1 (see Fig. 16).

Clinical Picture. Schmalhorst et al.[262] published the first paper drawing atten-tion to the clinical differences between centroblastic lymphoma and immunoblas-tic lymphoma. In the present context it is interesting that 6% of patients with

---

[259] Personal communication.
[260] deleted.
[261] Clausen, personal communication.
[262] 1979; see also Stewart et al. 1986.

Table 18. Relative frequency of the subtypes of centroblastic lymphoma (CBL) among the lymph node biopsies collected at the Lymph Node Registry Kiel in 1983

	% of CBL	% of all ML
Monomorphic	18.1	2.5
Polymorphic	49.4	6.8
Multilobated	12.5	1.7
Centrocytoid	19.9	2.7

centroblastic lymphoma and 6% of those with immunoblastic lymphoma showed a leukaemic blood picture or paraproteinaemia. Only 28% of patients with centroblastic lymphoma were in stage IV at the beginning of treatment. The reader may refer to BRITTINGER et al.[263] for further data concerning the similarities and differences between centroblastic and immunoblastic lymphomas. STEWART et al.[264] described the clinical findings in a relatively large series of cases collected in the United States.

Histology. The growth pattern is usually diffuse. In approximately 10% of cases, however, a follicular growth pattern is recognizable (Fig. 63). Occasional cases show follicular and diffuse proliferation of the tumour cells. Follicular variants are observed with about equal frequency among all four cytological subtypes of centroblastic lymphoma. The monomorphic and polymorphic types occasionally show scattered groups of epithelioid cells. A starry-sky pattern is sometimes observed. Follicular dendritic cells are rarely found (Fig. 64b).

There are a large number of mitotic figures (5–6/HPF). Most cases show a moderate number of reticulin fibres; but a large number of fibres may be seen in some cases, especially those of the multilobated type. PAS staining rarely reveals positive globular inclusions in the tumour cells.

Cytologically, the four subtypes have been characterized by HUI et al.[265] as follows:

I. Monomorphic Subtype (Fig. 64). More than 60% of the tumour cells are typical centroblasts, which gives the tumour a monotonous-looking appearance. The centroblasts may be medium-sized or large (10–14 μm). The nuclei are round and have fine chromatin, which makes them look relatively pale. About one-third of cases show pleomorphic nuclei, whose appearance is otherwise identical to that of the round nuclei. The nuclei have two to four small or medium-sized nucleoli, which are frequently marginal. Cytoplasm is scanty and basophilic.

The centroblasts may be interspersed with a few centrocytes, centrocytoid centroblasts and immunoblasts. When more than 10% of the tumour cells are immunoblasts, we classify the case as the polymorphic subtype of centroblastic lymphoma.

---

[263] 1984.
[264] 1986.
[265] 1987.

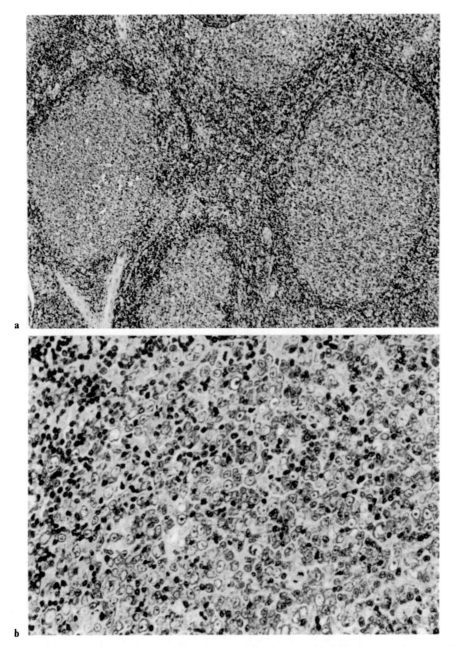

Fig. 63a, b. Centroblastic lymphoma, polymorphic subtype, with follicular growth pattern. The follicles contain more than 90% centroblasts and immunoblasts. Female, 65 years. Giemsa. **a** 70:1, **b** 440:1

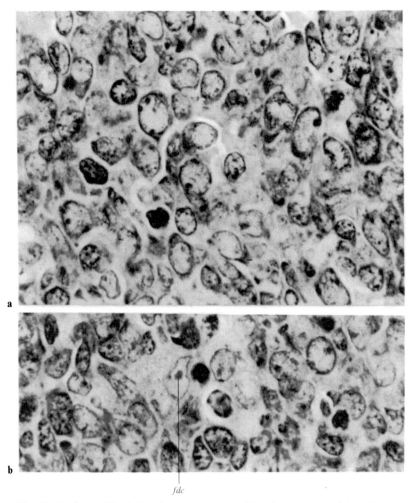

fdc

Fig. 64a, b. Centroblastic lymphoma, monomorphic subtype. Most of the cells are medium-sized to large centroblasts. The growth pattern is diffuse. A follicular dendritic cell (*fdc*) is seen in **b**. Female, 75 years. Cervical node. Giemsa. 1550:1

II. Polymorphic Subtype (Figs. 63, 65; cf. Fig. 1). Tumours of this subtype clearly consist of a mixture of cells. Immunoblasts are present in variable numbers. In most cases they catch the eye because of their size and morphology (large, central nucleoli; abundant, basophilic cytoplasm). All cases show typical centroblasts. In many cases there are centrocytoid centroblasts. There are often a few multilobated centroblasts as well. These cells are a strong indication of the germinal centre origin of the tumour.

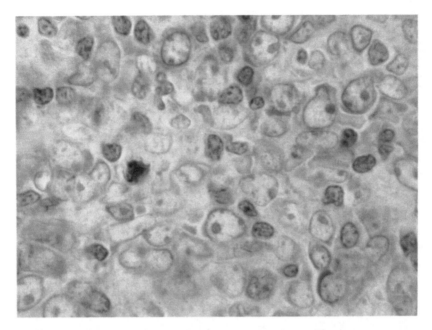

Fig. 65. Centroblastic lymphoma, polymorphic subtype, with Giemsa staining. Note the great variations in size and shape of the blast cells. One sees centroblast-like cells (nucleoli at the nuclear membrane; scanty, intensely basophilic cytoplasm), immunoblast-like cells (prominent, solitary, central nucleoli) and centrocyte-like cells (small, central nucleoli; cytoplasm is not visible). The small and large cells are interspersed with intermediate forms. Female, age unknown. Inguinal node. 1550:1

III. Multilobated Subtype (Fig. 66).[266] When more than 10%–20% of the tumour cells show lobated nuclei, i.e. when nuclear lobations are evident at first glance, we designate the tumour as the multilobated subtype. As a rule, the nuclei have three or four lobations. The cells are usually medium sized (11–13 μm). Occasionally, we have seen very large cells of otherwise identical appearance. The chromatin is fine. It is often difficult to recognize the nucleoli; when they are visible, they are usually medium sized and often marginal, like those of typical centroblasts. The cytoplasm is scanty to moderately abundant and moderately basophilic, but occasionally pale. Usually other types of germinal centre cells are also present in variable numbers and mixtures, viz. centroblasts, centrocytes, centrocytoid centroblasts and immunoblasts. Silver staining reveals that the tumour cells grow in narrow or large, compact complexes, which are surrounded by thick fibres (Fig. 67).

---

[266] See Baroni et al. 1987 for results of a thorough light and electron microscopic investigation and immunological data.

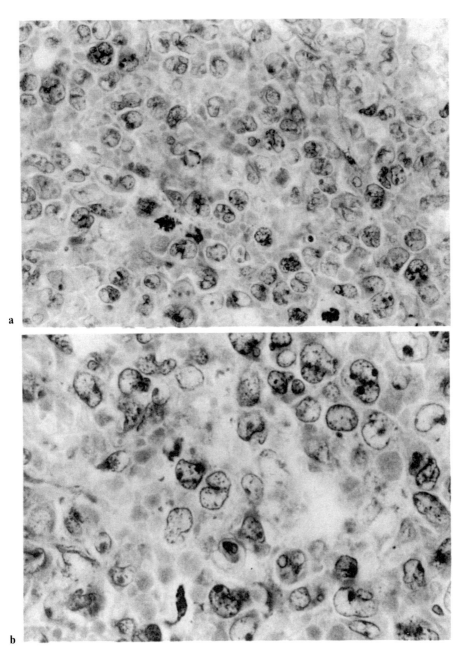

Fig. 66a, b. Centroblastic lymphoma, multilobated subtype. Male, 56 years. Inguinal node.
Giemsa. **a** 700:1, **b** 1024:1

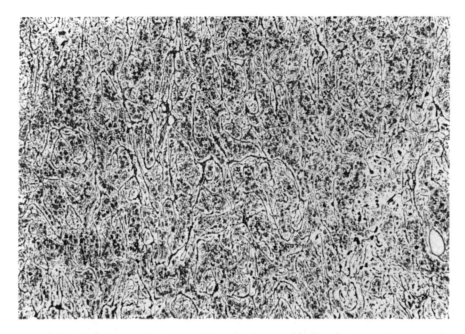

Fig. 67. Centroblastic lymphoma, multilobated subtype, with silver impregnation. Same biopsy as Fig. 66. The tumour cells form tightly packed complexes, which are surrounded and traversed by thick fibres. Gomori. 140:1

IV. Centrocytoid Subtype (Figs. 68–70). The term "centrocytoid centroblast" may be confusing, but we could not find a more appropriate name for a tumour cell that lies morphologically between a centrocyte and a centroblast. The cell is *relatively* small (9–11 μm); it has elongate or oval or even irregularly shaped nuclei with two to five small, basophilic, central nucleoli. Nuclear indentations are hardly ever seen. The chromatin is similar to that of centroblasts or somewhat coarser. The cytoplasm is scanty and slightly or moderately basophilic. These cells are always interspersed with a few other germinal centre cells (e.g. typical centroblasts and cells with multilobated nuclei) and immunoblasts. An imprint is very helpful in recognizing the various cell types (see below).

Cytology and Cytochemistry. By examining a lymph node imprint it is very easy to recognize a typical centroblast because of its scanty, markedly basophilic cytoplasm and round nucleus with multiple nucleoli. An imprint is especially important in the recognition of the centrocytoid subtype. Centrocytoid centroblasts show relatively small, oval or somewhat pleomorphic nuclei with one or more distinct nucleoli and scanty, deep grey or dark blue cytoplasm (centrocytes would have pale grey, more abundant cytoplasm!). The centrocytoid cells are interspersed with a few typical centroblasts.

A *cytochemical* analysis does not provide any diagnostically helpful information.

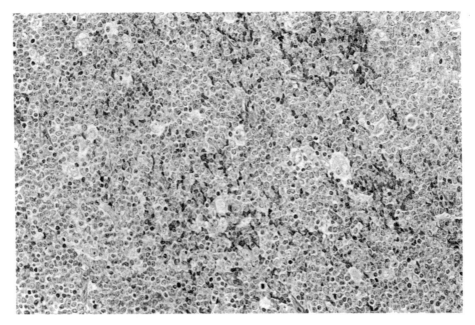

Fig. 68. Centroblastic lymphoma, centrocytoid subtype. Some "starry-sky cells" are recognizable. The tumour cells are uniform in appearance. Giemsa. 280:1

Diagnosis. Typical centroblasts and multilobated centroblasts are unmistakable signs of centroblastic lymphoma. For a diagnosis of this lymphoma type they must be present in at least small numbers (>10%). A follicular growth pattern is also proof of a centroblastic lymphoma when the tumour cells are of blastic nature. Such a growth pattern is not seen very often, however.

Differential Diagnosis. Centroblastic lymphoma has to be distinguished from centroblastic-centrocytic lymphoma with a high content of centroblasts and from other types of high-grade ML, particularly from immunoblastic lymphoma.

When we draw the line between *centroblastic-centrocytic lymphoma* and centroblastic lymphoma, the actual number of centroblasts is not the decisive factor. We diagnose centroblastic lymphoma only when solid foci of centroblasts have replaced at least one circumscribed area of a lymph node.

The indefinite borderline between centroblastic lymphoma and *immunoblastic lymphoma* is already evident from the existence of the polymorphic subtype of centroblastic lymphoma, in which there is a mixture of centroblasts and immunoblasts. This tumour has also been called centroblastic-immunoblastic lymphoma. We still include the polymorphic subtype in the group of centroblastic lymphomas when at least 10% of the tumour cells are definitely germinal centre cells (centroblasts, multilobated centroblasts). One justification for this definition is the fact that such cases may show a follicular growth pattern, which emphasizes the germinal centre nature of the tumour cells.

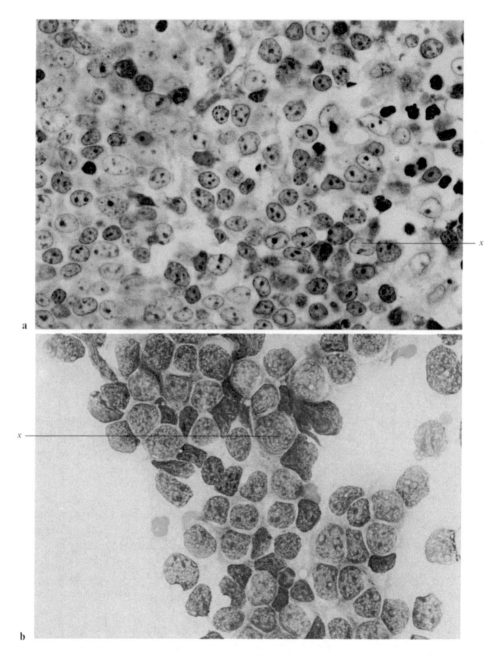

Fig. 69a, b. Centroblastic lymphoma, centrocytoid subtype. The tumour cells are medium-sized and relatively monotonous-looking. They have multiple nuclei that appear well demarcated in an imprint (**b**). Both the section and the imprint show some centroblasts of typical morphology (*x*). Male, 53 years. Inguinal node. **a** Section. Giemsa. **b** Imprint of the same node. Pappenheim. **a, b** 695:1

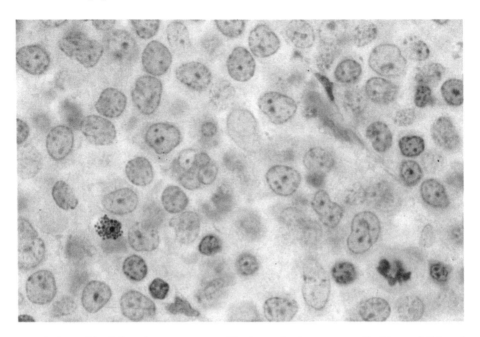

Fig. 70. Centroblastic lymphoma, centrocytoid subtype. In the *centre*, a cell with a multilobated nucleus is present. Male, 53 years. Inguinal node. Giemsa. 1094 : 1

Only the monomorphic subtype has to be distinguished from *Burkitt's lymphoma*. For this purpose it is absolutely necessary to use optimum techniques because inappropriate fixation and embedding of the tissue specimen can cause the central nucleoli of Burkitt's lymphoma to move to the nuclear membrane and hence to imitate those of centroblastic lymphoma. The nuclei of Burkitt's lymphoma cells are more intensely stained that those of centroblastic lymphoma cells and they have coarser chromatin. Cohesiveness is the most important criterion of Burkitt's lymphoma. A starry-sky pattern, on the other hand, can be found in a few cases of centroblastic lymphoma. There are certainly a few remaining cases that cannot be clearly classified as one or the other type with morphological methods alone.

An immunohistological analysis is the most reliable way to distinguish the *multilobated subtype* of centroblastic lymphoma from the type of T-cell lymphoma with the same name, which is comparatively rare. The reader may refer to BARONI et al.[267] for findings that are of help in making a differential diagnosis.

The *centrocytoid subtype* of centroblastic lymphoma must be distinguished from diffuse centroblastic-centrocytic lymphoma and centrocytic lymphoma. Diffuse centroblastic-centrocytic lymphoma can be recognized clearly because of the presence of centrocytes with pleomorphic, often indented nuclei and practically invisible cytoplasm and the presence of centroblasts with intensely basophilic

[267] 1987.

cytoplasm. The borderline between centrocytic lymphoma and the centrocytoid subtype of centroblastic lymphoma is less sharp. Centrocytoid cells are somewhat larger than centrocytes, and they show non-indented nuclei and clearly recognizable, slightly or moderately basophilic cytoplasm. Mitotic activity is higher in the centrocytoid subtype. Centrocytoid cells contain more and larger nucleoli. There are often a few multilobated centroblasts in the centrocytoid subtype. In contrast, centrocytic lymphoma is characterized by a monotonous appearance, absence of blast cells, practically invisible cytoplasm, small nucleoli, often hyalinized small vessels and thick fibres.

Prognosis. Patients with primary centroblastic lymphoma show a higher survival rate than do those with any other type of high-grade ML[268] (see Figs. 17, 71). A comparison of the subtypes reveals that the monomorphic subtype has a significantly better prognosis than do the polymorphic and centrocytoid subtypes.[269]

3.2.1.2 Secondary Centroblastic Lymphoma

As mentioned on p. 89, centroblastic-centrocytic lymphoma evolves into a centroblastic lymphoma in a considerable number of cases. All four subtypes of centroblastic lymphoma can develop secondarily. The transformation may occur at the same time as the development of centroblastic-centrocytic lymphoma; i.e. besides the typical follicular centroblastic-centrocytic lymphoma, there are monotonous-looking proliferations of blast cells in the same lymph node or elsewhere. We designate such cases as *simultaneously* developed, (in principle) secondary centroblastic lymphoma.

In other cases, a centroblastic lymphoma develops after a number of months or a few or even many years; this is called *subsequent* secondary centroblastic lymphoma. In such cases, a centroblastic-centrocytic lymphoma is no longer recognizable in the lymph node. Occasionally, however, one can still find the original centroblastic-centrocytic proliferation elsewhere, e.g. in the bone marrow. A subsequent secondary centroblastic lymphoma may also develop in cases of immunocytoma.

The *prognosis* of simultaneous secondary centroblastic lymphoma corresponds to that of primary centroblastic lymphoma (all subtypes taken together), whereas subsequent secondary centroblastic lymphoma shows a much poorer prognosis (Fig. 71).[270]

---

[268] Strauchen et al. 1978; Meusers et al. 1979.
[269] Brittinger et al. 1984. NB: the "special cases" of centroblastic lymphoma described by Brittinger et al. largely correspond to what is now called the centrocytoid subtype.
[270] Brittinger et al. 1984; H. Bartels, personal communication 1985.

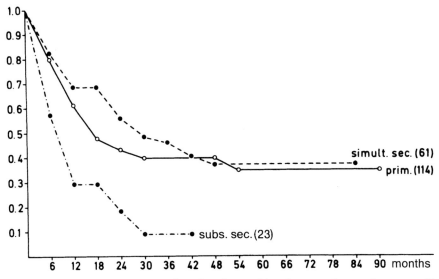

Fig. 71. Overall survival probability of patients with primary and secondary centroblastic lymphoma. Simultaneous secondary centroblastic lymphoma (*simult. sec*) shows about the same prognosis as does primary centroblastic lymphoma (*prim.*). In contrast, subsequent secondary centroblastic lymphoma (*subs. sec*) shows a much less favourable prognosis. (Based on data from H. BARTELS, personal communication 1985)

3.2.2 Immunoblastic Lymphoma of B-Cell Type

WF: Some cases of malignant lymphoma, large cell, immunoblastic ± plasmacytoid (H)

Lukes-Collins: B-immunoblastic sarcoma

Definition. We apply the term immunoblastic lymphoma to tumours that consist chiefly of immunoblasts of B or T type. This means that a majority of the cells are large and intensely basophilic and that they contain large, central, often solitary nulceoli. This definition does not apply to all cases of the T-cell type (see p. 226). In this section we shall deal with immunoblastic lymphoma of the B-cell type.

Immunoblastic lymphoma cells may show differentiation into plasma cells or plasmablasts; in such cases, the tumour can be identified morphologically as a B-immunoblastic lymphoma. Peroxidase–antiperoxidase (PAP) immunostaining of paraffin sections discloses monotypic cIg in many cases of immunoblastic lymphoma, indicating that they are of B-cell type. Some cases can be distinguished from non-neoplastic B-cell proliferations, e.g. viral infections, only by demonstrating monoclonality by immunohistochemical analyses of cryostat sections or even molecular genetic studies.

Immunology. sIg can be demonstrated in 80% of cases. Ig-negative cases can be recognized only with pan-B markers (CD19, CD22). The antigen profile largely corresponds to that of centroblastic lymphoma. CD5-positive cases are usually secondary immunoblastic lymphomas that have developed out of lymphoplasma-cytoid immunocytoma or B-CLL. The proliferation rate corresponds to that of centroblastic lymphoma (mean: 55%). The presence of a small number of resid-ual follicular dendritic cells is an exceptional finding. In 60%–70% of cases monotypic cIg (usually IgM; sometimes IgG or IgA) is demonstrable in paraffin sections. cIg is always found in immunoblastic lymphoma with plasmacytic dif-ferentiation.

Occurrence. Of all cases of NHL in our collection, 4.3% were diagnosed as B-immunoblastic lymphoma. The disease shows a peak incidence in the 7th decade of life. Our youngest patient was 43 months old, the oldest 91 years old. The male-to-female ratio is about 1.1:1 (see Fig. 16).

In about 20% of cases of immunoblastic lymphoma the tumour appears as a result of blast cell transformation of a low-grade ML, viz. B-CLL, immunocy-toma or (rarely) centrocytic lymphoma.

Clinical Picture. The clinical picture of B-immunoblastic lymphoma is very simi-lar to that of centroblastic lymphoma.[271] Superficial, often cervical, lymph nodes are involved most frequently. In many cases the lymph nodes on only *one* side of the diaphragm are enlarged. Bone marrow and liver are not infiltrated as often as they are in most other types of NHL.[272]

Patients with immunoblastic lymphoma rarely show a leukaemic blood pic-ture. Paraproteinaemia (usually IgM) is evident in about 10%–15% of cases.

Histology. All cases of B-immunoblastic lymphoma show a diffuse growth pat-tern. A starry-sky pattern is seen in a few cases. A majority of the tumour cells are large, basophilic immunoblasts, which usually have an oval nucleus contain-ing a large, usually solitary, central nucleolus. These cells may be interspersed with numerous reactive macrophages or even with groups of epithelioid cells (Fig. 72). The macrophages have abundant, pale cytoplasm, which frequently contains debris of phagocytosed tumour cells. In contrast, epithelioid cells show intensely acidophilic cytoplasm and no signs of apoptosis. There are numerous mitotic figures (7–8/HPF). Reticulin fibres are sparse in about half the cases; in the other half, there is a slight to moderate increase in the number of fibres (Fig. 73). Occasionally, the tumour cells contain globular or diffuse intracytoplas-mic PAS-positive deposits (=Ig).

The immunoblasts may be interspersed with plasma cells, plasma cell precur-sors, and numerous lymphocytes. Hence we distinguish three variants of B-im-munoblastic lymphoma:

1. B-Immunoblastic Lymphoma without Plasmacytic Differentiation (Figs. 74, 75). The immunoblasts are large (12–15 μm). Besides typical immunoblasts with large, central nucleoli, there are cells with multiple, medium-sized or large nucle-

---

[271] Schmalhorst et al. 1979; Brittinger et al. 1984.
[272] Mann et al. 1979.

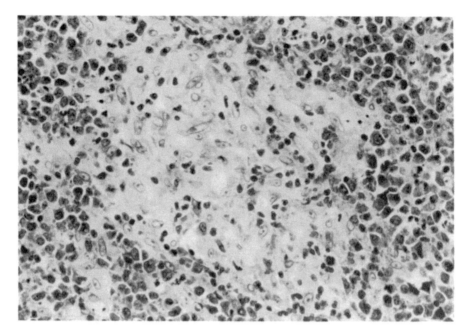

Fig. 72. B-immunoblastic lymphoma with plasmablastic differentiation and a cluster of epithelioid cells. The cytoplasm of epithelioid cells is oxyphilic and appears pale in this picture, whereas the cytoplasm of the surrounding tumour cells is basophilic and appears dark. Male, 75 years. Axillary node. Giemsa. 350 : 1

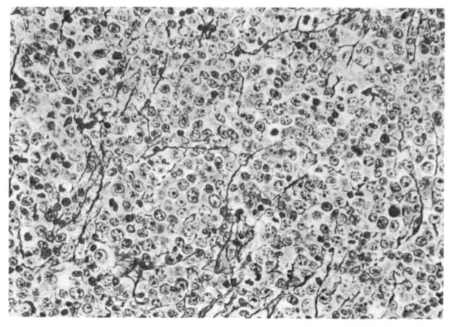

Fig. 73. B-immunoblastic lymphoma with plasmacytic differentiation with silver impregnation. The tumour cells are interspersed with a moderate number of reticulin fibres. Male, 42 years. Supraclavicular node. Gomori. 350 : 1

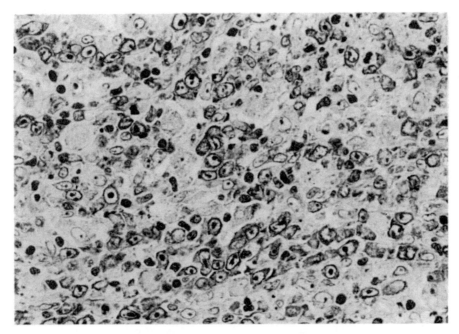

Fig. 74. B-immunoblastic lymphoma without plasmacytic differentiation. The tumour cells are large and intensely basophilic. They have prominent, usually solitary, central nucleoli. The tumour cells are interspersed with many non-neoplastic macrophages with abundant, pale cytoplasm and small nucleoli. Female, 66 years. Inguinal node. Giemsa. 560:1

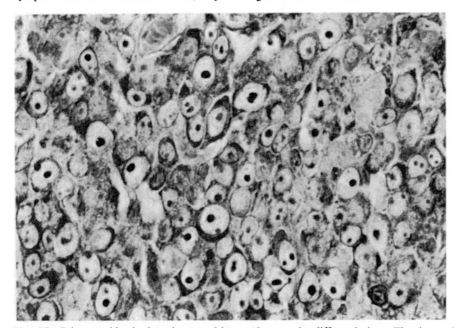

Fig. 75. B-immunoblastic lymphoma without plasmacytic differentiation. The intensely basophilic tumour cells contain prominent, mostly solitary, basophilic nucleoli, which are centrally located in the nucleus. Non-neoplastic macrophages are almost absent. Female, 81 years. Inguinal node. Giemsa. 875:1

oli. The cytoplasm is quite abundant and moderately or intensely basophilic. Germinal centre cells and cells of plasmacytopoiesis are not found. CIg is demonstrable less often than in the other subtypes.

2. B-Immunoblastic Lymphoma with Plasmacytic Differentiation (Figs. 76, 77). The immunoblasts are somewhat smaller (10–13 μm). The nuclei are round and sometimes eccentric. The nucleoli are large, basophilic and solitary or multiple; they are not in contact with the nuclear membrane. The cytoplasm is markedly basophilic and sometimes accumulated on one side of the nucleus. In the latter case, it often shows a perinuclear pale area (enlarged Golgi apparatus). One always finds plasma cells and all plasma cell precursors, which we used to call proplasmacytes and plasmablasts.[273] The occurrence of epithelioid cells with or without Langhans giant cells is more frequent in this subtype than in the first one. Monotypic Ig is found in the cytoplasm.

3. B-Immunoblastic Lymphoma with a High Content of Lymphocytes (Fig. 78). In this subtype some of the large immunoblasts lie together in dense groups, while others are spread about a lymphocytic background in large numbers. B-lymphocytes are sometimes interspersed with plasma cells or lymphoplasmacytoid cells showing monotypic Ig and, occasionally, intranuclear PAS-positive inclusions. This means that a secondary immunoblastic lymphoma has developed out of immunocytoma. In other cases there is no plasmacytic component. Such cases may represent B-CLL with development of Richter's syndrome. Another possibility is T-cell lymphoma. We have seen two cases of T-cell lymphoma of AILD type in which a B-immunoblastic lymphoma developed secondarily. This subtype of immunoblastic lymphoma has to be distinguished from large cell B-cell lymphoma with a high content of T cells (see p. 162).

Cytology and Cytochemistry. Cytological or cytochemical analyses do not provide any diagnostically helpful information.

Diagnosis. A majority of cells are B-immunoblasts. There may be an admixture of cells of the plasma cell series and lymphocytes. Centroblasts and other germinal centre cells are either missing or present in very small numbers (<10%).

Differential Diagnosis. B-immunoblastic lymphomas must be distinguished from hyperimmune reactions and virus infections, immunocytoma (with a high content of blast cells), anaplastic plasmacytoma, polymorphic centroblastic lymphoma, Burkitt's lymphoma, large cell anaplastic lymphoma, T-immunoblastic lymphoma, (genuine) histiocytic "lymphoma", undifferentiated carcinoma (especially lymphoepithelial carcinoma, also known as Schmincke's tumour or nasopharyngeal carcinoma) and other undifferentiated tumours (e.g. malignant rhabdoid tumour). In *hyperimmune reactions* and *viral infections*[274] (infectious mononucleosis, rubella) the number of immunoblasts may be so high that the pathologist's first guess is

---

[273] Lennert 1961.
[274] Lennert et al. 1981.

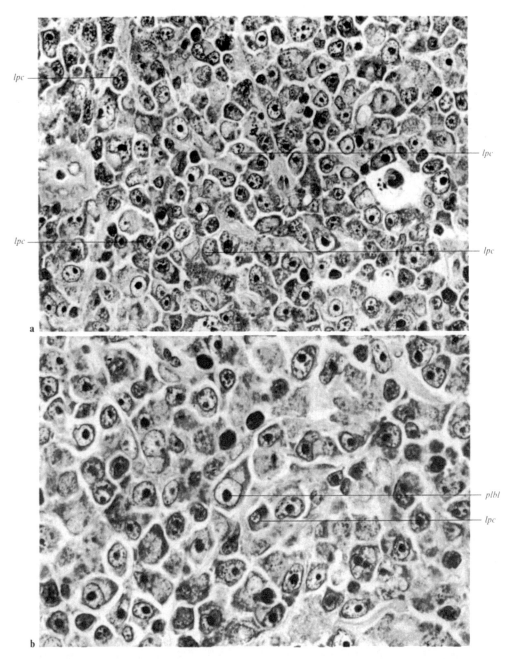

Fig. 76a, b. B-immunoblastic lymphoma with plasmacytic differentiation. The immunoblasts are large and show prominent, solitary, central, intensely basophilic nucleoli. Some lymphoplasmacytoid cells (*lpc*). One very large plasmablast-like cell (*plbl*) with a large perinuclear pale area. Same node as Fig. 73. Giemsa. **a** 560:1, **b** 875:1

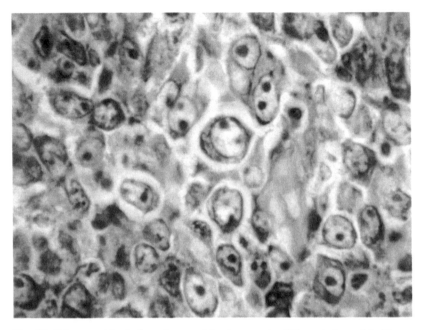

Fig. 77. B-immunoblastic lymphoma with plasmacytic differentiation with Giemsa staining. Tumour cells contain one or two prominent, central, basophilic nucleoli. Cytoplasm is intensely basophilic with some paler areas that probably represent Golgi bodies. Female, 67 years. Cervical node. 1550 : 1

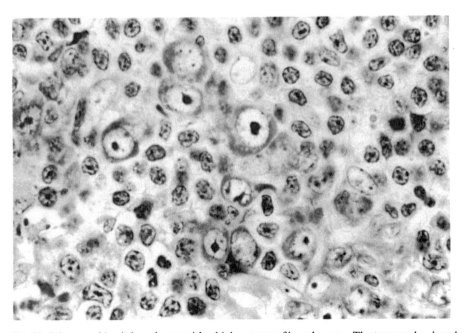

Fig. 78. B-immunoblastic lymphoma with a high content of lymphocytes. The tumour developed secondarily in a case of immunocytoma. Giemsa. 825 : 1

immunoblastic lymphoma (Fig. 79). This happens especially in cases that show large groups of blast cells in the sinuses. One may also be thrown off the scent by the apparently effaced lymph node architecture, whereby germinal centres are often absent or just small or occur only in part of the node. It is usually possible, however, to recognize the sinuses, at least in parts of the lymph node. Epithelioid venules are often abundant. Cytologically, there is usually a mixture of large immunoblasts and medium-sized lymphoid cells. In a case of infectious mononucleosis, for example, these can be interpreted as lymphocytes that are in the process of transformation into immunoblasts. As a rule, lymphoplasmacytoid cells and plasma cell precursors are also present. Occasionally, one finds large mononuclear and multinucleate blast cells that are very similar to, or even morphologically identical with, Hodgkin and Sternberg-Reed cells. In such cases an immunohistochemical analysis is often mandatory to demonstrate B and T cells and polyclonality of the B cells and to exclude the possibility of genuine Sternberg-Reed cells (which would be CD15+).[275]

All types of *immunocytoma* consist chiefly of small lymphocytes. In addition, a small or moderate percentage of the cells belong to the plasma cell series. Finally, one sees blast cells (centroblasts, immunoblasts, plasmablasts) loosely interspersed among the lymphocytes. The blast cells are not accumulated in groups and are much less abundant than in the subtype of B-immunoblastic lymphoma with a high content of lymphocytes.

The cells of *anaplastic plasmacytoma* show somewhat smaller nuclei and thus a slight resemblance to plasma cells. The tumour usually represents a metastasis of myeloma. Hence the cells mainly express IgG or IgA, whereas they rarely produce IgM. The reaction to L26 (CD20-like) is negative.

The borderline between *polymorphic centroblastic lymphoma* and immunoblastic lymphoma is not sharp. We diagnose the former when more than 10% of the cells are clearly recognizable germinal centre cells (centroblasts, multilobated cells). VAN DER VALK et al.[276] have developed exact morphometric criteria for distinguishing centroblastic and immunoblastic lymphomas.

The distinction between *Burkitt's lymphoma* and centroblastic lymphoma is discussed on p. 146.

In *large cell anaplastic lymphoma* the cells are larger and usually do not show the typical large, round, central nucleoli. The cytoplasm is usually more abundant and grey with Giemsa staining. The tumour cells are often arranged in groups or bands, especially in dilated sinuses. They are usually interspersed with numerous reactive macrophages and T lymphocytes. The immunohistochemical reaction for CD30 is always positive, whereas it is mostly negative in B-immunoblastic lymphoma.

T-immunoblastic lymphoma can be morphologically identical with B-immunoblastic lymphoma without plasmacytic differentiation. Usually, however, the tumour cells of the T type are less basophilic (grey with Giemsa staining) or

---

[275] Fellbaum et al. 1988.
[276] 1984a.

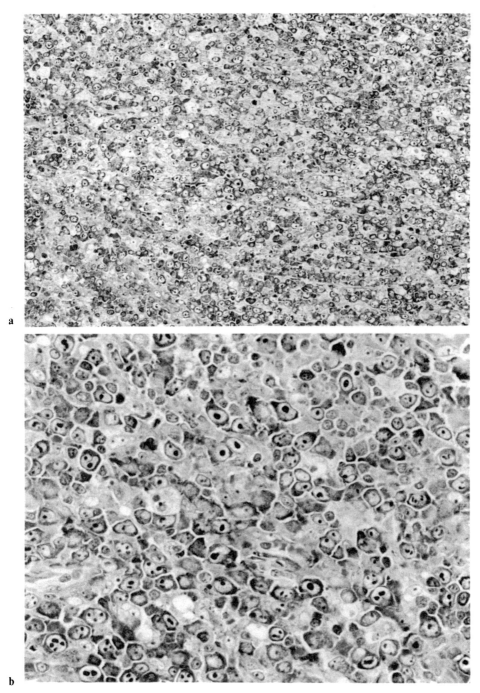

Fig. 79a, b. Infectious mononucleosis, serologically confirmed. *Warning:* This disorder can be confused with immunoblastic lymphoma or polymorphic centroblastic lymphoma. The nodal architecture is completely effaced. The lesion shows markedly basophilic blast cells of various (!) sizes and small lymphocytes that are in the process of transformation. There are also mononuclear and binucleate cells with giant nucleoli (resembling Hodgkin and Sternberg-Reed cells). Male, 16 years. Cervical node. Giemsa. **a** 220:1, **b** 560:1

pale ("clear"). In the first instance, an immunohistochemical analysis is essential to recognize the B-cell or T-cell nature of the tumour.

Histiocytic neoplasms[277] are still in need of a definitive characterization. They may look like large cell anaplastic lymphoma or like immunoblastic lymphoma without plasmacytic differentiation, or they may consist of large cells with oval nuclei and pale grey, abundant, esterase-positive (!) cytoplasm. In most cases tumour-forming monocytic leukaemia is probably the underlying disorder. In any event, malignant neoplasms of macrophages (other than monocytic leukaemia) are extremely rare and require systematic investigation with enzyme cytochemical (non-specific esterase), immunohistochemical and molecular genetic methods.

Lymphoepithelial carcinoma (Schmincke's tumour, nasopharyngeal carcinoma) is characterized by masses of large, moderately basophilic cells with strikingly pale nuclei (Fig. 80).[278] The nuclei contain large nucleoli, as do the nuclei of Hodgkin cells. The tumour complexes contain numerous T lymphocytes and interdigitating cells. Between the tumour cell clusters one often finds numerous inflammatory cells, especially eosinophils and plasma cells, and sometimes epithelioid cell granulomas as well. Even caseous necrosis is occasionally seen, and the conjunction of necrosis with epithelioid cell granulomas may simulate tuberculosis.[279] With silver impregnation the tumour cell clusters, which are free of fibres, are often sharply demarcated from the fibrous regions of the residual lymphoid tissue. The PAS reaction is always negative. As a rule, the patient's blood serum shows elevated EBV-antibody titres, especially IgA viral capsid antigens (VCA).[280]

Metastases of other undifferentiated malignant tumours can be excluded not only by morphology, but also by applying monoclonal antibodies to paraffin sections. KL1 (broad spectrum cytokeratin antibody) is very helpful for identifying carcinomas. KL1 is not an absolutely specific antibody, however. For instance, it is often found in a tumour whose nature has not yet been clarified and which rarely metastasizes to lymph nodes, viz. *malignant rhabdoid tumour*[281] (Fig. 81). This tumour is very similar to immunoblastic lymphoma, except that the cytoplasm of a few or numerous tumour cells contains eosinophilic, round inclusions, which are negative or very weakly positive with PAS staining. According to electron microscopic findings, these inclusions represent filament bundles of the intermediate type. Immunohistochemistry reveals vimentin as well as cytokeratin. The reader may refer to SCHMIDT et al.[282] for further immunohistochemical data. The tumour usually affects children and originates in the kidney, but it can also occur in soft tissue, especially in adults.[283] The course of the disease is very rapid.

---

[277] Lennert et al. 1984.

[278] Lennert et al. 1978.

[279] Rennke and Lennert 1973.

[280] Ho et al. 1981; Karpinski et al. 1981.

[281] Haas et al. 1981; Schmidt et al. 1982, 1989; Seo et al. 1988; Weeks et al. 1989.

[282] 1989.

[283] Balaton et al. 1987.

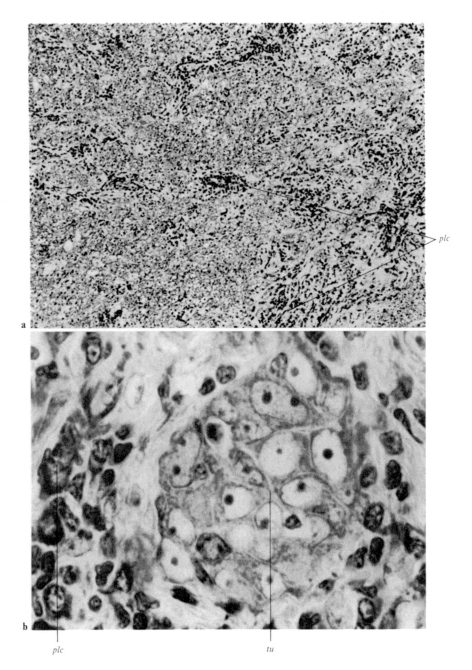

Fig. 80a, b. Lymphoepithelial carcinoma (Schmincke's tumour, nasopharyngeal carcinoma). The tumour cells (*tu*) have pale nuclei with very conspicuous, basophilic nucleoli and form compact masses. Between the tumour cell clusters there are strands and accumulations of plasma cells (*plc*) that are even more basophilic than the tumour cells (dark blue versus deep greyish blue). Female, 62 years. Cervical node. Giemsa. **a** 140:1, **b** 1550:1

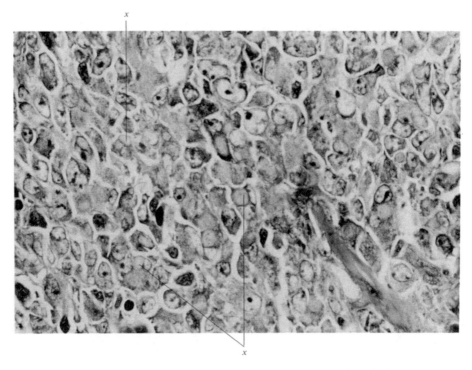

Fig. 81. Malignant rhabdoid tumour showing some globular cytoplasmic inclusions (*x*). H & E. 700:1

Prognosis. The prognosis for adult patients with immunoblastic lymphoma is poorer than that of most other types of high-grade ML of B-cell type. The 5-year survival rate is approximately 50% or less.

Addendum: Angio-endotheliotropic (Intravascular) Lymphoma[284]

Recently, immunophenotypic studies showed that the entity "malignant angioendotheliomatosis" is not a neoplasm derived from endothelial cells. Rather, in the vast majority of cases it is a high-grade malignant B-cell lymphoma. Exceptional cases may be of T-cell type. Some cases can be classified as B-immunoblastic lymphoma, while others cannot be classified. The tumours spread exclusively by way of blood vessels and involve predominantly the central nervous system and the skin. Some patients respond well to chemotherapy for high-grade ML.

---

[284] Stroup et al. 1990.

3.2.3 Burkitt's Lymphoma (BL)

WF: Malignant lymphoma, small non-cleaved cell, including Burkitt's (J)

Lukes-Collins: Small non-cleaved FCC, Burkitt and non-Burkitt variants

Terminology. Burkitt's lymphoma (BL) is the only type of NHL that we have not named after the proliferating cell type or the morphological structure, but rather after the person who discovered the tumour, namely, DENNIS BURKITT. The reason for this exception is our ignorance of the cellular origin of this lymphoma type. Is it a germinal centre cell, as indicated by LUKES and COLLINS' term "small non-cleaved FCC"? If so, *which* of the germinal centre cells in our cytological scheme would be a possible candidate? Typical centroblasts are certainly not a possibility, because they show a different nuclear configuration (peripheral nucleoli!). Perhaps it is the cells with multiple, central nucleoli that accumulate in the dark, lower zone and may be interpreted as precursors of centroblasts ("precentroblasts"). Some immunophenotypic data favour the view that BL is of germinal centre origin, e.g. the expression of common ALL antigen and CD77. The CD77 antigen is expressed by germinal centre cells and not by any other cell compartment.[285] It is also possible, however, that BL cells are related to the medium-sized blast cells of B type that infiltrate the lymph node pulp in infectious mononucleosis.

Before entrenching an unproven hypothesis in the terminology of our classification, we should like to keep the neutral term BL, which was the stated preference of the authors of the article published in *Lancet* in 1988.[286] We consider the term "small non-cleaved cell" used in the WF to be unacceptable for various reasons. At least it does not make any sense unless, at the least, FCC (follicular centre cell) is appended, as in the Lukes and Collins classification, because (1) the cells are not small, but rather medium sized or large, and (2) "non-cleaved" is not a suitable criterion for characterizing a lymphoma cell, since almost all types of lymphoma show cells with "non-cleaved" nuclei.

In the WF table[287] the word "Burkitt's" stands below the term "small non-cleaved cell". In the explanatory text, however, there is mention of a lymphoma of a similar "small non-cleaved cell" type that is to be differentiated from "Burkitt's lymphoma". A similar distinction is made in many other publications, in which the old category "undifferentiated" ML (term coined by RAPPAPORT) is separated into a Burkitt type and a non-Burkitt type.[288]

In collaboration with HUI,[289] we re-examined our series of high-grade malignant B-cell lymphomas after re-embedding the biopsy specimens in resin. We tried to sort them in a reproducible manner. We found a group of lymphomas that looked very similar to BL, but still showed certain differences. The tumour cells were more pleomorphic and exhibited some features of plasma cell differentia-

---

[285] Fellous et al. 1985.
[286] Stansfeld et al. 1988.
[287] The Non-Hodgkin's Lymphoma Pathologic Classification Project 1982.
[288] E.g. Berard et al. 1969; Cossman 1985; Felman et al. 1985a, b; Kelly et al. 1987.
[289] Hui et al. 1988.

tion. The cohesiveness was less pronounced and a starry-sky pattern was not a constant feature. This type of tumour evidently corresponds to the "small non-cleaved cell" category of the WF that is not additionally designated as "Burkitt's" and to RAPPAPORT's "undifferentiated ML, non-Burkitt's". Our immunohisto-chemical data also indicated that it belongs in a special category: the cytoplasm of tumour cells always contains Ig (usually IgM), and, in contrast to typical BL, the tumour cells do not express CD10. Hence we proposed the designation "with plasmablastic differentiation",[290] "with cIg" or "with Ig secretion". This seemed all the more appropriate since MAGRATH et al.[291] found monoclonal IgM bands in blood serum samples from many American patients with "undifferentiated" ML of Burkitt and non-Burkitt types. In that study they used an improved electroimmunofixation technique. In contrast, the investigators were unable to demonstrate monoclonal Ig in African BL. They reported similar findings on cell lines derived from African BL and American "undifferentiated" lymphomas of Burkitt and non-Burkitt types.[292] The very subtle studies performed by PAYNE et al.[293] provided more evidence in favour of differentiating a special variant of BL. Nevertheless, the picture is not black and white. There is overlapping of the immunohistochemical reactions. Furthermore, the diagnostic reproducibility of such a distinction still appears to be uncertain. This is evident, for example, from the results of a study by the Children's Cancer Study Group.[294] Several pathologists examined 159 cases of "undifferentiated" lymphoma collected between 1977 and 1983, and they were unable to classify them unanimously as "Burkitt's" or "non-Burkitt's". After re-examining the slides twice, they were able to reach a consensus in only 67% of cases, and did so more frequently in cases of the "Burkitt's" type (82%) than in those of the "non-Burkitt's" type (54%).

We had a similar experience at a workshop of the European Lymphoma Club, at which an updated Kiel classification was discussed and an attempt was made to reproduce the subtypes HUI had distinguished. We had rather limited success, even though we had HUI's brilliant slides to work with. For this reason, we did not distinguish two subtypes of BL in the classification scheme we published after the workshop.[295]

Nonetheless, the immunohistochemical findings, and evidently some clinical findings[296] as well, indicate that there may be a variant of BL that differs from classical BL and particularly from Epstein-Barr virus (EBV)-positive cases. Prospective studies are necessary, however, to ascertain whether it is sensible to draw a borderline on the basis of immunohistochemical criteria.

In the following we shall first treat typical BL and then discuss the cIg-positive BL variant. We used to use the term "Burkitt type" to distinguish non-endemic BL from endemic BL. This has turned out to be unnecessary, because there

---

[290] Hui et al. 1988.
[291] 1983.
[292] Benjamin et al. 1982.
[293] 1987.
[294] Wilson et al. 1987.
[295] Stansfeld et al. 1988.
[296] Wilson et al. 1987.

are no constant morphological differences between African BL and American or European BL. Hence we no longer use the term "Burkitt type" in this sense.

In the updated Kiel classification we have taken BL out of the group of lymphoblastic lymphomas (cf. p. 15). Although this may be confusing at first, we felt obliged to do so, because BL differs from the other lymphoblastic (precursor cell) lymphomas on account of its special morphological, immunohistochemical and cytogenetic features.

In Vitro Studies on BL Cell Lines. Important information has been provided by studies on BL cell lines in vitro[297] using superior morphological techniques. There turned out to be remarkable cytological differences between the cell lines, but they did not directly match the histological pictures in vivo. The morphology ranged from "small non-cleaved cells" to large immunoblast-like cells. This spectrum is reflected in biopsies, though not quite so extremely.

Rowe et al.[298] presented another study on the in vitro behaviour of BL cell lines. They found differences in growth pattern and immunohistochemical features between endemic BL and sporadic forms of EBV-positive BL. Furthermore, not only was there a difference in phenotypic expression between the cell lines and tumour biopsies, but the expression also changed during the time of cell culture.

Definition. The lymphoma is mostly composed of medium-sized, markedly basophilic, cohesive cells with multiple, central nucleoli. There is also a starry-sky pattern, at least focally. EBV can be detected in more than 90% of African cases of BL,[299] but in only about 10% of the cases in our collection.[300] There is no regular morphological difference between EBV-positive and EBV-negative BL. BL is the fastest growing tumour, with a potential doubling time of 25.6 h.[301]

Immunology. The tumour cells are characterized by constant expression of sIg, usually IgM; IgA is expressed in exceptional cases. In most cases both light and heavy Ig chains are detectable, but occasionally only heavy chains or only light chains are found. A reaction for cIg in paraffin sections (and, accordingly, Ig secretion in vitro) is apparently not found in African BL, but cIg has been seen in some American or European cases. We define the cIg-positive cases as a variant of BL (see p. 146). In cryostat sections the expression of common ALL antigen (CD10) and of CD19 and CD22 is a virtually constant feature. CD23 is not expressed in tumour biopsies. Follicular dendritic cells are not detectable within the infiltration. The number of proliferating cells (Ki-67 +) reaches the highest figures in this lymphoma type, with a median of about 80% positive cells.[302] The monoclonal antibody 38.12 is not specific for BL.[302a]

---

[297] E.g. Felman et al. 1985a,b; Kelly et al. 1987.
[298] 1985; c.f. Rooney et al. 1986.
[299] Zur Hausen 1979.
[300] Demonstrated by in situ hybridization by C. H. Trautmann (unpublished data).
[301] Iversen et al. 1974.
[302] See Garcia et al. 1986 for further immunohistochemical data.
[302a] Pallesen and Zeuthen 1987.

Cytogenetics. Cytogenetic and molecular genetic studies of BL have provided fundamental impulses for tumour research.[303] An early event in the development of BL is usually a reciprocal translocation between chromosomes 8 and 14. Because of this, the oncogene *c-myc* of chromosome 8 is transposed into the vicinity of a gene on chromosome 14 that codes for the constant region of heavy Ig chains. Less common is the translocation 8; 22, least common a translocation 8; 2. Based on cytogenetic findings and other criteria, a new concept for understanding the origin and development of BL in Africa and in non-African countries has been proposed by LENOIR and BORNKAMM.[304]

Occurrence. In the areas of Africa where BL (and malaria!) is endemic, it shows an incidence of 1–12 cases per 100000 children per year. SCHMAUZ[305] has observed that the percentage of BL cases varies according to the incidence of malaria from 23.2% to 44.6% of all ML in his series. In the United States LEVINE et al.[306] calculated a frequency of 1.4 cases per 1000000 white males and 0.4 cases per 1000000 white females. In our collection, BL of the lymph node, including the CIg-positive cases, accounts for 2.6% of the NHL. If one includes the extranodal cases, which make up about 50% of the cases of BL, one reaches a figure of about 3%. Among children in Germany BL of the lymph node accounts for at least 25%, and at most 40%, of the NHL (see p. 44).

The age peak is somewhat earlier in Africa (between the 3rd and 6th year of life) than in the United States. In our collection, as in the American studies,[307] there are several adults, whereas in African studies adult cases are a rarity. Nodal cases of BL in our collection (Fig. 82) show a first peak in the first two decades, a second peak in the 5th decade and a third peak in the 7th–8th decade. Our youngest patient was 3 years old, our oldest 87. In the first two decades males predominate highly, whereas in the 8th decade females are affected more frequently. Altogether the male-to-female ratio is 1.5 : 1.

Clinical Picture. In earlier reports on African BL the most frequent site of primary manifestation was the jaw,[309] but in the meantime the incidence of primary manifestation in the abdomen has increased markedly.[310] In the United States only about 33% of patients show involvement of the jaw; instead, the lymphoma usually develops as an abdominal tumour (ileocaecal region, abdominal lymph nodes, retroperitoneum or ovaries).[311] A leukaemic blood picture develops in about 5%–10% of the non-endemic cases of BL (accounting for approx. 2%–3% of cases of "ALL" type L3 according to the FAB classification).

---

[303] Zech et al. 1976; reviewed by Klein and Klein 1985.
[304] 1987.
[305] Personal communication 1990.
[306] 1985.
[307] Arseneau et al. 1975; Banks et al. 1975.
[308] deleted.
[309] Wright 1970.
[310] R. Schmauz, personal communication 1990.
[311] Arseneau et al. 1975; Banks et al. 1975; Levine et al. 1975.

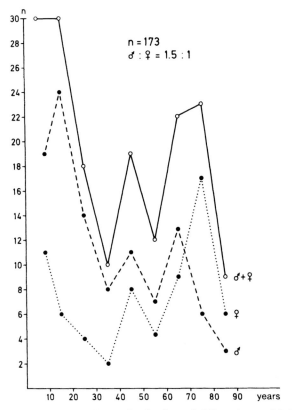

Fig. 82. Age and sex distribution of 173 patients with Burkitt's lymphoma (including the CIg-positive variant). Data from nodal cases collected at the Lymph Node Registry, 1983–1987

Histology. The tumour cells are "cohesive", i.e. they lie close together (Fig. 83) and thereby appear to form compact masses. The tumour cells have a monotonous appearance because of their uniform morphology and size. They are usually medium sized. They do not show any signs of maturation into plasmablasts or plasma cells. The nuclei are round and show intensely stained chromatin and two or three medium-sized, central, basophilic nucleoli. The cytoplasm is scanty or moderately abundant, markedly basophilic and often vacuolated (Sudan red positive). Some cases show tumour cells that are large *and cohesive*, and their nuclei have large, solitary nucleoli. Such cells have been described in the literature as "immunoblastic" variants. They have also been found in HIV-positive patients and in BL cell lines in vitro.[312] As a rule, the tumour cells are interspersed with numerous starry-sky cells, i.e. large macrophages that have phagocytosed many tumour cells, including intact tumour cells and even those in mitosis (Fig. 84). The cell death is interpreted as apoptosis. Mitotic activity is high (> 10/HPF). Reticulin fibres are very sparse. Occasionally, we have observed proliferation of BL

---

[312] E.g. Felman et al. 1985a,b.

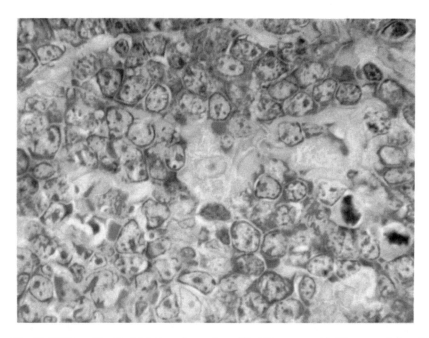

Fig. 83. EBV-positive Burkitt's lymphoma from West Germany with Giemsa staining. Note the basophilic, "cohesive", relatively large tumour cells. Two mitotic figures. Most of the nucleoli are centrally located. In the *centre* of the picture, a large macrophage (starry-sky cell) with a weakly stained nucleus, one medium-sized, weakly basophilic nucleolus and abundant, pale cytoplasm. Female, 6 years. Cervical node. 1550:1

in follicles resembling germinal centres; this has also been described in the literature.[313] PALLESEN[314] described two cases in which infiltration of the mantle zone appeared to precede infiltration of the germinal centres.

Cytochemistry. In blood smears or lymph node imprints the acid phosphatase reaction is granular (not focal). The PAS reaction is negative. Most of the vacuoles can be identified with Sudan red staining as fat droplets.

Diagnosis. Monotony, basophilia, *cohesiveness* and a starry-sky pattern are the main diagnostic criteria. These features can be recognized only in well-fixed and well-embedded biopsy material. Frequently, the cohesiveness and the typical cytology can be seen only in outer parts of the slides. In such cases a well-fixed band, which is often very narrow, surrounds the undiagnosable central areas.

The starry-sky pattern may be lacking in some parts of a biopsy, especially if it is from an extranodal site. Nevertheless, a starry-sky pattern is still an important diagnostic criterion. Admittedly, it is not specific to BL, since it occurs in a large number of high-grade malignant NHL.

---

[313] E.g. Mann et al. 1976.
[314] 1983.

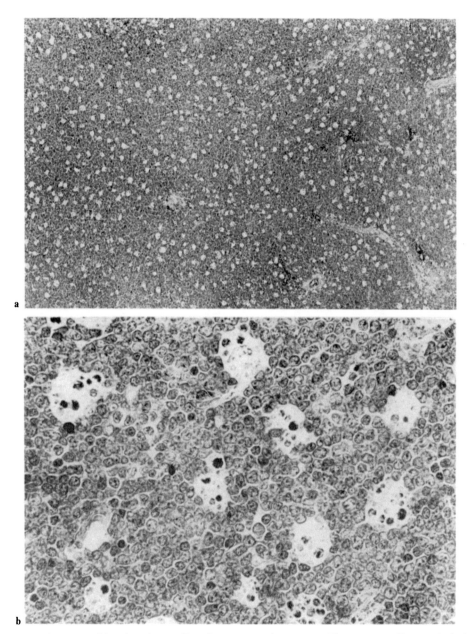

Fig. 84a, b. Burkitt's lymphoma. Prominent starry-sky pattern. The tumour cells are relatively small. The starry-sky cells contain much tumour cell debris. Male, 7 years. Patient had high EBV antibody titres. Axillary node. Giemsa. **a** 56:1, **b** 560:1

Differential Diagnosis. The borderline between BL and other high-grade malignant B-cell lymphomas cannot always be drawn sharply, especially if the slides are not of optimum quality. For example, slight technical flaws may cause artificial displacement of the nucleoli toward the nuclear membrane, resulting in the erroneous diagnosis of *monomorphic centroblastic lymphoma.* The danger of a false diagnosis is high, because a starry-sky pattern is also occasionally observed in monomorphic centroblastic lymphoma. In such cases, cytological examination of optimum-quality slides is absolutely necessary.

It is also occasionally difficult to distinguish *B-immunoblastic lymphoma* from BL. Immunoblastic lymphoma can contain a certain number of medium-sized cells with multiple, central nucleoli, which are suggestive of BL. The decisive factor, however, is the presence of large immunoblasts with relatively abundant, basophilic cytoplasm and large, often solitary, central nucleoli. Both the large cell variant of BL and immunoblastic lymphoma often show diffuse cIg. There are two other distinguishing features, however, viz.: the large cell variant of BL shows cohesive growth (in the outer regions of the lymph node) and, in most cases, rearrangement of *c-myc.*

Prognosis. There appears to be a fundamental difference between EBV-positive and EBV-negative cases of BL. EBV-positive BL patients who have a defect in the T-cell immune reaction (e.g. due to malaria, AIDS or Purtilo's syndrome, or following organ transplantation) occasionally show spontaneous remission and respond well to treatment. BL patients who are EBV-negative and have a normal T-cell system (but with the same chromosomal aberration) do not show spontaneous remission. RIEHM[315] reported full remission in 80% of children with BL, as long as there was no widespread metastasis in the abdomen ("patients at risk").

3.2.3.1 Burkitt's Lymphoma with Cytoplasmic Immunoglobulin

The borderline between BL without cIg and BL with cIg is not sharp and must be drawn somewhat arbitrarily. Even cases of classic BL may show some cIg in nuclear clefts. In this section, however, we consider only the cases in which a large number of, or even all the tumour cells clearly show intracytoplasmic Ig deposits. Morphologically, this accumulation of Ig proceeds along with transformation of the tumour cells into immunoblasts, plasmablasts or plasma cells (the latter but rarely and then only in small numbers). A similar process has been observed in tissue culture: as time goes by, the classic BL cells transform into immunoblasts and plasma cells.[316]

Immunology. In the variant discussed here cIg can be detected in formalin-fixed tissue. This is not true in classical BL, with a few exceptions that underline the

---

[315] Personal communication.
[316] O. Gentilhomme, personal communication.
[317] deleted.
[318] deleted.

continuous spectrum of BL. Conversely, in BL with cIg common ALL antigen (CD10) is expressed only in exceptional cases, while in BL without cIg it is expressed almost invariably. In addition, CD23 expression is occasionally found in cIg-positive BL. PAYNE et al.[319] described CD10 expression in only three of ten cases and IgG instead of IgM on the surface of tumour cells in four cases. Otherwise the antigenic profile of cIg-positive BL corresponds to that of typical BL.

Occurrence. In our collection the cIg-positive BL was found in lymph nodes less frequently than typical BL, viz. in about 1% of the cases of ML (collected in 1983). The average age of our patients is 54 years; the youngest patient was 5, the oldest 82. The tumour appears to occur most frequently in the 6th–8th decades of life. Males and females are affected with approximately equal frequency.

Clinical Picture. The cIg-positive variant seems to occur somewhat less frequently in extranodal sites (especially in the terminal ileum) than cIg-negative BL. It appears to be associated more often with a leukaemic blood picture.[321]

Histology (Figs. 85, 86). A majority of the tumour cells are medium-sized and basophilic, but there are both larger and smaller basophilic forms as well. Mononuclear and multinucleated giant cells with the same morphology are also occasionally found. Small and medium-sized cells are often suggestive of cells of plasmacytopoiesis, particularly by virtue of their large, pale perinuclear halo (Golgi apparatus) and their more abundant and perhaps even more strongly basophilic cytoplasm. This explains why HUI et al.[322] spoke of a plasmablastic subtype of BL. We usually find several small or medium-sized nucleoli. In some cases the cells are large and have large, solitary nucleoli. Although such cells are indistinguishable from immunoblasts, they show a cohesive growth pattern.

Diagnosis. The decisive factor is the impression that one is dealing with a case of BL, except that the cytology does not quite fit. The cells are more pleomorphic. According to our definition, they occasionally show plasmablastic differentiation and are accordingly cIg positive.

Differential Diagnosis. See p. 146.

Prognosis. In the American "BL-like lymphoma" the prognosis is supposed to be much worse than in typical BL.[323] We do not yet have any data of our own on the course of the disease.

---

[319] 1987.
[320] deleted.
[321] Watanabe et al. 1973.
[322] 1987.
[323] Miliauskas et al. 1982; Oviatt et al. 1983; Payne et al. 1987.

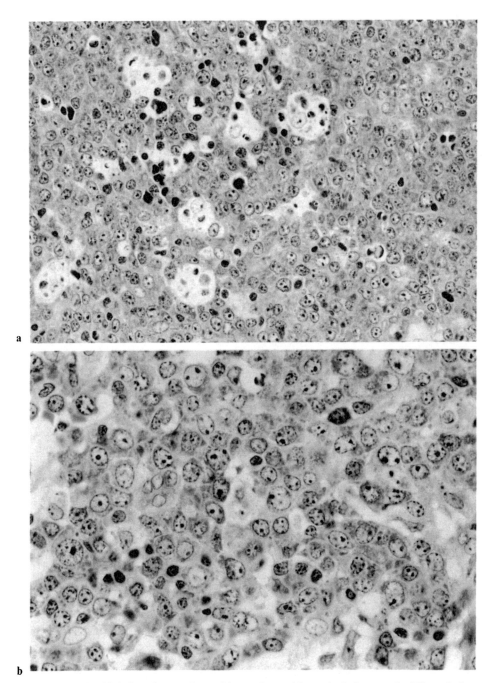

Fig. 85a, b. Burkitt's lymphoma, cIg-positive variant, with marked plasmacytic differentiation. Male, 80 years. Axillary node. Giemsa. **a** 440:1, **b** 695:1

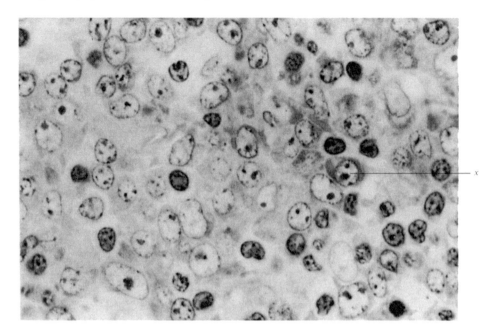

Fig. 86. Burkitt's lymphoma, cIg-positive variant. Plasmablast (x). Male, 74 years. Axillary node. Giemsa. 1094:1

Addendum: Malignant Lymphomas in Immunocompromised Patients

Malignant tumours have been observed to develop following organ transplantation and subsequent immunosuppressive treatment. In 1972 PENN and STARZL[324] described 76 malignant tumours in about 8000 organ transplant recipients. About 55% of them proved to be epithelial tumours, while approximately 40% were ML. It also turned out that patients who were intravenous drug users with the concomitant risk of HIV infection run 40 times as great a risk of developing ML. The lymphomas that develop in patients with HIV infection are largely high-grade malignant NHL, with a large share of BL. The t(8;14) and t(8;22) translocation that is typical of HIV-positive BL cases was described as early as 1983.[325] If one looks at the group of BL in isolation, the risk of developing BL is 1000 times as great in this group of patients as in the normal population.[326] In areas where BL is endemic the frequency amounts to about 10% of the ML, whereas in non-endemic regions BL makes up 1%–2% of the NHL. Following transplantation the frequency increases to 4%–10%, and after HIV infection to about

---

[324] 1972.
[325] Chaganti et al. 1983.
[326] Ernberg 1989.

30%. If we extrapolate from these data, we can assume that in about 10–20 years ML occurring in immunosuppressed or immunodeficient patients will account for a major number of the cases of ML as a whole.

Lymphomas with a similar morphological picture, a similar localization and a similar clinical course have been found in patients who had received organ transplants and subsequent immunosuppressive treatment and in immunodeficient patients with HIV infections.[327] In addition to classical BL, lymphomas resembling BL have been described,[328] and in some cases the EBV genome was detected in the tumour cells.[329] B-immunoblastic lymphoma has been described in a similar number of cases.[330] We should like to point out, however, that there is an immunoblast-like variant of BL that is recognizable from the cohesiveness of the tumour cells (by taking a good look at the well-fixed outer zones of the biopsies!). In the literature many of the lymphomas were described as "undifferentiated" ML, "diffuse large cell" ML or polymorphic B-cell lymphoma.[331] Most of the lymphomas were of high-grade malignancy, and they were almost exclusively of B-cell origin.[332] The percentage of verified low-grade malignant NHL lies below 10%. Among these a few cases of germinal centre cell lymphoma and immunocytoma have been described. Whether these low-grade ML happened by chance to occur in connection with immunodeficiency, or whether they were causally related to the same, is a question that must remain open. At present it does not appear likely that there is a connection. A varying percentage (10%–20%) of cases of Hodgkin's lymphoma have been reported, some of which were classified as the nodular sclerosis subtype and others as the mixed cellularity subtype.[333] Many cases, however, have a distinct morphological appearance (low content of lymphocytes, etc.).

The ML occurring in immunodeficient patients following transplantation or with HIV infections have another feature in common, viz. their characteristic localizations. They are very predominantly found in extranodal sites. The CNS is affected in an unusually large percentage of cases.[334] In patients who are not immunodeficient, primary ML very seldom occurs in the CNS. Other unusual sites of primary involvement are the liver[335] and the transverse colon[336] (the ML in such cases have been histologically classified as Hodgkin's lymphoma). Further localizations are the lungs and the soft tissue at the site of injection of antilymphocyte sera.[337]

---

[327] Monfardini et al. 1990; Hamilton-Dutoit et al. 1991; Raphael et al. 1991.
[328] Ziegler et al. 1982.
[329] Hamilton-Dutoit et al. 1989; Borisch-Chappuis et al. 1990.
[330] Levine et al. 1984.
[331] Frizzera et al. 1981.
[332] Egerter and Beckstead 1988.
[333] Ioachim et al. 1985; Tirelli et al. 1988.
[334] Ziegler et al. 1984; Ioachim et al. 1985; Kalter et al. 1985; Egerter and Beckstead 1988; Tirelli et al. 1988.
[335] Frizzera et al. 1981.
[336] Cerilli et al. 1977.
[337] Weintraub and Warnke 1982.

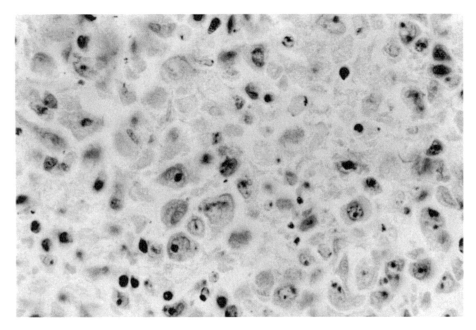

Fig. 87. Polymorphic B-cell proliferation after kidney transplantation and clinically verified EBV infection 3 weeks ante-mortem. The Ig in the tumour cells proved to be polyclonal. It is likely that this was a virulent EBV infection and not yet ML. Giemsa. 695:1. (Specimen kindly provided by G. FRIZZERA)

Histopathological, immunohistological and molecular genetic findings in high-grade ML that developed after organ transplantation have been described by FRIZZERA et al.,[338] who coined the term "polymorphic B-cell lymphoma". They applied this term to a proliferation of large blast cells, including typical immunoblasts and some immunoblasts with plasmacytoid differentiation. So-called multilobated cells were also found. A few Sternberg-Reed cells, smaller lymphoid cells and mature plasma cells were described as well. Large necrotic areas were frequently recognized within the infiltrations, as is typical of fulminating EBV infections (Fig. 87).

In 1981, FRIZZERA et al.[339] described diffuse polymorphic B-cell hyperplasia and so-called polymorphic B-cell lymphoma in renal transplant recipients. They concluded that the monoclonal lymphoma developed gradually out of an initially polyclonal B-cell proliferation. Similar findings on the development of monoclonality have been reported by other research groups.[340] It has been demonstrated that tissue samples taken simultaneously from different tumour sites showed

---

[338] Frizzera et al. 1981; Hanto et al. 1981, 1983.
[339] Frizzera et al. 1981.
[340] Cleary and Sklar 1984; Pelicci et al. 1986; Barriga et al. 1988; Lippman et al. 1988.

different rearrangements of the Ig genes. Hence a multifocal origin was postulated for these lymphomas and, together with other factors, held responsible for their rapid progression.[341] Furthermore, at about the same time EBV was successfully detected in the genome of the tumour cells from many of the investigated tumours. It was not possible to demonstrate this in *all* cases, however. The investigators concluded that EBV is not the only agent responsible for the development of the lymphomas they examined.[342]

In questionable cases, the gradual transition from "polymorphic B-cell hyperplasia" to "polymorphic B-cell lymphoma" described by FRIZZERA et al. makes it impossible to distinguish fatal EBV infections from high-grade malignant B-cell lymphomas. Although the presence of polytypic (polyclonal) plasma cells and plasma cell precursors is an indication of virus-related hyperplasia, this finding does not rule out the possibility that a high-grade malignant B-cell lymphoma has already developed at another site.

3.2.4 Large Cell Anaplastic Lymphoma of B-Cell Type (Ki-1 +)

WF: Not listed

Lukes-Collins: Not listed

Large cell anaplastic lymphoma (LCAL) could be identified by means of the antibody Ki-1, which is directed against CD30.[343] The tumour is chiefly derived from T cells and was originally named Ki-1 lymphoma. In a small percentage of cases, however, tumours that have the same morphology and are also positive for CD30 are derived from B cells. For a description of the morphology the reader may refer to the section on LCAL of T-cell type (p. 234). The tumour cells are large and have moderately abundant, grey cytoplasm (Fig. 88). Giant cells occasionally occur. In LCAL of B-cell type the carcinoma-like appearance predominates, whereas the impression of histiocytosis is less common. The CD30 expression is weaker than the reaction seen in the T-cell type, and it is more often intracytoplasmic in contrast to the surface expression observed in the T-cell type.

In addition, there are large cell lymphomas of B type that we designate as *unclassified*, because they do not correspond exactly to any of the categories we have distinguished. They can be recognized as B-cell lymphomas only on the basis of the demonstration of B-cell antigens (CD19, CD22). They can be classified as being high-grade malignant, because they are composed only of large, basophilic cells. In general, they are CD30 negative. The exceptional CD30-positive cases should probably be included in the group of LCAL.

---

[341] Cleary and Sklar 1984.
[342] Cleary et al. 1988.
[343] Stein et al. 1985.

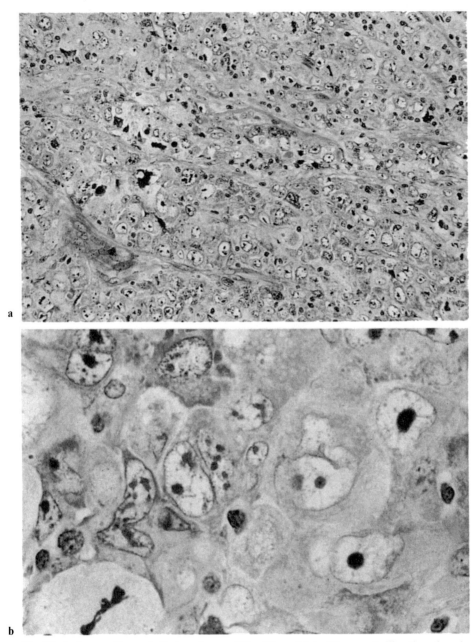

Fig. 88a, b. Large cell anaplastic lymphoma of B-cell type. Male, 75 years. Axillary lymph node. Giemsa. **a** 205:1, **b** 1024:1

3.2.5 Lymphoblastic Lymphoma of B-Cell Type

WF: Malignant lymphoma, lymphoblastic, convoluted cell and non-convoluted cell (I)

Lukes-Collins: Not listed

Definition. We apply the term "lymphoblastic lymphoma" to all high-grade malignant neoplasms that consist chiefly of medium-sized "blast cells" with scanty, more or less basophilic cytoplasm. The nucleus of these cells shows fine chromatin and is usually round, but sometimes gyrate or "convoluted". The neoplasia may appear in tumour form and/or as leukaemia (acute lymphoblastic leukaemia [ALL]).

When we say "lymphoblasts" we do not mean the blast cells of peripheral lymphoid tissue (lymph nodes, tonsils, gastrointestinal tract) but rather the precursor cells in the bone marrow (B and T precursor cells) and thymus (T precursor cells).

Lymphoblasts express B or T antigens. Early B-cell or T-cell features can now be demonstrated even in cells whose B or T nature was not initially recognized ("null type"). Among the lymphoblasts of B type we can distinguish three variants on the basis of their immunocytological phenotype:

1. "Pre-pre-B lymphoblasts" express B antigens (CD19) on the surface and in the cytoplasm, but are negative for sIg and cIg
2. "Pre-B lymphoblasts" contain μ chains but no light chains in their cytoplasm
3. (Mature) B lymphoblasts express sIg (μ/*kapppa* or *lambda*)

Immunology. All lymphoblastic lymphomas of B-cell type express the B cell-associated antigen CD19; approximately 90% simultaneously show CD22. Usually, when CD22 is missing, sIg is also not detectable. About 60% of the lymphoblastic lymphomas of B type express common ALL antigen (CD10). The proportion of proliferating cells lies between 40% and 80%. Follicular dendritic cells cannot be detected.

In paraffin sections the intracytoplasmic μ chains of pre-B lymphoblasts cannot be recognized. The reaction for Ki-B3 (which reacts with antigen related to CD45) is positive, but this is not a suitable feature for differentiating B-lymphoblastic lymphoma from T-lymphoblastic lymphoma, since the latter shows a positive reaction in some cases. Hence L26 (CD20-like) and anti-CD3 antibodies should also be applied.

Occurrence. The pure tumour form of B-lymphoblastic lymphoma is rare. Most cases occur as (B-)ALL. In 1983 (see Table 11) we were able to substantiate only 11 cases (= 0.9% of all ML) of B-lymphoblastic lymphoma by immunohistochemistry. Bucsky et al.[344] found only 2.1% cases of B type among 188 cases of

---

[344] 1988.

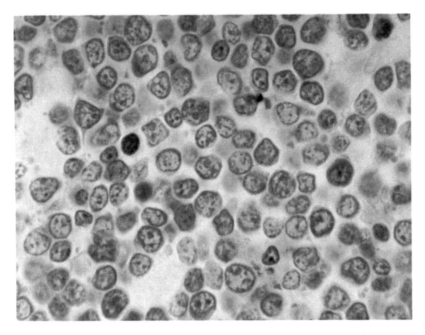

Fig. 89. B-lymphoblastic lymphoma with Giemsa staining. Relatively small tumour cells with a narrow rim of moderately basophilic cytoplasm. There is marked similarity to T-lymphoblastic lymphoma, but the acid phosphatase reaction was negative. Male, 11 years. Mediastinal node. 1550:1

non-leukaemic NHL in the first 18 years of life (in contrast to 25.5% cases of T type and 7.4% unclassified lymphoblastic lymphomas).

We cannot make any definite statements about the age and sex distribution of non-leukaemic B-lymphoblastic lymphoma. It occurs in all age groups. We saw patients up to an age of 77 years.[345]

Histology. The lymph node is infiltrated by a very monotonous-looking population of medium-sized lymphoblasts (9–11 μm; see Fig. 89). The nuclei are round, oval, indented or gyrate ("convoluted"). They have very fine chromatin and one to three small or medium-sized, basophilic nucleoli. The cytoplasm is scanty and stains greyish blue or blue with Giemsa. Mitotic figures are plentiful (approx. 10/HPF). Occasionally there is a starry-sky pattern, but it is not very pronounced. The trabeculae and capsule, especially in the leukaemic variant, are sometimes heavily infiltrated, but still clearly distinguishable from the sinuses (Fig. 90).

---

[345] Hui et al. 1987.

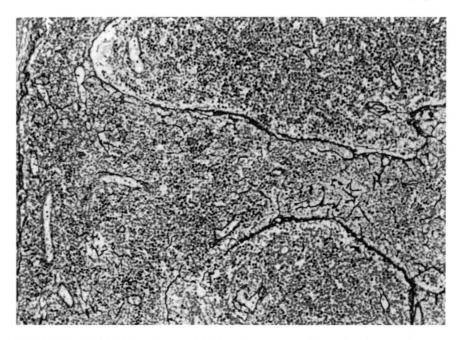

Fig. 90. B-lymphoblastic lymphoma with silver impregnation. The trabecula and adjacent capsule are heavily infiltrated and expanded, but not effaced. In most parts they are sharply demarcated from the sinuses and infiltrated pulp. Female, 4 years. Supraclavicular node. Gomori. 140:1

Cytology and Cytochemistry. The slightly to moderately basophilic, scanty cytoplasm is easier to recognize in imprints. The acid phosphatase reaction is negative or shows a few positive granules. One never finds the typical focal reaction pattern seen in T-lymphoblastic lymphoma. The non-specific esterase reaction is negative or, if positive, somewhat granular. The chloroacetate esterase reaction is negative in all cells.

Diagnosis. The diagnosis of lymphoblastic lymphoma (without subtyping) is simple. The monotonous appearance of the medium-sized blast cells gives the decisive clue even at a low magnification. It is not possible to distinguish between T and B types by morphology alone, however. At present, an immunological examination of fresh biopsy material (frozen sections or smears of an aspirate or blood) is indispensable. The lack of a focal acid phosphatase reaction is an indication of a B-cell lymphoma, but does not exclude a T-lymphoblastic lymphoma.

Differential Diagnosis. A differential diagnosis must include not only T-lymphoblastic lymphoma (see p. 244), but also acute myeloid leukaemia, myelomonocytic leukaemia and centrocytic lymphoma (see pp. 101 f.).
    Acute myeloid leukaemia or myelomonocytic leukaemia infiltrates lymph nodes fairly frequently and is therefore sometimes submitted for histological examination. These types of leukaemia may also show medium-sized blast cells

that can hardly be distinguished from lymphoblasts. In acute myeloid leukaemia the blast cells are occasionally somewhat more basophilic and larger than those of lymphoblastic lymphoma. If a monocytic component occurs, the nuclei show an irregular, occasionally bean-shaped configuration. In the differential diagnosis silver impregnation is helpful, as are cytochemical analyses of paraffin sections and imprints and an immunohistochemical study of paraffin sections.

Fibres are more numerous in acute myeloid leukaemia and myelomonocytic leukaemia than in lymphoblastic lymphoma or ALL. Sections stained with silver impregnation reveal the most important feature, viz. a considerable increase in capillaries, which is more pronounced in myelomonocytic leukaemia than in acute myeloid leukaemia.

Cytochemically, myelocytes and promyelocytes that are positive for chloro-acetate esterase can usually be found in paraffin sections from both myelogenic leukaemias. These cells often lie together in groups, especially in the sinuses and connective tissue of the node. In imprints the same cells can be found easily with the aid of the chloroacetate esterase or peroxidase reaction. The non-specific esterase reaction reveals diffusely positive monocytes.

Immunohistochemically, neoplastic myeloid cells and monocytes may express CD15 (3C4, Leu-M1), CD68, lysozyme and Ki-M1p.

Prognosis. About 75% of the children with pre-B and pre-pre-B types of ALL and lymphoblastic lymphoma treated by RIEHM[346] showed remission. For the "mature cell" B-lymphoblastic type the figure was even 80%. Immunologically verified data on lymphoblastic lymphomas of the three B-cell subtypes in adults are not available. There is a strong correlation between distinct chromosomal abnormalities and the prognosis of lymphoblastic lymphoma.[347]

3.3 Rare and Ambiguous Types of B-Cell Lymphoma

3.3.1 Large Cell, Sclerosing B-Cell Lymphoma of the Mediastinum

History. Since 1978 large cell ML other than lymphoblastic lymphoma have been described in the mediastinum, particularly in the upper anterior region.[348] In general they show a characteristic type of sclerosis.[349] The site of origin is probably the thymus,[350] which normally contains B cells of various shapes and sizes.[351] From here the tumour cells infiltrate and destroy the mediastinum and

---

[346] Personal communication 1989.

[347] Fletcher et al. 1991; Pui et al. 1991.

[348] Miller et al. 1978; Lichtenstein et al. 1980; Levitt et al. 1982; Trump and Mann 1982; Yousem et al. 1985; Addis and Isaacson 1986; Menestrina et al. 1986; Möller et al. 1986, 1987; Leahu and Niculescu 1987; Jacobson et al. 1988; Lamarre et al. 1989.

[349] Miller et al. 1978; Lichtenstein et al. 1980; Menestrina et al. 1986; Perrone et al. 1986.

[350] Addis and Isaacson 1986; Menestrina et al. 1986.

[351] Hofmann et al. 1988.

grow into large vessels, the lungs, the heart, the wall of the chest, etc. They do not metastasize to extrathoracic lymph nodes or bone marrow, whereas the kidneys, adrenal gland, brain and other organs are frequently involved. The patients are usually young and mostly female. Cytologically, the lymphomas have been designated as "large cleaved", "large non-cleaved", "small non-cleaved", "histiocytic", "clear cell" or simply as "large cell". PERRONE et al.[352] classified 35 cases as follicular centre cell lymphoma, 13 cases as T-immunoblastic lymphoma and seven cases as B-immunoblastic lymphoma, although they did not draw on immunological data. Only in the past few years has it been possible to define the lymphoma as a derivative of B cells.[353]

Definition. We apply the term "large cell, sclerosing B-cell lymphoma of the mediastinum" to a tumour that fulfils the following criteria:

1. The tumour is located in the mediastinum, specifically in the upper anterior region.
2. The tumour cells are large and often show certain features of centroblastic lymphoma cells.
3. Between the tumour cells there are loose networks or wide bands of fibres.
4. Immunohistochemical staining usually does not reveal Ig, but pan-B markers are expressed.

The tumour must be classified as a high-grade malignant B-cell lymphoma. It probably does not originate in a lymph node, but instead is derived from B lymphocytes of the thymus. Hence, strictly speaking, it should be interpreted as an extranodal lymphoma.

Immunohistochemistry.[354] In more than 70% of the cases the tumour cells express the B-cell antigens CD22 and CD20. The B-cell antigen CD19, however, is detectable in only about half the cases. Another characteristic of this lymphoma type is the constant absence of cIg expression. sIg can be detected only in exceptional cases. Whereas the common leucocyte antigen can be demonstrated regularly, expression of HLA class II antigens is lacking in about 30% of cases. More than 90% of the investigated cases were positive for PC1 (plasma cell-associated antigen). This antigen is not expressed exclusively on plasma cells, however, and thus does not allow any conclusion as to the degree of differentiation of those lymphomas. The reaction demonstrating common ALL antigen (CD10) is generally negative. Follicular dendritic cells cannot be demonstrated.

---

[352] 1986.

[353] Yousem et al. 1985; Addis and Isaacson 1986; Menestrina et al. 1986; Möller et al. 1986, 1987.

[354] Menestrina et al. 1986; Möller et al. 1987; Lamarre et al. 1989.

Occurrence. The tumour is uncommon, but not extremely rare. We see about two out of every 1000 cases of nodal lymphoma.

The mean age is 39 years, with a difference between the sexes.[355] Women show a lower mean age and are affected about $2^1/_2$ times as often as men.[356] The youngest patient was 10 years old, the oldest 63.[357] Similar data on age and sex are found in all other studies. The predominance of young women is frequently mentioned.

Clinical Picture. The patients are usually in stage I_E or II_E when they consult their physician. Symptoms that are attributable to the mediastinal tumour are most prominent, viz. shortness of breath, superior vena cava syndrome, cough and pain in the breast, neck and arms.

Histology. The tumour is composed of large cells (Fig. 91) with strands of fibres intertwined around them or enclosing them. This gives the fibre pattern a rather characteristic appearance (Fig. 92) that does not occur in this form in nodal NHL. The fibres may also form wide hyalinized bands. Sometimes there is merely focal development of sclerosis; hence it may be overlooked in a given portion of the tumour. Occasionally, one sees remnants of the thymus or fibrous structures that remind one of thymus tissue. In addition, there are sometimes band-like accumulations of lymphocytes with or without plasma cells.

The tumour cells themselves vary in appearance. In many instances there is a similarity to polymorphic or centrocytoid centroblastic lymphoma. The cells with "multilobated" nuclei already described by PERRONE et al.[358] also tally with this. Most investigators have related the lymphoma cells to germinal centre cells ("cleaved" and "non-cleaved" cells). MÖLLER[359] designated the tumour cells as "clear". We always found slightly or moderately basophilic cytoplasm, however, not the transparent-looking cytoplasm of T-cell lymphomas. Sporadically, we saw tumours that showed very large nuclei and a marked tendency to form giant cells. Mitotic figures are usually plentiful. Occasionally there are also necrotic areas.

Despite their great similarity to nodal germinal centre cell lymphomas, we eschew defining these lymphomas according to the criteria of the Kiel classification. We consider them to be independent tumours, which are probably of thymic origin and should not be subsumed under the nodal lymphomas.

Diagnosis. The large size of the tumour cells, sclerosis, the mediastinal localization of the tumour, and the age and sex of the patient are generally sufficient criteria for identifying this type of lymphoma. The demonstration of B-cell antigens on the tumour cells substantiates the diagnosis.

---

[355] Lamarre et al. 1989.
[356] Perrone et al. 1986.
[357] Perrone et al. 1986.
[358] 1986.
[359] Möller et al. 1986; 1987.

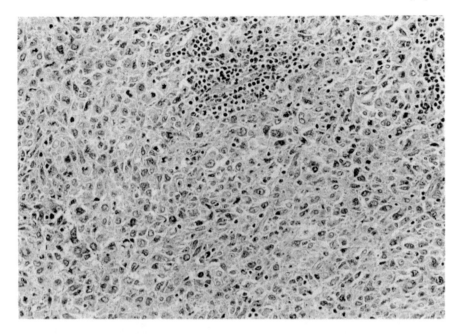

Fig. 91. Large cell, sclerosing B-cell lymphoma of the mediastinum. Female, 26 years. Giemsa. 220:1

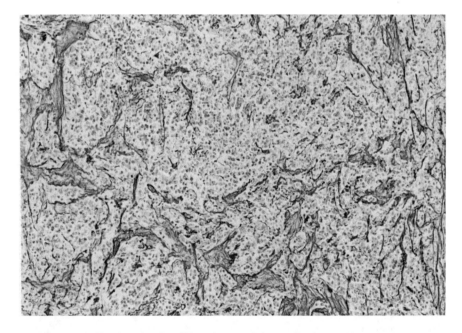

Fig. 92. Large cell, sclerosing B-cell lymphoma of the mediastinum. Male, 28 years. Gomori. 110:1

Differential Diagnosis. The following tumours must be considered in a differential diagnosis.

1. *Hodgkin's lymphomas* do not show pure B-cell populations, since there is an admixture of Sternberg-Reed cells or lacunar cells and often of eosinophils and neutrophils. The band-forming or diffuse sclerosis is frequently more pronounced.

2. *Large cell anaplastic lymphomas* (LCAL) show larger cells with somewhat more abundant cytoplasm. The cells express CD30, but they are often negative for B-cell antigens.

3. *Carcinomas of the thymus* do not show marked sclerosis and are positive for epithelial markers.

4. Other large cell NHL of nodal origin, viz. *centroblastic lymphoma* and *immunoblastic lymphoma of B and T types*, do not show sclerosis. Large cell, sclerosing B-cell lymphoma of the mediastinum may be very similar in morphology to one of these lymphoma types. There are immunohistochemical differences, however, since the mediastinal lymphoma frequently exhibits a loss of Ig and of HLA class II antigen; but these are not absolute criteria.

5. Other epithelial or non-epithelial (soft tissue) tumours located in the thorax, including seminoma and solitary fibrous tumour of the mediastinum.[360]

Prognosis. At first, large cell sclerosing B-cell lymphoma of the mediastinum was considered to have a poor prognosis, but there are now more reports that the lymphoma can usually be brought into remission with chemotherapy with or without radiotherapy.[361] Favourable prognostic factors are the patient's age (older than 25 years at the time of diagnosis), the stage (I_E or II_E), highly pronounced tumour sclerosis and a favourable response to the initial treatment.[362]

3.3.2 Microvillous, Large Cell Lymphoma

Since 1980[363] there have been a number of reports of large cell lymphomas in which electron microscopy revealed that the tumour cells had a villous surface. Like LCAL, these lymphomas frequently showed intrasinusoidal growth. The tumour cells have been given various descriptive names: porcupine, anenome or filiform.[364]

KINNEY et al.[365] investigated seven "microvillous" lymphomas with light and electron microscopic and immunohistochemical methods and compared them with LCAL. It was usually impossible to make a distinction by morphology alone. The immunohistochemical and electron microscopic characteristics of the microvillous lymphomas and LCAL also overlapped. The distinguishing feature of the microvillous lymphomas, viz. the numerous villous cytoplasmic

---

[360] Witkin and Rosai 1989.

[361] Jacobson et al. 1988.

[362] Perrone et al. 1986.

[363] Osborne et al. 1980, 1983; Sibley et al. 1980.

[364] See Kinney et al. 1990.

[365] 1990.

processes, was recognizable only on electron microscopy. Immunohistochemically, it was almost always possible to prove that the tumours were B-cell lymphomas (Ki-1–, EMA–). Only 21% of the cases of LCAL (Ki-1+) showed numerous cytoplasmic processes.

3.3.3 B-Cell Lymphomas with a High Content of T Cells

There have been several reports of cases showing a predominant T-cell proliferation together with a mostly large cell, monotypic B-cell proliferation.[366] It has become obvious that neoplastic T cells can induce a monotypic B-cell proliferation since it was discovered that monoclonal gammopathy can develop in mycosis fungoides[367] and a monotypic immunoblastic or large cell anaplastic B-cell proliferation can be seen in the AILD (LgX) type of T-cell lymphoma (cf. p. 207).

RAMSAY et al.[368] published five cases of B-cell lymphoma in which the morphology and initial immunohistochemistry suggested a diagnosis of T-cell neoplasia because more than 90% of the tumour cells were T cells. Genetic analysis, however, did not show evidence of monoclonality in either the (large) T-cell fraction or the (small) B-cell fraction. Unfortunately, we cannot interpret the morphology of these cases satisfactorily from these authors' descriptions and photomicrographs. Case 3 may have been an AILD (LgX) type of T-cell lymphoma. The other cases may have included other types of low-grade malignant T-cell lymphoma. None of the cases appeared to be identical with those described by SCARPA et al.[369] or OSBORNE et al.[370]

OSBORNE et al.[371] published seven cases of large cell, B-cell lymphoma with a high content of T cells simulating a T-cell lymphoma. The authors demonstrated monoclonal proliferation of the B cells (rearrangement for heavy and light chain genes) by Southern blot analysis, in contrast to the absence of rearrangement of the T-cell receptor β gene. Unfortunately, we cannot recognize from the photomicrographs and descriptions whether there were any cases of the AILD (LgX) type of T-cell lymphoma (rare cases of which do not show rearrangement of the TcRβ gene) among the cases published by OSBORNE et al. There was also no mention of CD30 expression. A similar case of large cell, B-cell lymphoma was reported by SCARPA et al.[372] In that case the number of T cells had decreased dramatically in a second biopsy. The authors concluded that this was "not a new entity, but rather a peculiar presentation of a large B-cell lymphoma".

We have also observed a number of cases in which a large cell, B-cell lymphoma was associated with a T-cell proliferation that was sometimes pleomorphic and showed mitotic activity. Do these represent two different clones (a B-cell clone and a T-cell clone), i.e. a combination of a B-cell neoplasm and a

---

[366] Ramsay et al. 1988; Scarpa et al. 1989; Osborne et al. 1990.
[367] Kövary et al. 1977.
[368] 1988.
[369] 1989.
[370] 1990.
[371] 1990.
[372] 1989.

T-cell neoplasm?[373] Or did the T-cell neoplasm induce a monotypic proliferation of blast cells of B type? Or were the T cells of non-neoplastic nature, even when they were pleomorphic, atypical and actively dividing? The morphological and immunohistochemical findings alone do not provide an answer in such cases and similar ones described in the literature. Only by analyzing the T cells for gene rearrangement is it possible to make a decision, or at least a guess. Recently, a genotypic analysis of 15 such cases was performed.[373a] In three specimens clonal amplification products were detected in a PCR reaction with primers for the TcRγ-chain genes. There was no obvious correlation between T-cell pleomorphism and T-cell clonality.

---

[373] Hu et al. 1987.
[373a] H. Griesser, personal communication.

4 T-Cell Lymphomas

Lymphoblastic lymphoma of T-cell type, originally known as the "convoluted cell type", was recognized quite early. It was soon apparent that the tumour has its origin in the thymus or bone marrow and represents a lymphoma of immature T cells, i.e. a pre-thymic or thymic lymphoma.[374] Lymphoblastic lymphoma of T-cell type must be distinguished clearly from peripheral T-cell lymphomas. In order to reflect this in the Kiel classification, we have placed T-lymphoblastic lymphoma at the very end of the list of high-grade ML. Hence all T-cell lymphomas listed above this last group should be regarded as peripheral T-cell lymphomas.

In contrast to the relatively early identification of T-lymphoblastic lymphoma,[375] it took more than 10 years before the peripheral T-cell lymphomas could be sorted into groups to some extent. Over the years, increasingly complicated classifications of T-cell lymphomas have been proposed.[376] Only LUKES' group[377] combined most of the peripheral T-cell lymphomas under the term "immunoblastic sarcoma of T type". The stream of news about HTLV-1-induced "adult T-cell leukaemia/lymphoma" (ATLL) in Japan and the Caribbean also led to a seemingly boundless flood of publications.[378] ATLL had to be compared with the HTLV-1-negative T-cell lymphomas. Such a comparison was made in 1984 at a workshop of Japanese and European lymphoma experts, and the results were published in the *International Journal of Cancer*.[379]

Subsequently, we worked out a classification with several Japanese colleagues (T. SUCHI, M. KIKUCHI, E. SATO), the Chinese pathologist L. Y. TU† and A. G. STANSFELD.[380] Our classification was intended to reflect the progress of the past decade. It has been included in the updated Kiel classification. We are aware, however, that this is merely an attempt and certainly of a preliminary nature, since there is extraordinary diversity in the appearance of the lymphomas and in

---

[374] Lukes and Collins 1974a,b.
[375] Lukes and Collins 1974a,b.
[376] Waldron et al. 1977; Collins et al. 1979; Palutke et al. 1980; Watanabe et al. 1981; Lennert et al. 1982; Catovsky et al. 1982b; Collins 1982; Jaffe 1985, 1988; Schneider et al. 1985; Stansfeld 1985; Weisenburger et al. 1985a, 1987a; Jones et al. 1986; Norton and Isaacson 1986.
[377] Schneider et al. 1985.
[378] Takatsuki et al. 1976a, 1982; Uchiyama et al. 1977; Tokunaga et al. 1978; Hanaoka et al. 1979, 1982; Kikuchi et al. 1979, 1986; Suchi et al. 1979; Tokunaga and Sato 1980; Hattori et al. 1981; Hanaoka 1984.
[379] Lennert et al. 1985.
[380] Suchi et al. 1987.

the course of the disease. Moreover, the borderline between low-grade and high-grade malignant T-cell lymphomas is not as sharp as that between low-grade and high-grade malignant B-cell lymphomas. The simultaneous presence of low-grade malignant and high-grade malignant areas within one tumour is much more common in cases of T-cell lymphoma than in B-cell lymphomas.

Peripheral T-cell lymphomas have certain characteristics that lead the pathologist to suspect a neoplasm of peripheral T lymphocytes (Table 19). The T zones are infiltrated first. There is often a marked, but sometimes merely a moderate increase in the number of epithelioid venules.[381] In the high-grade malignant T-cell lymphomas, the endothelial cells of the venules are flatter than normal, or there is incomplete development of endothelium. In low-grade ML, especially T-CLL and T-zone lymphoma, epithelioid venules are of typical morphology. T-lymphoblastic lymphomas, on the other hand, do not show an increase in venules (!). The tumour cells of peripheral T-cell lymphomas usually vary greatly in size and shape. The nuclei usually look more pleomorphic than monomorphic. Sometimes there are clear cells (PAS-negative!). These come in all sizes and are almost specific to T-cell lymphomas. Occasionally, one finds giant cells, including those of the Sternberg-Reed type. The tumour cells are often interspersed with a few, and sometimes many, eosinophils. Epithelioid cells are also sometimes found. They usually form small groups in which Langhans giant cells may develop. Epithelioid cell granulomas like those seen in sarcoidosis do not occur. In a few types of T-cell lymphoma the tumour cells are interspersed with a relatively large number of polytypic plasma cells. In rare cases the neoplastic T cells induce monotypic B-cell proliferation (B immunoblasts, plasma cells and plasma cell precursors). In such cases the patient's blood may show monoclonal gammopathy.[382]

Clinically, a lymph node is the main site of most peripheral T-cell lymphomas. Frequently, the skin and/or mucosa of the gastrointestinal tract and the lungs and/or pleura are involved. JAFFE[383] has reported that the risk of infiltration of the blood (30%) is closely associated with infiltration of the skin. It is not uncommon for Waldeyer's ring to be the primary site or a site of metastasis of a peripheral T-cell lymphoma, e.g. lymphoepithelioid lymphoma. Clinical trials have shown that peripheral T-cell lymphomas, with the exception of T-CLL and mycosis fungoides, should be treated like high-grade malignant NHL. Some intestinal T-cell lymphomas constitute a special category,[384] even though the allegedly specific antibody HML-1 does not appear to be as specific as was first assumed.[385]

The monoclonality of B-cell proliferations is usually easy to recognize on the basis of immunohistochemical demonstration of light chain restriction. There is no such simple marker in T-cell lymphomas. A molecular genetic analysis is needed to demonstrate rearrangement of the T-cell receptor genes. Immunohisto-

---

[381] Kittas et al. 1985.
[382] Kövary et al. 1977; Matsuzaki et al. 1985.
[383] 1985.
[384] Spencer et al. 1988; Stein et al. 1988.
[385] Pallesen and Hamilton-Dutoit 1989.

Table 19. Histological characteristics of peripheral T-cell lymphomas

1. Primary infiltration of T regions

2. Epithelioid venules are often increased in number and sometimes atypical

3. Tumour cells
   Mostly pleomorphic (to a variable degree)
   Rarely basophilic
   Occasionally "clear" cells
   Occasionally giant cells, including Sternberg-Reed type

4. Sometimes admixture of:
   Interdigitating cells
   Epithelioid cells
   Eosinophils
   Plasma cells (polytypic)

5. Low-grade ML frequently transforms into high-grade ML

chemically, it is sometimes possible to distinguish benign T-cell proliferations from malignant ones on the basis of an aberrant immunophenotype.[386] For example, characteristic antigens of peripheral T cells, such as CD2, CD3, CD4 or CD8, may be missing in a neoplasm, especially if it belongs to one of the high-grade malignant categories..

Peripheral T-cell lymphomas are characterized by a marked tendency to change in morphology and immunophenotype. Whereas B-cell lymphomas show only further development from low-grade to high-grade ML, we have observed several cases of large cell anaplastic lymphoma of T-cell type that transformed into lymphomas composed of smaller cells, e.g. pleomorphic, small cell T-cell lymphoma (see Figs. 144, 145). Different grades of malignancy can also be observed at the same time in various localizations, but this is not a feature unique to T-cell lymphomas.

4.1 Low-Grade Malignant Lymphomas of T-Cell Type

4.1.1 Lymphocytic: Chronic Lymphocytic Leukaemia of T-Cell Type (T-CLL)

WF: Malignant lymphoma, small lymphocytic, consistent with CLL (A)

Lukes-Collins: Small lymphocyte T; knobby, cytopenic and prolymphocytic subtypes

Definition. There are three subtypes of chronic lymphocytic leukaemia of T-cell type (T-CLL). The subtypes have distinct morphological and immunological features and show considerable clinical differences.[387] They have been named the knobby type (I), the azurophilic type (II) and the pleomorphic type (III). In

---

[386] Lennert et al. 1986; Knowles 1988; Feller 1989; Pallesen and Hamilton-Dutoit 1989.
[387] Lennert et al. 1982; Suchi et al. 1987.

Table 20. Cytological and immunological features of the various subtypes of T-CLL and T-PLL

	I Knobby type	II Azurophilic type	III Pleomorphic type	T-PLL
Nuclei	Humped	Round	Pleomorphic	Somewhat larger, round or pleomorphic
Azurophil granules	−	+	−	+/−
Nucleoli	Small	Small	Small	Medium-sized
CD4	+	−	−	+/−
CD8	−	+	+	+/−
CD57	−	+/−	−	−
CD7	+/−	−	−	+

addition, there is a prolymphocytic leukaemia of T-cell type (T-PLL; see p. 172). The three subtypes of T-CLL show the following features in blood or lymph node smears (Table 20).

Type I: In the first subtype, the nuclei have irregular and often multiple protrusions. Hence it has been called the *knobby type* in accordance with a suggestion made by LUKES.[388] The cells are only slightly larger than normal blood lymphocytes and have greyish blue, scanty, non-granulated cytoplasm.

Type II: The *azurophilic type* is characterized by round nuclei and abundant, greyish blue cytoplasm, which contains azurophil granules. Such cells were recognized long ago in normal blood and account for approximately 5% of the T lymphocytes. In Germany they have been called "azure granulated lymphocytes". In the international literature they are now known as "large granular lymphocytes".

Type III: The *pleomorphic type*[389] shows very irregularly shaped nuclei with deep indentations. Cytoplasm is moderately abundant and greyish blue, and it does not contain azurophil granules. Type III is similar to the HTLV-1-induced Japanese T-cell leukaemia (ATLL),[390] but the latter shows even more marked pleomorphism. The cases of type III in our collection are HTLV-1 negative.

Immunology.[391] All three subtypes of T-CLL show the phenotype of mature T cells (CD3+, CD2+, CD5+). In addition, the so-called knobby type expresses CD4, whereas the azurophilic and pleomorphic types express CD8. ATLL, which is cytologically similar to the pleomorphic type, expresses CD4 and is thereby distinguishable from the latter type (which is CD8+). In some cases the azurophilic type shows expression of CD57 (Leu-7). The expression of comple-

---

[388] Levine 1981.
[389] Hui et al. 1987.
[390] Hanaoka 1984.
[391] Reinherz and Schlossman 1981.

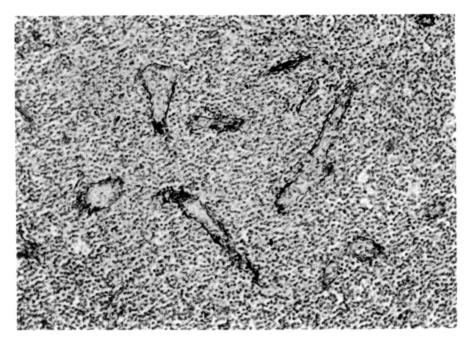

Fig. 93. T-CLL. Numerous PAS-positive epithelioid venules. Male, 69 years. Axillary node. PAS. 175:1

ment receptors is variable and not constant in any type. About 50% of cases of the knobby type are CD7 positive; this antigen is invariably expressed in T-PLL.

An analysis of T-cell receptor genes, especially of the TcRβ-chain gene, has shown that a majority of cases with an increase in so-called azure granulated lymphocytes ("lymphocytosis of large granular lymphocytes with granulocytopenia"[392]) must now be considered to be clonal T-cell proliferations and can be interpreted as T-CLL of large granular lymphocytes.[393]

Occurrence. The relative frequency of T-CLL among all cases of CLL is about 3%. T-CLL generally occurs in middle and old age, but it has been observed in one 19-year-old patient.[394]

Clinical Picture. Infiltration of the bone marrow is not always present, and when it occurs, it is not as heavy as in B-CLL. On the other hand, infiltration of the skin is frequently observed ("dermatotropism" of T lymphocytes). Involvement of lymph nodes is often slight and is most common in type I. In contrast, marked splenomegaly is seen in almost all patients. Blood counts in cases of type II often disclose granulocytopenia.

---

[392] McKenna et al. 1977; Bom-van Noorloos et al. 1980b; Aisenberg et al. 1981.; Loughran et al. 1988.
[393] Aisenberg et al. 1985; Loughran and Hammond 1986; Semenzato et al. 1987.
[394] McKenna et al. 1979.

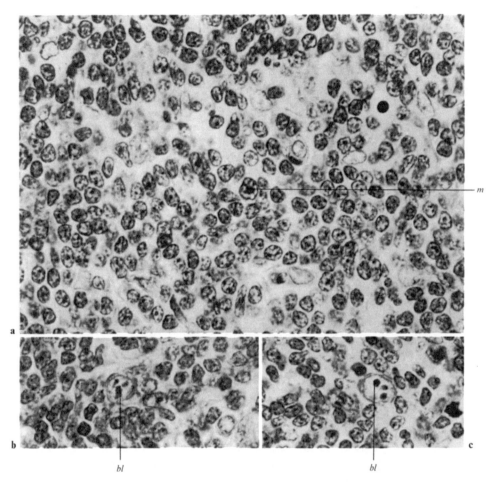

Fig. 94a–c. T-CLL. **a** Note the medium-sized cell (*m*) with a prominent nucleolus and a convoluted nucleus. **b, c** Two large blast cells (T immunoblasts, *bl*). Male, 41 years. Inguinal node. **a**
PAS, **b, c** Giemsa. 875:1

Histology. There is always a marked increase in the number of epithelioid venules
in T-CLL (Fig. 93), whereas in B-CLL it is less pronounced or not seen at all. The
nuclei of the lymphocytes are more variable in shape than those of B-CLL. The
few blast cells often have multiple, large, central nucleoli (Fig. 94). In contrast to
B-CLL, T-CLL does not show a pseudofollicular pattern (proliferation centres).
The T lymphocytes migrate through the walls of the venules and partially destroy
them. When this happens, the venules can be recognized better from their fibres
and basement membranes (see Fig. 93). Occasionally, we have seen a marked
increase in the number of so-called plasmacytoid T cells (once with IgA paraproteinaemia).

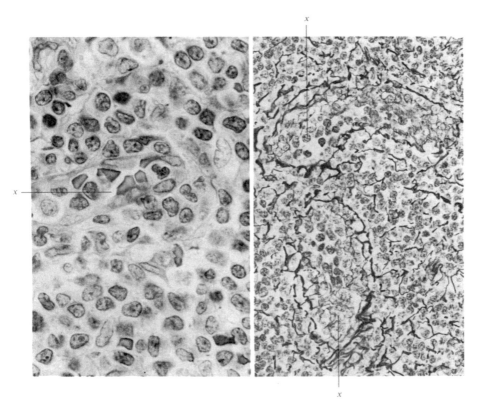

Fig. 95a, b. Prolymphocytic leukaemia of T-cell type. **a** Same magnification as Fig. 94 (T-CLL). There is no significant morphological difference. Nucleoli are recognizable in some cells. Also same magnification as Fig. 24 (prolymphocytic leukaemia of B-cell type). Venules (*x*) are invaded and effaced by neoplastic prolymphocytes. Hence it is more difficult to identify the venules with Giemsa staining (**a**) than with silver impregnation (**b**). Male, 71 years. Axillary node. **a** Giemsa. 875:1. **b** Gomori. 345:1

Cytology and Cytochemistry. In blood smears or lymph node imprints from cases of the azurophilic type, the lymphocytes show a granular reaction for acid phosphatase.

The non-granular lymphocytes, especially in cases of type I, often exhibit a small or large spot of acid non-specific esterase activity. In addition, there is often a focal acid phosphatase reaction. Most cases of type I also show small or large dipeptidylpeptidase IV-positive (CD26+) granules,[395] which are proof of the T-cell origin of a case of CLL.

Development into a Lymphoma of High-Grade Malignancy. T-CLL may transform into a T-immunoblastic lymphoma.[396]

---

[395] Feller et al. 1982b, 1983a; Lennert et al. 1982.
[396] Palutke et al. 1980.

Prognosis. The prognosis is most favourable in cases of the azurophilic subtype; the disease often exists for many years without treatment. The pleomorphic subtype shows the poorest prognosis.

Addendum: Prolymphocytic Leukaemia of T-Cell Type (T-PLL)

In the prolymphocytic variant (T-PLL) the leukaemic cells are somewhat larger and have round or pleomorphic nuclei. These contain medium-sized, very prominent, solitary nucleoli. Cytoplasm is abundant and markedly basophilic (in contrast to the greyish blue cytoplasm in all types of T-CLL!). The cases of T-PLL in our collection include fewer variants than did those presented by Catovsky's group.[397]

Immunologically, T-PLL can be CD4 or CD8 positive. In rare cases both CD4 and CD8 are expressed.[398] CD7 is always demonstrable. In contrast, the thymic cortex antigen is missing; this makes it possible to distinguish T-PLL from T-lymphoblastic lymphoma. Other antigens constantly expressed in T-PLL are CD2, CD3 and CD5.

Histologically, T-PLL is almost identical to T-CLL, but the nuclei look somewhat larger. We do not make a diagnosis on sections, however, but rather on imprints or blood smears (Fig. 95).

4.1.2 Small Cell, Cerebriform T-Cell Lymphomas: Mycosis Fungoides and Sézary's Syndrome

WF: Mycosis fungoides

Lukes-Collins: Cerebriform T

Definition. Mycosis fungoides[399] is a T-lymphocytic lymphoma that primarily involves the skin. Primary involvement of lymph nodes and internal organs is not observed. The T lymphocytes of mycosis fungoides have "cerebriform" nuclei (so-called Lutzner cells), i.e. nuclei with deep indentations resembling the sulci on the surface of the brain. These cells often show positive focal reactions for acid phosphatase and acid non-specific esterase, which are typical of CD4-positive helper/inducer T cells. Neoplastic T lymphocytes with features of suppressor cells have been described, however, in a few cases.[400] Such cells cause a different clinical picture. We avoid using the term "cutaneous T-cell lymphoma" as a synonym for small cell, cerebriform lymphomas, because there are other primary T-cell lymphomas of the skin that differ from mycosis fungoides and Sézary's syndrome.

Sézary's syndrome is a variant of mycosis fungoides. It is characterized by the triad erythroderma, lymphadenopathy and a leukaemic blood picture (Lutzner cells in the blood). In contrast to B-CLL, the leukaemic cells of Sézary's syndrome

---

[397] Matutes et al. 1986.
[398] Catovsky et al. 1982b,c.
[399] Reviews: Kerl and Kresbach 1979; Sterry 1985; Slater 1987; Geerts 1988.
[400] Kansu and Hauptman 1979.

do not infiltrate the bone marrow until later stages of development, and the marrow may remain free of infiltration up to the time of death.

Immunology. The neoplastic T cells show the phenotype of mature T cells (CD2 +, CD3 +, CD5 +). In addition, they express CD4. The interspersed CD8-positive cells may be considered to be reactive. Only as an exception does the neoplastic cell population consist of CD8-positive cells. The number of Ki-67-positive cells in skin infiltrates is less than 5% in small cell mycosis fungoides and Sézary's syndrome. In mycosis fungoides, the lymph node infiltrates are permeated with accumulations of interdigitating cells (CD1 +), which can also be recognized in paraffin sections with stainings for S100 protein.

Clinical Picture. In the skin one can distinguish a premycotic, an infiltrative and a tumour phase. The infiltrative phase is the earliest point at which lymph nodes may be involved by the neoplastic process. The helper cell function of Lutzner cells occasionally results in a monoclonal increase in Ig in the patient's blood.[401]

Occurrence. A pathologist rarely has an opportunity to examine a lymph node biopsy from a patient with mycosis fungoides or Sézary's syndrome. In 1983, 0.9% of the cases in our collection were diagnosed as mycosis fungoides or Sézary's syndrome. The patients were mostly between the ages of 50 and 90 years, and there was a slight predominance of males.

Histology.[402] It is easier to make a diagnosis on a *skin* biopsy than it is on a lymph node biopsy. In the infiltrative phase a band-shaped infiltrate is found in the *upper* dermis, with involvement of the lower epidermis. Pautrier's microabscesses are highly characteristic of this type of lymphoma; they consist of Lutzner cells, S100-positive interdigitating cells, and Langerhans cells (which are indistinguishable from interdigitating cells on light microscopy).

At first, *lymph nodes* show only dermatopathic lymphadenitis with a marked increase in the number of interdigitating cells, including Langerhans cells, in T regions (Fig. 96). Later, the specific cells of mycosis fungoides are also found in T regions (Fig. 97), viz.: (1) Lutzner cells, i.e. T lymphocytes with cerebriform nuclei (it is easier to recognize this nuclear configuration on electron microscopy than it is in routine paraffin sections; Fig. 98), and (2) so-called mycosis cells, i.e. giant cells of variable nature and morphology. Mycosis cells have only a few nuclei and slightly to intensely basophilic cytoplasm, which may be scanty or abundant. Their nucleoli are medium sized or large, but not as large as those of typical Sternberg-Reed cells. In general, interdigitating cells or Langerhans cells are seen in relatively large numbers as remnants of dermatopathic lymphadenitis, even after a relatively long period of infiltration.

In the tumour phase, the neoplastic cells become larger, whereby all variants of high-grade malignant peripheral T-cell lymphomas may develop, viz. medium-

---

[401] Kövary et al. 1977.
[402] Review: Matthews 1985.

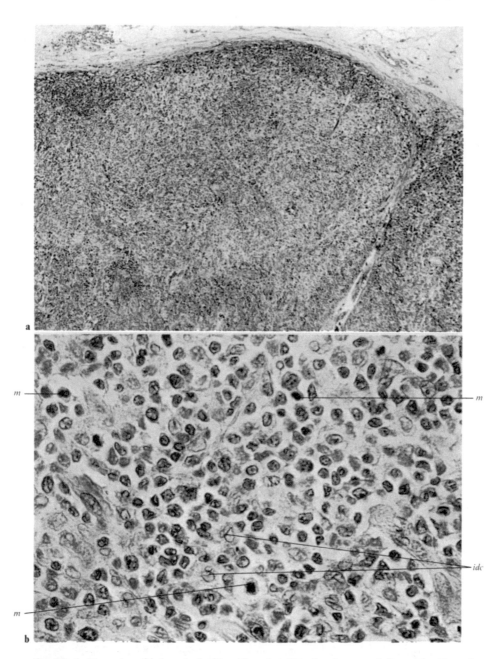

Fig. 96a, b. Dermatopathic lymphadenitis with early infiltration by mycosis fungoides. Note the very large T nodule in **a** and the large number of pleomorphic cerebriform lymphocytes, three mitotic figures (*m*) and some interdigitating cells (*idc*) in **b**. Female, 59 years. Inguinal node. **a** Giemsa. 70:1. **b** H & E. 560:1

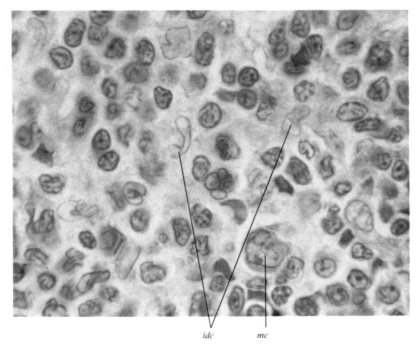

idc   *mc*

Fig. 97. Mycosis fungoides with Giemsa staining. Numerous cerebriform lymphocytes (Lutzner cells). Many (at least eight) interdigitating cells (*idc*). One so-called mycosis cell (*mc*). Female, 79 years. Clinically, the patient had leukaemia, but did not have Sézary's syndrome. Inguinal node. 1550:1

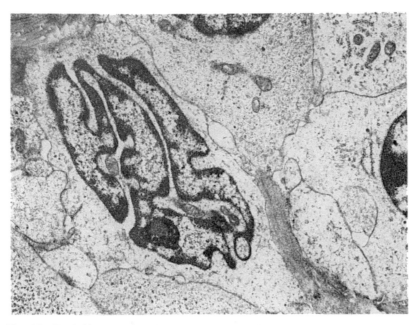

Fig. 98. Cerebriform nucleus in a "Lutzner cell" in mycosis fungoides. 5100:1. (Electron micrograph provided by E. KAISERLING)

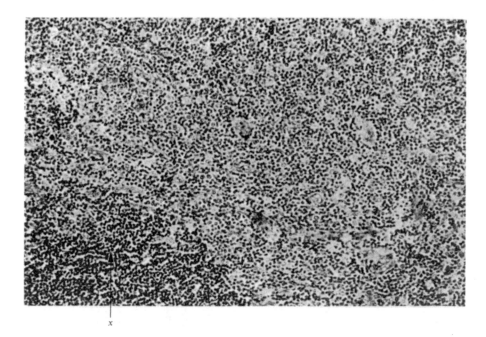

Fig. 99. Sézary's syndrome, first diagnosed 10 years earlier. At the *lower left*, remnant of non-infiltrated lymphoid tissue (*x*). Here the lymphocytes are smaller, and they appear to lie closer together than do those in the infiltrated area. Female, 64 years. Supraclavicular node. Giemsa. 140:1

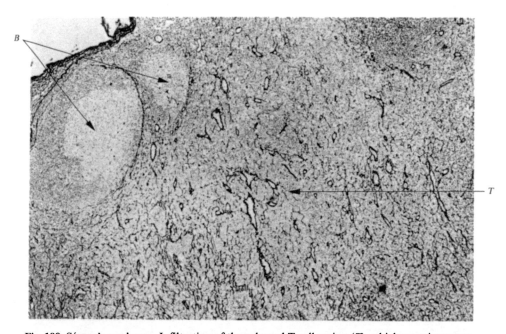

Fig. 100. Sézary's syndrome. Infiltration of the enlarged T-cell region (*T*), which contains many epithelioid venules and fibres. In the cortex there are remnants of lymph follicles with germinal centres (*B*). Female, 55 years. Inguinal node. Gomori. 56:1

sized or large cell, pleomorphic lymphoma, immunoblastic lymphoma or large cell anaplastic lymphoma.

In Sézary's syndrome, the skin infiltration corresponds to that of mycosis fungoides. In contrast, the lymph node is characterized by greater monotony. Evidently, a pronounced dermatopathic lymphadenitis usually does not precede the specific infiltration. Correspondingly, the T zones are largely infiltrated by small cerebriform lymphocytes (Fig. 99), whereas interdigitating cells are interspersed in small numbers.[403] Since a marked increase in the number of venules is also present, the picture is reminiscent of T-CLL (Fig. 100).

Cytochemistry. In blood smears or lymph node imprints, the lymphoid cells (Lutzner cells) often contain up to three large, acid non-specific esterase-positive granules. The granules are sometimes very large ("spot-like") and isolated. The acid phosphatase reaction is less typical (granular or focal activity).

Diagnosis. It is often extraordinarily difficult, or even impossible, to recognize infiltration of a lymph node by mycosis fungoides or Sézary's syndrome at an *early* stage. Sparse infiltrates in the large T nodules of dermatopathic lymphadenitis are often particularly difficult to identify. Several investigators have applied quantifying methods that demonstrate neoplastic involvement of a lymph node earlier than is possible by morphological examination. SCHEFFER et al.[404] used DNA cytophotometry, and WEISS et al.[405] analysed DNA extracts for rearrangement of the β-chain genes of the T-cell receptor.

Early infiltration by a small cell, cerebriform lymphoma must be assumed when large *accumulations* or clusters of small lymphocytes with pleomorphic nuclei are recognized histologically at the edge of T nodules or in the pulp. Isolated cells with pleomorphic nuclei or abnormally large blast cells within T nodules are not diagnostic features by themselves.

In the *skin*, T-cell infiltration of the upper dermis and lower epidermis, with invasion into the epithelium, and Pautrier's pseudo-abscesses are highly characteristic findings. The same is true of HTLV-1-positive Japanese T-cell lymphomas. Other T-cell lymphomas of the skin are localized in the dermis and may not infiltrate the epidermis, at least not at the beginning.[406]

Differential Diagnosis. T-CLL and pleomorphic, small cell T-cell lymphomas are more monotonous in appearance and do not show remnants of dermatopathic lymphadenitis. They also do not contain so-called mycosis cells (giant cells).

Prognosis. As long as mycosis fungoides is confined to the skin, the prognosis is relatively favourable (the median survival time is longer than 10 years[407]). When the disease spreads to extracutaneous organs, however, the prognosis becomes

---

[403] Willemze et al. 1985.
[404] 1980.
[405] 1985b.
[406] Jaffe 1985.
[407] Hoppe et al. 1990.

poor (the median survival time is approx. 1 year[408]). The degree of lymph node infiltration has been used as a prognostic indicator.[409] Otherwise, one may say that the course is more or less slow as long as the proliferating cells remain small. The prognosis worsens when there is transformation into one of the large cell types of T-cell lymphoma.

4.1.3 Lymphoepithelioid Lymphoma ("Lennert's Lymphoma")

WF: Malignant lymphoma, large cell, immunoblastic [!], with epithelioid cell component (H)

Lukes-Collins: Lymphoepithelioid lymphoma

History. In the course of a cytological investigation of Hodgkin's disease and Piringer's lymphadenitis in 1952,[410] one of the authors (K. L.) noticed three cases in which small focal accumulations of epithelioid cells completely destroyed the lymph node architecture and the patients died within a relatively short time. The author considered the disease to be a variant of Hodgkin's lymphoma and called it "epithelioid cellular lymphogranulomatosis" (ECLg).

In 1968, the author and MESTDAGH[411] studied a larger series of cases and distinguished ECLg from *Hodgkin's lymphoma with a high content of epithelioid cells.* ECLg usually contained no, or at most very few, Sternberg-Reed cells and showed small, focal accumulations of epithelioid cells. In contrast, Hodgkin's lymphoma with a high content of epithelioid cells exhibited moderate to large numbers of Sternberg-Reed cells and irregular, often diffuse epithelioid cell infiltrates.

Because of the frequent absence of typical Sternberg-Reed cells in ECLg, the interpretation of the lesion as Hodgkin's lymphoma was open to question. Furthermore, we have observed two cases in which a "sarcoma" developed, differing in morphology from so-called Hodgkin's sarcoma. For this and other reasons, we recommended in 1973[412] the neutral term "lymphoepithelioid lymphoma" (LeL) and considered the possibility that the neoplasm is a form of NHL.

Shortly thereafter, DORFMAN[413] and LUKES and TINDLE[414] suggested the term "Lennert's lymphoma" and saw differential diagnostic problems with immunoblastic lymphadenopathy. BURKE and BUTLER[415] then published 16 cases of LeL. DIEBOLD et al.[416] and BEDNÁŘ[417] observed further cases in Europe. Since

---

[408] Hoppe et al. 1990.
[409] E.g. Matthews 1985.
[410] Lennert 1952.
[411] Lennert and Mestdagh 1968.
[412] Lennert 1973; Lennert et al. 1975.
[413] Dorfman and Warnke 1974; Dorfman 1975.
[414] 1975.
[415] 1976.
[416] 1977.
[417] 1979.

Table 21. Diagnostic analysis of 367 cases that showed a marked, focal epithelioid cell reaction and could be interpreted as lymphoepithelioid lymphoma (LeL) or were suspected to be LeL. (Data from PATSOURIS et al. 1988)

	n	[%]
LeL	110	**30.0**
Angioimmunoblastic lymphadenopathy	97	**26.4**
Hodgkin's lymphoma, mixed cellularity type	99	**27.0**
Nodular paragranuloma	12	3.3
Immunocytoma	39	**10.6**
Other B-cell lymphoma	4	1.1
High-grade malignant T-cell lymphoma	2	0.5
Inflammation	4	1.1
	367	100.0

then, a lively discussion of this lymph node lesion has been conducted in the literature.[418]

At the end of the 1970s, NOËL[419] investigated our collection of cases, which had by then become very large. He found that he could diagnose LeL of the Hodgkin type, i.e. ECLg in the actual sense, in only 44.5% of the 114 cases that had been interpreted originally as ECLg or as suspicious for ECLg. In 31.5% of the cases, NOËL considered the lesion to be a variant of lymphogranulomatosis X (LgX). In 8% of the cases another ML of the Hodgkin's or non-Hodgkin's type was found to be present. A final diagnosis could not be reached in 16% of the cases.

Recently, PATSOURIS et al.[420] have performed morphological and immunological investigations of the new cases of LeL and the suspected cases collected at the Lymph Node Registry in Kiel since the time of NOËL's studies. The results are listed in Table 21. Immunohistochemical, cytogenetic and molecular genetic findings obtained at the same time[421] proved that LeL is a T-cell lymphoma, which was assumed earlier by other investigators on the basis of less sound arguments.[422] Since LeL occasionally contains typical Sternberg-Reed cells, it is understandable that it is not always easy to distinguish LeL from Hodgkin's lymphoma. LeL is indeed an eloquent example showing that the morphological borderline between Hodgkin's lymphoma and NHL is not sharp.

As shown in Table 21, PATSOURIS et al. examined 367 cases that were morphologically identical with LeL. Only 30% proved to be LeL. Almost as many cases (26.4%) were T-cell lymphomas of AILD (LgX) type with a high content of

---

[418] Editorial in Lancet 1976; Robb-Smith 1976; Tindle and Long 1977; Kim et al. 1978b, 1980; Hayes and Robertson 1979; Nanba et al. 1987a.

[419] Noël et al. 1979, 1980.

[420] Patsouris et al. 1988, 1989a,b, 1990.

[421] Feller et al. 1986a; Gödde-Salz et al. 1986; O'Connor et al. 1986a.

[422] Green et al. 1975; Klein et al. 1977; Belpomme et al. 1978; Delsol et al. 1978; Lukes et al. 1978a,b; Palutke et al. 1978; Kikuchi et al. 1979; Mann et al. 1979; Suchi et al. 1979; Bom-van Noorloos et al. 1980a; De Waele et al. 1981; Bogomoletz et al. 1983.

epithelioid cells. The third large group (27.0%) comprised cases of Hodgkin's lymphoma of mixed cellularity type with a high content of epithelioid cells. In addition, there was a small group (3.3%) with the lymphocyte predominance subtype of Hodgkin's lymphoma, viz. paragranuloma. The fourth large entity (10.7%) was immunocytoma with a high content of epithelioid cells. Then there were a few cases of NHL and, finally, the group of inflammatory lymph node diseases (1.1%), including one case of miliary tuberculosis and one case of Whipple's disease.

Definition. LeL is a T-cell lymphoma with CD4 expression. It is characterized by a focal epithelioid cell reaction. It consists chiefly of T lymphocytes and always contains at least a few T immunoblasts with occasional atypical large cells. Typical Sternberg-Reed cells occur in only a small number of cases and then only sparsely (no more than one or two cells per section!). In order to distinguish LeL from immunocytoma with a high content of epithelioid cells, an immunohistochemical analysis of paraffin sections for CIg is essential.

Immunology. The proliferating cells (Ki-67+) show the phenotype of mature T cells (CD2+, CD3+, CD5+). In addition, they constantly express CD4, whereas the CD8 antigen is missing on proliferating cells.[423] A partial loss of antigens can occur when the lymphoma shows transformation into a high-grade ML.

In paraffin sections there are only relatively few plasma cells with a polytypic pattern (no light chain restriction).[424] Giant cells corresponding or similar to Hodgkin or Sternberg-Reed cells may be positive for antibodies (3C4, Leu-M1) against the X-hapten antigen CD15.[425]

The DNA analysis of T-cell receptor genes shows a rearrangement pattern similar to that of peripheral T-cell lymphomas, with rearrangement of TcRγ and β-chain genes.[426]

Occurrence. LeL is a rare disease. It makes up 1.4% of the NHL in our collection, which is definitely selected. LUKES et al.[427] found six cases among 425 cases of NHL. The tumour is found chiefly in elderly patients; the age curve shows a peak between the 6th and 8th decades (Fig. 101). There is a slight male preponderance.

Clinical Picture.[428] Generalized lymphadenopathy is found more often than localized lymphadenopathy at the time of the first clinical examination. When lymph node enlargement is localized, it is usually seen in the cervical region. Splenomegaly was reported in 43% of the patients in our series and hepatomegaly in 23%. In some cases the palatine tonsils were enlarged and infiltrated at the onset of the disease. Fever was observed in about 50% of our cases and pruritus

---

[423] Feller et al. 1986a.
[424] Patsouris et al. 1988.
[425] Patsouris et al. 1988.
[426] Feller et al. 1986a; O'Connor et al. 1986a.
[427] 1978a.
[428] Based on data published by Noël et al. 1979 and Patsouris et al. 1989a,b, 1990.

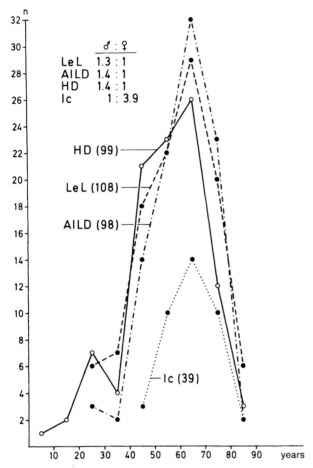

Fig. 101. Age distribution and sex ratio of lymphomas with a high content of epithelioid cells. *LeL* = lymphoepithelioid lymphoma. *AILD* = T-cell lymphoma of AILD (LgX) type with a high content of epithelioid cells. *HD* = Hodgkin's lymphoma of mixed cellularity type with a high content of epithelioid cells. *Ic* = immunocytoma with a high content of epithelioid cells. (Based on PATSOURIS et al. 1988, 1989a,b, 1990)

in 18%. In contrast to patients with the AILD (LgX) type, only 7% of those with LeL showed a skin rash. Spontaneous remission occurred in 14% of the cases.

Blood counts frequently reveal lymphopenia and, occasionally, eosinophilia or monocytosis (up to 29%). The ESR is seldom elevated. Usually, serum Ig levels are normal and the tuberculin reaction is negative. Some other clinical findings are listed in Table 22.

Histology. The normal structure of the lymph node is replaced by a neoplasm, which, at a low magnification, resembles Hodgkin's lymphoma more than it resembles NHL (Fig. 102). Germinal centres or remnants of germinal centres are found only rarely. The lymph node capsule and surrounding tissue are infiltrated focally (57%), diffusely (23%) or not at all (20%).

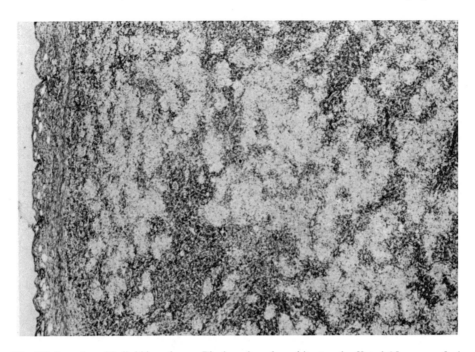

Fig. 102. Lymphoepithelioid lymphoma. The lymph node architecture is effaced. Numerous foci of epithelioid cells are scattered about the node. There are no germinal centres. Female, 74 years. Cervical node. Giemsa. 56:1

Table 22. Clinical features of lymphoepithelioid lymphoma (LeL) and other lymphomas with a high content of epithelioid cells. (Data from PATSOURIS et al. 1988, 1989a, b, 1990)

	LeL	AILD type	Hodgkin's lymphoma, mixed cellularity	Immuno-cytoma
	(n=108) [%]	(n=98) [%]	(n=99) [%]	(n=39) [%]
Generalized lymphadenopathy	71	84	57	73
B-symptoms (Ann Arbor)	60	67	52	65
Pruritis	18	46	12	17
Skin rash	7	38	3	9
Haemolytic anaemia	–	18	–	14
Sjögren's syndrome	–	–	–	31
Other autoimmune diseases	2	16	3	15
Allergies to antibiotics	5	24	3	4
Allergies to chemotherapeutic drugs	–	10	–	–
Paraproteinaemia	–	–	–	38
Bence-Jones proteinuria	–	–	–	25

The neoplasm consists especially of lymphocytes and epithelioid cells. The lymphocytes are somewhat larger than normal lymphocytes and have round or somewhat pleomorphic nuclei. A few cases of LeL show lymphocytes with abundant, pale cytoplasm ("clear cells").

The lymphocytes are interspersed with medium-sized lymphoid cells with round, pale nuclei, small nucleoli and scanty, weakly basophilic cytoplasm (Fig. 103). There are also typical immunoblasts with large, solitary nucleoli and basophilic cytoplasm (Figs. 103, 104). These can be interpreted as T immunoblasts, although they cannot be distinguished from B immunoblasts by morphology alone.

We interpret the medium-sized and large cells as stimulated lymphocytes that either are in the process of transforming or have already done so. They are probably responsible for the production of lymphokines, which cause attracted blood monocytes to transform into epithelioid cells. This assumption is supported not only by the close proximity of the medium-sized and large "transformed lymphocytes" to the groups of epithelioid cells, but also by an observation published by SCHWALBE et al.: [429] They determined the highest index in the direct leucocyte migration test with serum from a patient with T-cell lymphoma with a high content of epithelioid cells. The index was much lower in ten cases of Hodgkin's lymphoma and seven cases of NHL of other types.

Mitotic figures are usually sparse, but some cases show moderate mitotic activity, and a few may even show high mitotic activity.

The epithelioid cells are mostly accumulated in small foci (Fig. 105), as they are in Piringer's lymphadenitis (toxoplasmosis). Epithelioid cells are rarely seen in larger masses in LeL, but solitary epithelioid cells, or pairs of them, are often found among the lymphocytes. The nuclei of some epithelioid cells are oval, others are elongate and arched or bent. They contain relatively large, pale reddish violet nucleoli. The chromatin is so fine that it is barely recognizable with Giemsa staining. The cytoplasm is acidophilic, but its periphery may be basophilic (violet with Giemsa staining). The epithelioid cells exhibit considerable polymorphism and may even have giant nuclei, but they rarely show mitotic activity. They are occasionally multinucleate like Langhans giant cells.

Besides lymphocytes and epithelioid cells, solitary, typical Sternberg-Reed cells and Hodgkin cells are seen in 2%–4% of the cases of LeL. More often, however, there are a few solitary mononuclear and multinucleate cells with a similar morphology (Fig. 103). These cells do not correspond to classic Sternberg-Reed cells or Hodgkin cells, because their chromatin is coarser, the nucleoli are more basophilic and not as large, and the cytoplasm is also more basophilic.

A small, or sometimes moderate, number of eosinophils are often interspersed among the other cells. Plasma cells are usually scanty. There is hardly ever an increase in the number of neutrophil granulocytes or mast cells.

The number of epithelioid venules is modest or, at most, moderately increased. There is no significant increase in the number of fibres; in particular, one does not find any large areas of sclerosis, even after the patient has been treated. Occasionally there are small areas of necrosis, but hardly ever large ones.

---

[429] 1978.

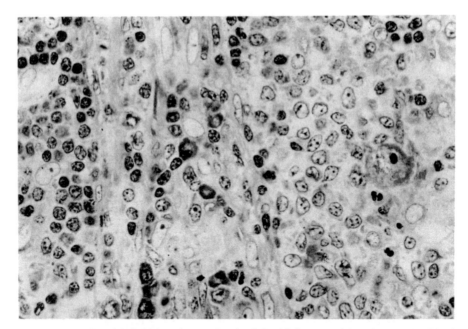

Fig. 103. Lymphoepithelioid lymphoma. On the *left*, chiefly normal lymphocytes (residual B lymphocytes?). On the *right*, somewhat larger, paler lymphocytes (CD4+) and one giant cell resembling a Sternberg-Reed cell. Male, 53 years. Axillary node. Giemsa. 512:1

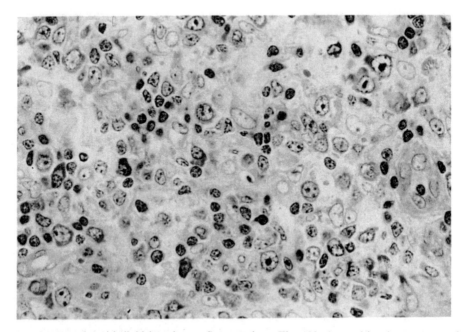

Fig. 104. Lymphoepithelioid lymphoma. Same node as Fig. 103. Area with a low content of epithelioid cells, some immunoblasts and a few plasma cells. Giemsa. 512:1

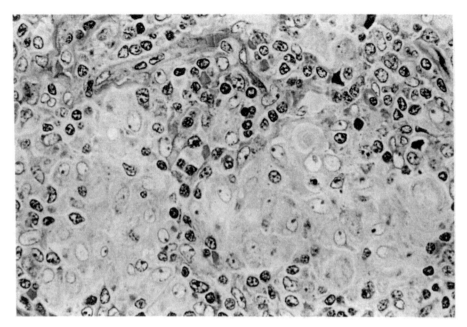

Fig. 105. Lymphoepithelioid lymphoma. Two foci of epithelioid cells. They are surrounded by lymphocytes (CD4+) and some plasma cells. Same node as Figs. 103 and 104. Giemsa. 512:1

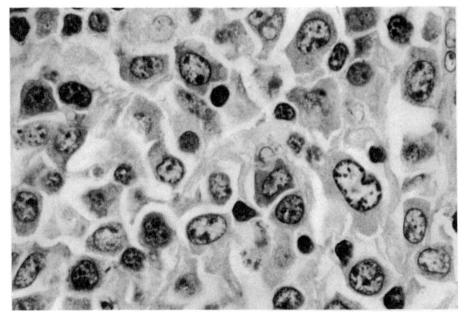

Fig. 106. Same case as Figs. 103–105 after a period of years in which spontaneous remissions occurred. The neoplasm has developed into T-immunoblastic lymphoma without epithelioid cells. Giemsa. 1024:1

Development into a High-Grade Malignant Lymphoma. In 1968, one of the authors (K. L.) and MESTDAGH[430] reported on the development of one case of LeL into a large cell lymphoma. PALUTKE et al.[431] have reported a similar case. In the large series investigated by PATSOURIS et al.[432] there were eight cases of large cell T-cell lymphoma, which could be classified as pleomorphic lymphoma, immunoblastic lymphoma (Fig. 106) or large cell anaplastic (Ki-1 +) lymphoma of T type. In those cases the epithelioid cell component had almost completely disappeared. It is conceivable that the tumour cells were no longer able to produce lymphokines. Since 1968, there have been several reports of development of such large cell ("histiocytic", "immunoblastic") lymphomas in alleged cases of LeL.[433] It is likely that some of these cases should not be interpreted as LeL, but rather as the AILD (LgX) type of T-cell lymphoma or immunocytoma with a high content of epithelioid cells.[434] The latter two types of lymphoma can transform into B-immunoblastic lymphoma.

Diagnosis. LeL is characterized by a mostly focal epithelioid cell reaction against a relatively monotonous-looking lymphocytic background. In general, Sternberg-Reed cells are not found, but one or two giant cells of this type may be seen now and then. There is no sclerosis. When the tissue specimen is skilfully embedded in resin, the pathologist can clearly see that the neoplastic lymphocytes are larger than residual normal lymphocytes (Fig. 103).

Differential Diagnosis. LeL has to be distinguished from T-cell lymphoma of AILD (LgX) type with a high content of epithelioid cells, from Hodgkin's lymphoma with a high content of epithelioid cells (chiefly mixed cellularity type, sometimes paragranuloma), from immunocytoma with a high content of epithelioid cells, from other NHL and from focal epithelioid cell reactions of inflammatory type. The most important distinguishing features are summarized in Tables 22–25.

1. The differential diagnostic significance of *T-cell lymphoma of AILD (LgX) type with a high content of epithelioid cells* (Fig. 107) was recognized early by DORFMAN and WARNKE,[435] LUKES and TINDLE[436] and DELSOL et al.[437] It was confirmed by the investigations of NOËL et al.[438] and substantiated in a thorough study by PATSOURIS et al.[439] At first, however, it was not clear that the tumour was a T-cell lymphoma. The investigators diagnosed it merely as (angio)immunoblastic lymphadenopathy. According to our concept, the type with a high content of epithelioid cells was just *one* of five cytological types of LgX.[439a]

---

[430] Lennert and Mestdagh 1968.
[431] 1980.
[432] 1988.
[433] Klein et al. 1977; R. J. Lukes, personal communication.
[434] E.g. Miller et al. 1979.
[435] 1974.
[436] 1975.
[437] 1977a,b.
[438] 1979, 1980.
[439] 1989a.
[439a] Lennert et al. 1979.

Table 23. Histological features of lymphoepithelioid lymphoma (LeL) and other lymphomas with a high content of epithelioid cells. (Data from Patsouris et al. 1988, 1989 a, b, 1990)

	LeL	AILD type	Hodgkin's lymphoma, mixed cellularity	Immuno-cytoma
	(n = 108) [%] or degree	(n = 98) [%] or degree	(n = 99) [%] or degree	(n = 39) [%] or degree
Total effacement of nodal architecture	100	100	**89**	100
Germinal centres				
active	3	–	11	–[a]
remnants	6	–	–	2
"burnt out"	–	**24**	–	–
Intercellular PAS-positive material	–	**34**	–	–
Cell density	High	Relatively low	High	High
Trabeculae partially intact	8	45	18	17
Epithelioid venules				
sparse	**8**	–	–	–
modest	68	–	47	72
abundant	24	100	53	28
PAS-positive, thickened basement membrane and perivascular hyalinisation	–	Marked	–	Slight
Reticulin fibres				
sparse	**48**	–	–	20
modest	52	39	37	54
abundant	–	**61**	**63**	26
Necrosis	3	6	**20**	4

[a] In an earlier study (Noël et al. 1979) there were five cases with florid germinal centres.

According to Patsouris et al.,[440] the most important distinguishing features of the AILD type of T-cell lymphoma are the following. The most prominent feature is the high content of small vessels (Figs. 108, 109). Together with the predominantly lymphocytic proliferation, these vessels diffusely permeate the lymph node and also the capsule and surrounding tissue. The vessels are largely epithelioid venules. They often have atypical features, such as sparse, flat endothelial cells, and they are frequently branched (so-called arborizing vessels) and usually show a PAS-positive, enlarged basement membrane (cf. AILD type of T-cell lymphoma, p. 204). Hence PAS staining is especially useful in the differential diagnosis. It also reveals amorphic PAS-positive material between the cells in

---

[440] 1989a.

Table 24. Cytological features of lymphoepithelioid lymphoma (LeL) and other lymphomas with a high content of epithelioid cells. (Data from PATSOURIS et al. 1988, 1989 a, b, 1990)

	LeL (n=108) [%]	AILD type (n=98) [%]	Hodgkin's lymphoma, mixed cellularity (n=99) [%]	Immuno-cytoma (n=39) [%]
"Clear" cells	2	13	–	–
Lymphoplasmacytoid cells	–	–	–	100
Numerous plasma cells and precursors	26	64	23	79
PAP reaction	Polytypic	Polytypic	Polytypic	Monotypic
Intranuclear PAS+ inclusions	–	–	–	11
Mitotic figures				
sparse (0–4/HPF)	67	78	98	9
modest (5–9/HPF)	28	13	2	72
abundant (>9/HPF)	5	9	–	19
Sternberg-Reed cells	2 } solitary	3 } solitary	100 } numerous	2 } solitary
Hodgkin cells	4	7	100	6
Sternberg-Reed cell-like giant cells	14	11	34	16
Hodgkin cell-like giant cells	26	27	40	57
Epithelioid cells				
focal	84	93	69	57
diffuse	16	7	31	43
Epithelioid cell tubercles	–	–	7	–
Langhans giant cells	8	10	14	13
Numerous eosinophils	34	61	50	11
Numerous neutrophils	1	2	26	6
Numerous mast cells	1	1	1	8

about one-third of the cases of the AILD type, but not in LeL. Another essential criterion is the absence of florid germinal centres. Sometimes, however, one sees so-called burnt-out germinal centres. This phenomenon is actually a result of hyperplasia of the follicular dendritic cells, which are hardly recognizable among the variegated cell population of the AILD type with standard stainings (Fig. 110). With immunohistochemical stainings, however, the follicular dendritic cells stand out, as they are accumulated in large groups (see Fig. 120). The fibre content is generally much higher, but the cell density usually appears to be much lower than that of LeL. Cytological examination of the AILD type reveals the on average higher content of plasma cells (and plasma cell precursors) and eosinophils. In contrast, there is no essential morphological difference between

Table 25. Further features of lymphoepithelioid lymphoma (LeL) and other lymphomas with a high content of epithelioid cells. (Data from PATSOURIS et al. 1988, 1989a, b, 1990)

	LeL	AILD type	Hodgkin's lymphoma, mixed cellularity	Immuno-cytoma
	(n = 108)	(n = 98)	(n = 99)	(n = 39)
Peak in age curve	7th decade	7th decade	7th decade and low peak in 3rd decade	7th decade
Age range	21–87 years	22–82 years	8–82 years	48–89 years
Male-to-female ratio	1.3 : 1	1.4 : 1	1.4 : 1	**1 : 4**
Development into high-grade malignant lymphoma	7%	13%	–	26%
Carcinoma	–	11% (3 before, 5 after)	6% (before)	15% (2 before, 2 after)

the T-cell proliferation of AILD type and that of LeL, except that the so-called clear cells occur somewhat more frequently in the AILD type. The Sternberg-Reed cells and other giant cells correspond in morphology and frequency to those of LeL. Development into a high-grade malignant T-cell lymphoma is somewhat more common (13%) in the AILD type than in LeL (7%).

There are also certain clinical differences between the AILD type and LeL.[441] Pruritus, skin rashes and bacterial infections occur much more frequently in the AILD type. Allergic or hyperimmune reactions (autoimmune diseases, including haemolytic anaemia; allergies to antibiotics or chemotherapeutics) are found almost exclusively in the AILD type. We should like to emphasize the high incidence of carcinoma before or after manifestation of T-cell lymphoma of the AILD type, whereas we have never found development of carcinoma in a case of LeL. The age and sex distribution of the AILD type is almost identical with that of LeL (Fig. 101).

In spite of all the morphological and clinical differential diagnostic criteria, there are still a small number of cases that can be placed in one of the two categories only with difficulty. This shows how closely related these two types of T-cell lymphoma are.[441a]

2. Many years ago, one of the authors (K. L.)[442] showed that focal epithelioid cell reactions are a characteristic early feature of *Hodgkin's lymphoma*, especially that of the mixed cellularity type. They are also frequently seen in the lymphocyte predominance type. Such cases were called the "L & H type" by LUKES et al.,[443]

---

[441] Patsouris et al. 1989a.
[441a] Nakamura and Suchi 1991.
[442] Lennert 1953a,b.
[443] 1966.

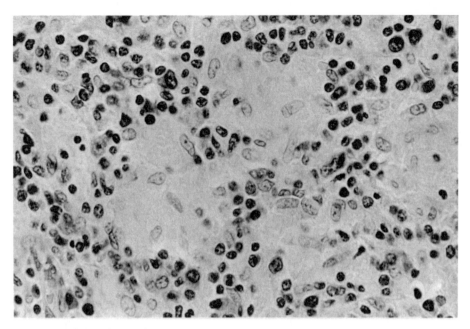

Fig. 107. T-cell lymphoma of AILD (LgX) type with a high content of epithelioid cells. Several groups of epithelioid cells (with "skinny" nuclei). Male, 26 years. Inguinal node. Giemsa. 785 : 1

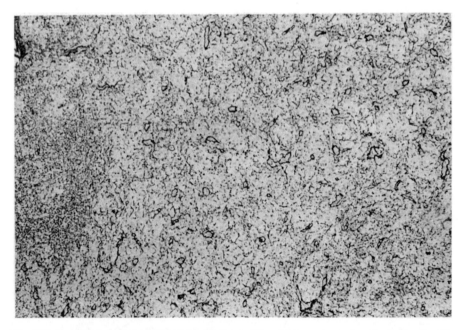

Fig. 108. T-cell lymphoma of AILD (LgX) type with a high content of epithelioid cells. The lymph node architecture is effaced and replaced by numerous small foci of epithelioid cells. These are interspersed with numerous vessels (venules). Male, 54 years. Inguinal node. Gomori. 110 : 1

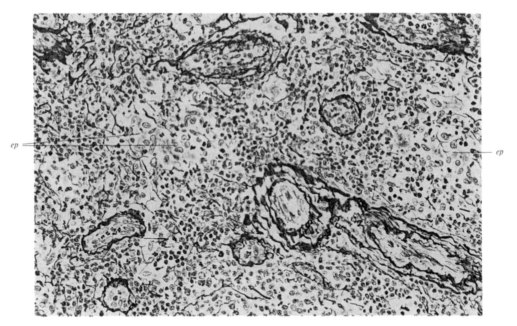

ep   *ep*

Fig. 109. T-cell lymphoma of AILD (LgX) type with a high content of epithelioid cells. Groups of epithelioid cells (*ep*). Vessels with wide mantles of argyrophilic structures (fibres, basement membrane). Male, 56 years. Inguinal node. Gomori. 205:1

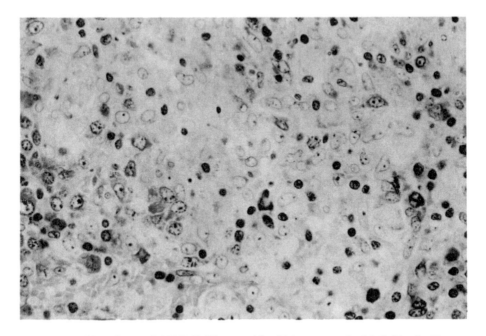

Fig. 110. T-cell lymphoma of AILD (LgX) type with a high content of epithelioid cells. Numerous follicular dendritic cells with vesicular nuclei. Male, 54 years. Lymph node. Giemsa. 440:1

whereby "H" stood for "histiocytic".[444] Early stages of infiltration in cases of Hodgkin's lymphoma of mixed cellularity type can usually be diagnosed correctly because the epithelioid cell reaction develops in the T regions and is accompanied by a few typical Sternberg-Reed cells. Large, uninfiltrated areas of the lymph node, including lymph follicles, with or without germinal centres, are still recognizable at this stage.

After the lymph node has been completely replaced by Hodgkin's lymphoma, the epithelioid cells usually disappear. This does not happen in what we used to call "epithelioid cell-*rich* lymphogranulomatosis", which we now designate as the *mixed cellularity type of Hodgkin's lymphoma with a high content of epithelioid cells*, in conformity with the Rye classification. In that type of Hodgkin's lymphoma, epithelioid cells are the predominant type of cell (Fig. 111a). They often form large masses, sometimes with clusters of epithelioid cells at the edges. In contrast to LeL, this type of Hodgkin's lymphoma always shows *some* typical Sternberg-Reed cells among the predominant epithelioid cells and the less prominent lymphocytes (Fig. 111b). It occasionally occurs in younger patients, but shows the same peak in the 7th decade of life as does LeL (see Fig. 101). There is no significant difference in the sex ratio.

It has been known for a long time that epithelioid cell granulomas with the appearance and size of tubercles may be found in Hodgkin's lymphoma.[445] They were found in 7% of the cases of Hodgkin's lymphoma in addition to the focal and diffuse increases in epithelioid cells, but do not occur in the other types of lymphoma with a high content of epithelioid cells.

In paragranuloma,[446] which we consider to be a special variant of the lymphocyte predominance type of Hodgkin's lymphoma, epithelioid cells may be seen in small foci, or else they are interspersed among the lymphocytes. In nodular paragranuloma the epithelioid cells are frequently arranged like a wreath around the nodules. Moreover, the nodularity helps the pathologist to make a correct diagnosis, since it is almost always recognizable in at least part of the lymph node; silver impregnation is especially helpful. In contrast to LeL, paragranuloma shows predominantly B lymphocytes and a few giant cells of the L & H type, which differ somewhat in morphology from classic Sternberg-Reed cells, chiefly because of their nuclei with multiple protrusions, their smaller nucleoli and their basophilic, relatively scanty cytoplasm (so-called popcorn cells). These giant cells represent multinucleate B immunoblasts.[447] In addition, a few classic Sternberg-Reed cells are often found.

3. *Immunocytoma* is one type of NHL that can be associated with a pronounced focal epithelioid cell reaction. The number of exemplary cases published in the literature is increasing, although the tumours are sometimes given a differ-

---

[444] Epithelioid cells probably develop out of monocytes (and macrophages?), but they should no longer be called "histiocytes" or "macrophages" because they are practically incapable of phagocytosis and are able to secrete (!) monokines instead. Hence we distinguish them from macrophages, whose main function is phagocytosis.

[445] Jackson and Parker 1947; Lennert 1953b; Sacks et al. 1978.

[446] Poppema et al. 1979; Lennert and Hansmann 1987.

[447] Poppema et al. 1979; Lennert and Hansmann 1987.

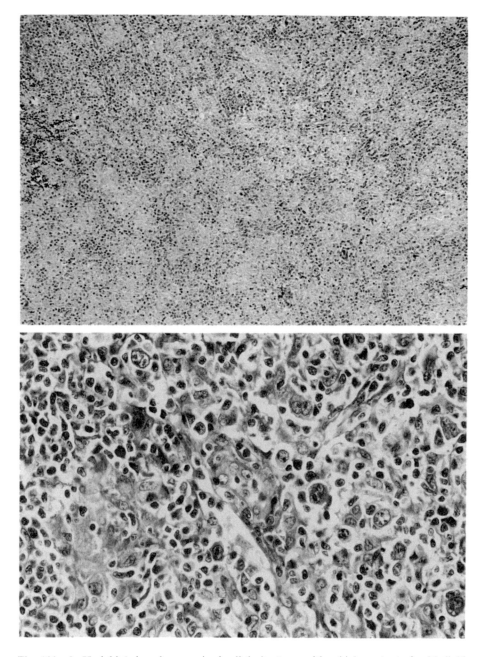

Fig. 111a, b. Hodgkin's lymphoma, mixed cellularity type, with a high content of epithelioid cells. Numerous Sternberg-Reed cells and one group of epithelioid cells (*lower left*) are recognizable in **b. a** Male, 44 years. Paracervical node. Giemsa. 110:1. **b** Male, 56 years. Cervical node. H & E. 440:1

ent name.[448] The areas between the epithelioid cell foci contain B lymphocytes with round nuclei *and* lymphoplasmacytoid cells (Fig. 113) or plasma cells, a few immunoblasts and centroblasts (Fig. 112). On immunohistochemical analysis of paraffin sections, immunocytoma is characterized by monoclonality of the CIg in plasma cells and plasma cell precursors.

The series studied by NoËL et al.[449] contained five cases with florid germinal centres and simultaneous "myoepithelial sialadenitis", which could probably be interpreted as immunocytoma. According to the *clinical* reports on the cases studied by PATSOURIS et al.,[450] 31% of the patients with immunocytoma with a high content of epithelioid cells showed Sjögren's syndrome, 15% had other autoimmune diseases, 38% had paraproteinaemia, and 25% had Bence-Jones proteinuria. The patients showed the same age peak as do those with LeL, but immunocytoma did not develop in patients younger than 48 years. Women were affected by immunocytoma four times as frequently as men, whereas there was a slight male predominance in all other types of lymphoma with a high content of epithelioid cells (Fig. 101).

4. In a few other cases of *NHL* (centroblastic-centrocytic lymphoma, centroblastic lymphoma, B-immunoblastic lymphoma, peripheral T-cell lymphoma) we have found a focal epithelioid cell reaction, which had led to a false diagnosis or supposition of LeL. Hence a focal epithelioid cell reaction is not specific to the types of Hodgkin's lymphoma and NHL mentioned above and should not lead to a diagnosis of LeL without further critical examination.

5. The most important type of *lymphadenitis* with focal epithelioid cell reactions is Piringer's lymphadenitis. This is usually the lymph node lesion seen in toxoplasmosis, but it may also occur in chronic infectious mononucleosis, leishmaniasis and brucellosis. The lymph node architecture is preserved, the follicles contain highly active germinal centres, the sinuses show so-called immature histiocytosis (sinusoidal B-cell reaction[451]), and the pulp exhibits polymorphic hyperplasia. The focal epithelioid cell reactions are seen in the pulp and in *germinal centres*. The small foci are irregularly distributed in the lymph node and are often confined to circumscribed areas of the cortex.

Another type of lymphadenitis with focal epithelioid cell reactions is seen in syphilis in stages I and II. Lymph nodes with this lesion show a toxoplasmosis-like picture and vasculitis in the septa, capsule and surrounding tissue.

Another disease to be considered in a differential diagnosis is *chronic miliary tuberculosis*. It can be diagnosed easily when acid-fast rods are demonstrable. The groups of epithelioid cells are somewhat larger than those found in LeL. We have seen a few other cases in which the epithelioid cell groups were larger than in LeL or toxoplasmosis, but smaller than in tubercles. We could not clarify their aetiology, but consider them to be of inflammatory origin.

---

[448] Scheurlen and Hellriegel 1971; Chirife 1979; Stiller et al. 1980; Spier et al. 1988.
[449] 1979, 1980.
[450] 1988, 1989a,b, 1990.
[451] De Almeida et al. 1984; Sheibani et al. 1984; Stein et al. 1984b; van den Oord et al. 1985.

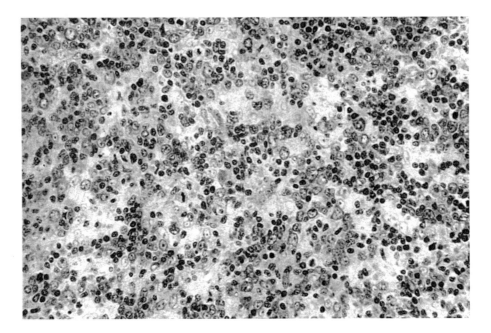

Fig. 112. Immunocytoma. The tumour cells are interspersed with numerous, very small groups of epithelioid cells (pale). Female, 64 years. Axillary node. Giemsa. 280 : 1

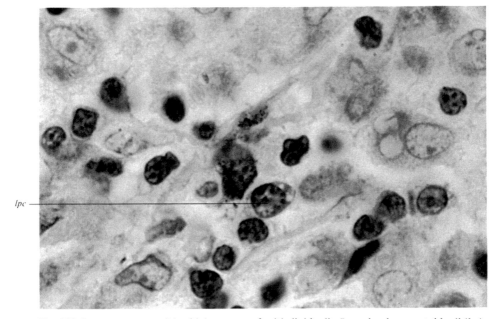

Fig. 113. Immunocytoma with a high content of epithelioid cells. Lymphoplasmacytoid cell (*lpc*). Note the mast cell above it. Giemsa. 1300 : 1

Finally, there were two cases in which we diagnosed LeL, but then electron microscopy revealed rod-shaped bacteria, which in one case were probably pathogens of *Whipple's disease* (Fig. 114).[452] In a second biopsy from the latter case the pathogens of Whipple's disease could be found on light microscopy with PAS staining. After PATSOURIS et al. finished their study, we observed two other cases of Whipple's disease that showed features of LeL. So far, we have found it almost impossible to clearly distinguish such cases from LeL on light microscopy when we do not find the PAS-positive pathogens. In questionable cases, a clearly focal increase in fibres suggests the bacteriogenic nature of the lesion. Other, chiefly electron microscopic criteria have been presented by KAISERLING et al.[453]

This discussion of the differential diagnosis would not be complete without noting that there will always be a few cases that cannot be identified with good morphological techniques alone. Depending on the differential diagnostic question, immunological analyses of fresh tissue, electron microscopy, bacteriological analyses and/or molecular genetic studies are advisable in such cases.

Prognosis. The life expectancy of the patients with LeL in our collection was relatively short. Patients presenting in stages I or II survived a median of 18 months, those in stages III or IV only 11 months. In some cases this poorer prognosis was definitely a result of insufficiently aggressive treatment. For example, many of the patients were treated according to an unsuitable protocol for Hodgkin's lymphoma. If one were to treat the patients more aggressively with chemotherapy from the very beginning, one might achieve better results, similar to those reported by SUCHI et al.[454] It is remarkable that the other three types of lymphoma with a high content of epithelioid cells do not differ significantly in prognosis (Fig. 115). As one would expect, patients in earlier stages always show a significantly higher survival rate than do those in later stages. This is especially true of the Hodgkin type.

4.1.4 T-Cell Lymphoma of AILD (LgX) Type

WF: Not listed

Lukes-Collins: IBL-like T-cell lymphoma

History and Terminology. In 1971, at a workshop of an American and Japanese lymphoma study group in Nagoya,[455] DORFMAN presented a characteristic histological lesion that he had observed in four patients. This observation was published a year later by LIAO et al.,[456] who called the lesion "malignant histiocytosis with cutaneous involvement and eosinophilia". At the same workshop two of the participating pathologists reported similar lesions, but under different names. One of the authors (K. L.) called the lesion "lymphogranulomatosis X" (LgX)

---

[452] Kaiserling et al. 1989.
[453] 1989.
[454] 1987.
[455] Akazaki et al. 1973.
[456] 1972.

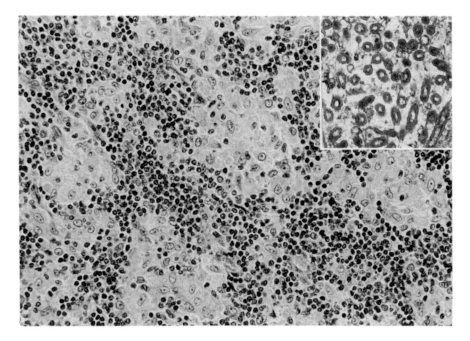

Fig. 114. Focal epithelioid cell reaction that looks like lymphoepithelioid lymphoma. On electron microscopy (inset) it proved to be Whipple's disease. Male, 40 years. Inguinal node. H & E. 256:1. Inset: 5000:1. (Electron micrograph provided by E. KAISERLING)

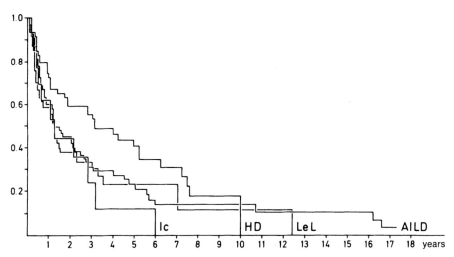

Fig. 115. Overall survival probability of patients with the four types of lymphoma with a high content of epithelioid cells. *Ic*=immunocytoma with a high content of epithelioid cells. *HD*=Hodgkin's lymphoma of mixed cellularity type with a high content of epithelioid cells. *LeL*=lymphoepithelioid lymphoma. *AILD*=AILD (LgX) type of T-cell lymphoma with a high content of epithelioid cells. (Based on data from E. PATSOURIS, personal communication)

because its morphology resembled that of Hodgkin's lymphoma (also called "lymphogranulomatosis" in German).[457] LUKES[458] named it "immunoblastic lymphadenopathy" (IBL). Later, FRIZZERA and RAPPAPORT[459] proposed the term "angioimmunoblastic lymphadenopathy with dysproteinaemia" (AILD), and SUCHI[460] called it "immunodysplastic disease". All of the authors interpreted the disease as an abnormal immune reaction. Transformation into immunoblastic sarcoma has been described in a number of publications, however, although with varying frequency.[461] Hence LgX was eventually interpreted as a pre-lymphoma.[462]

In 1979, SHIMOYAMA et al.[463] of Tokyo described a lymph node lesion that they regarded as similar to IBL but interpreted as a peripheral T-cell lymphoma. They called it "IBL-like T-cell lymphoma" and interpreted it as a "suppressor" T-cell lymphoma.[464] LUKES[465] examined the original slides in the Tokyo collection and did not consider them to be identical with the histological picture that he had described as IBL. He also noted that, in the past years, he had not observed more than two cases of IBL, and he concluded that IBL hardly occurred any more. In addition, LUKES[466] repeatedly pointed out that his IBL did not correspond to the AILD of FRIZZERA et al.[459] or NATHWANI et al.[467] For instance, he never saw "burnt-out" germinal centres, in contrast to the experience of FRIZZERA et al.[468] and our group.[469]

Meanwhile, investigations using classic cytogenetic[470] and molecular genetic methods[471] have proven that, at least in a vast majority of cases, LgX (AILD) is a clonal proliferation and thus probably corresponds to an ML. The cytogenetic anomalies closely resemble those seen in peripheral T-cell lymphomas[472] (often trisomy 3 or 5). Molecular DNA analysis of the TcR genes reveals rearrangement of the TcRγ and TcRβ-chain genes and sometimes rearrangement of an Ig heavy chain gene as well.[473] Not all cases that show rearrangement of the T-cell receptor genes β and γ simultaneously reveal a chromosomal anomaly. The reason for this may be that the tumour cell clone is too small. Histologically confirmed cases of

---

[457] Published later: Lennert 1973.

[458] Lukes and Tindle 1973, 1975, 1978.

[459] Frizzera et al. 1974, 1975.

[460] 1974.

[461] Lukes and Tindle 1978; Nathwani et al. 1978; Lennert et al. 1979.

[462] Lukes and Tindle 1978; Lennert et al. 1979.

[463] 1979, 1987; Watanabe et al. 1980.

[464] 1987.

[465] Personal communication 1984

[466] Lukes and Tindle 1978.

[467] 1978.

[468] 1974, 1975.

[469] Lennert et al. 1979.

[470] Hossfeld et al. 1976; Kaneko et al. 1982, 1988; Schwarze et al. 1982; Gödde-Salz et al. 1987; Schlegelberger et al. 1990.

[471] Fujita et al. 1986; Griesser et al. 1986a,b; O'Connor et al. 1986b; Weiss et al. 1986; Lipford et al. 1987; Suzuki et al. 1987; Feller et al. 1988; Toninai et al. 1988.

[472] Hossfeld et al. 1976; Kaneko et al. 1982; Schwarze et al. 1982; Gödde-Salz et al. 1987.

[473] Fujita et al. 1986; Griesser et al. 1986a,b; O'Connor et al. 1986b; Weiss et al. 1986; Lipford et al. 1987; Suzuki et al. 1987; Feller et al. 1988.

LgX, however, hardly ever lacked clonality in our molecular genetic studies.[474] There may be various reasons for the lack of clonal rearrangement of the β-chain gene of the T-cell receptor repeatedly described in the literature.[475] Perhaps there are cases of LgX that represent polyclonal T-cell proliferations or whose clones are too small to be detected within a polyclonal cell proliferation using the Southern blot hybridization technique.

Quantitative DNA analyses have also been performed in cases of LgX and revealed "abnormal stem cell lines".[476] According to SANDRITTER, this is proof of a malignant tumour.

Hence we think the term "T-cell lymphoma of AILD (or LgX) type", as defined by SHIMOYAMA et al.,[477] is justified for the great majority of cases that we previously designated as LgX.

There is still uncertainty as to the nature of the "bona fide" IBL of LUKES and TINDLE, if it is to be recognized as a separate entity. Our collection is also supposed to include non-neoplastic cases diagnosed as LgX. But what do they look like? It is not possible to determine whether the cases described by WEISS et al.[478] and O'CONNOR et al.,[479] which were not identified as being clonal by molecular genetics, were actually non-neoplastic cases of LgX (cf. p. 200). Perhaps we should consider a case to be non-neoplastic when it shows a marked increase in plasma cells and plasma cell precursors in the blood and lymph nodes, and when it is also associated with hyperimmune phenomena, such as immunohaemolytic anaemia. Such cases were described many years ago by FORSTER and MOESCHLIN[480] in an article entitled "*Extramedulläres, leukämisches Plasmocytom mit Dysproteinämie und erworbener hämolytischer Anämie*". FLANDRIN et al.[481] presented a similar condition that they called "*sarcomatoses ganglionnaires diffuses à différenciation plasmocytaire avec anémie hémolytique auto-immune*". In those cases the plasma cells were polyclonal. For many years, however, we have not seen the morphological picture associated with such a leukaemoid condition. From autopsy reports on cases in our collection[482] it is obvious that there must be a non-neoplastic "LgX". In several cases, the lymph nodes were "burnt out", i.e. there was a paucity of cells, but an abundance of fibres and vessels. The lymphoid cell proliferation had disappeared without a trace, even without chemotherapy.

A favourable course over a period of years or spontaneous remission does not necessarily mean, however, that there is no underlying T-cell lymphoma. For example, we know of a patient in spontaneous remission for 3 years, although the case met all the criteria for assuming the presence of ML, viz. a clonal chromo-

---

[474] Fujita et al. 1986; Griesser et al. 1986a,b; O'Connor et al. 1986b; Weiss et al. 1986; Lipford et al. 1987; Suzuki et al. 1987; Feller et al. 1988.
[475] O'Connor et al. 1986b; Weiss et al. 1986; Toninai et al. 1988.
[476] Sandritter and Grimm 1977; Common et al. 1980.
[477] 1979.
[478] 1986.
[479] 1986b.
[480] 1954.
[481] 1972; Flandrin 1978.
[482] Knecht et al. 1985.

some aberration and rearrangement of the β and γ chains of the T-cell receptor[483] (we must not forget that these criteria are not *absolute*!).

Definition. Although a small number of non-neoplastic cases of LgX (AILD) remain to be clarified, we now diagnose a T-cell lymphoma of AILD (LgX) type when the following criteria are fulfilled:

1. Absence of germinal centres
2. Variegated cytology, including T cells that are larger and more pleomorphic than normal T lymphocytes
3. Large, irregularly shaped accumulations of follicular dendritic cells
4. Marked increase in the number of venules, which have thickened basement membranes containing PAS-positive material

When we diagnose a T-cell lymphoma of AILD (LgX) type, clinicians who co-operate with us treat the patient with corticosteroids only briefly (on a trial basis). If the patient does not respond quickly, aggressive chemotherapy is started as soon as possible.[484] We no longer wait for the results of classic and molecular cytogenetics, because, so far, we have always obtained positive ones, i.e. results that favour ML.

Immunology and Molecular Genetics. The variegated infiltration shows a predominance of T cells with the phenotype of mature T cells. The CD4-to-CD8 quotient was 3.9 ± 2.7.[483] Simultaneous demonstration of the proliferation-associated antigen Ki-67 shows that CD4-positive cells proliferate almost exclusively in about two-thirds of the cases (group I), whereas in the other third (group II) there is an increased number of proliferating CD8-positive cells in addition to CD4-positive cells. Small numbers of B cells occur, usually arranged in foci interspersed among the T cells. These B cells show a polyclonal Ig pattern and are Ki-67 negative. In about 80% of cases there is an extensive, irregularly defined network of follicular dendritic cells (CD35+, Ki-M4+, CD23+), expression of CD35 being most prominent. This can be regarded as a diagnostic feature of the AILD (LgX) type of T-cell lymphoma.

DNA analysis of the T-cell receptor genes shows that clonal T-cell proliferations are present, at least in a vast majority of cases of the AILD type. Two different rearrangement patterns can be demonstrated. Group I shows a pattern like that seen in other peripheral T-cell lymphomas (rearrangement of TcRγ and TcRβ), while in group II the Ig heavy chain genes are rearranged as well. These two groups correlate with immunophenotypic and clinical parameters (cf. p. 210).

Occurrence. T-cell lymphoma of AILD (LgX) type accounts for 20.9% of the peripheral T-cell lymphomas in our collection and is thus the most frequent type of peripheral T-cell lymphoma. It makes up 3.6% of all ML in our collection. In

---

[483] Feller et al. 1988.
[484] Kiel Lymphoma Study Group, cf. Siegert et al. 1989.

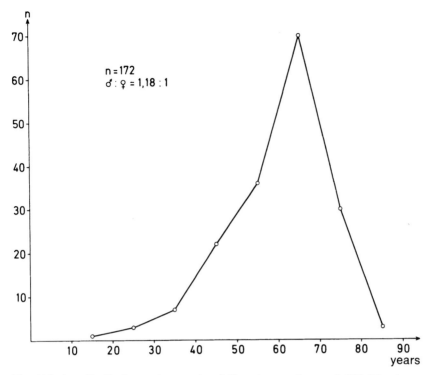

Fig. 116. Age distribution and sex ratio of "lymphogranulomatosis X". The data probably correspond for the most part to those of T-cell lymphoma of AILD (LgX) type. (Based on data from KNECHT and LENNERT 1981a)

a prospective study of unselected cases by the Kiel Lymphoma Study Group[485] there were 1127 patients with NHL plus 32 patients with "LgX", or about 2.7% of a total of 1159 patients. The age and sex distributions of the AILD type correspond, or at least come very close, to our data on LgX.[486] There is a steep peak in the 7th decade of life. Our youngest patient was 16 years old, the oldest was 84 (Fig. 116). One should be extremely careful with a diagnosis of T-cell lymphoma of AILD (LgX) type in childhood; as a rule, these cases are likely to be viral infections (e.g. rubella!). There is a slight male preponderance (the male-to-female ratio is approx. 1.18:1).

Clinical Picture.[487] This section is based on data we collected with KNECHT[488] in 172 cases of LgX. "B symptoms" were recorded in the medical histories of all patients. Half the patients had pruritus, and about 20% were susceptible to infections. Generalized lymphadenopathy was usually (80%) observed. Hep-

---

[485] Brittinger et al. 1984.
[486] Radaszkiewicz and Lennert 1975; Knecht and Lennert 1981a.
[487] Radaszkiewicz and Lennert 1975; Knecht and Lennert 1981a,b.
[488] Knecht and Lennert 1981a.

atomegaly and splenomegaly were seen in two-thirds of the patients. Fever was reported in 80% of cases. A third of the patients showed a remarkable tendency to develop oedema, particularly in the upper extremities and the face. Pleural effusions, ascites, lung infiltrates and enlargement of the parotid gland were seldom observed. In almost half the patients we noted skin lesions, especially exanthema. Two-thirds of the patients were anaemic; 23% had a positive Coombs' test, in which case the patients could be said to have either haemolytic anaemia or, if the marrow was depleted and reticulocytosis was missing, aplastic anaemia.[489] Leucocytosis was found in 29% of the patients, usually due to an increase in the number of granulocytes. Lymphopenia ($< 1 \times 10^9$/l) was reported in 25% of cases, eosinophilia in 28% and plasmacytosis (> 3%) in 8%. An analysis of blood smears in our laboratory[490] showed that the numbers of large granular lymphocytes (CD8+), hyperbasophilic cells (plasma cells, proplasma-cytes, plasmablasts) and basophil granulocytes (!) were increased. The basophil granulocyte count was up to 1×10^9/l. Histologically, lymphoma infiltration has been detected in the bone marrow by examination of trephine biopsies.[491] The ESR varied within a wide range; in 11% of cases it was normal, in 23% highly elevated. There was almost always a polyclonal increase in γ-globulins in the blood; only three times was monoclonality found terminally (IgM in two cases, IgG in one case).[492] Rheumatoid factors, cryoglobulin and antibodies against smooth muscle cells (vimentin) were reported in a few cases in our collection. DELLAGI et al.[493] found antivimentin autoantibodies in 75% of their patients with AILD. Circulating immune complexes appear to be a frequent phenomenon associated with T-cell lymphoma of AILD (LgX) type.[494] An important feature is drug hypersensitivity (chiefly antibiotics, antiphlogistics and cytostatic drugs), which is not uncommon and can appear prior to, simultaneously with or during the course of the disease and then leads to the skin lesions described above. In 11 of our 172 cases another malignant tumour (as a rule carcinoma) was found in addition to the lymphoma.[495] HTLV-1 antibodies are not detectable.

Histology.[496] The lymph node architecture is effaced. It is replaced by a highly vascularized infiltration, which frequently bypasses the capsule and spreads into the surrounding adipose tissue (Fig. 117). As a rule, follicles and germinal centres are missing. Usually, one still sees a few poorly defined foci of B lymphocytes, but they eventually disappear completely.

In most cases the number of follicular dendritic cells is markedly increased. They sometimes form concentrically arranged, pale foci, which were initially interpreted as "burnt-out" germinal centres (Fig. 118).[497] We now know that,

---

[489] Schoengen et al. 1976.
[490] Zankowich et al. 1984.
[491] Brearley et al. 1979; Schnaidt et al. 1980a,b; Hill and Burkhardt 1984.
[492] Cf. Klajman et al. 1981.
[493] 1984.
[494] Coupland et al. 1985; Euler et al. 1987.
[495] Knecht et al. 1985.
[496] Cf. Toninai et al. 1988.
[497] Frizzera et al. 1974, 1975; Lennert et al. 1979.

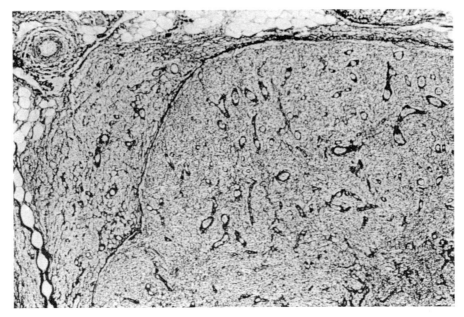

Fig. 117. T-cell lymphoma of AILD (LgX) type. Numerous venules with thickened walls in all of the lymphoid tissue in the node and in the surrounding tissue. The capsule remains intact. Male, 56 years. Cervical node. Gomori. 51:1

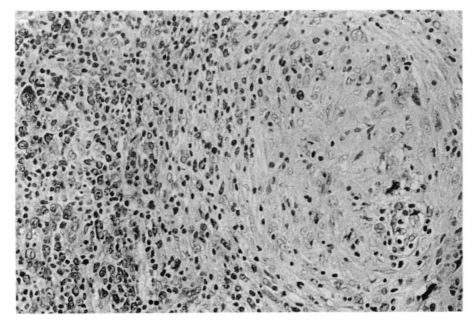

Fig. 118. T-cell lymphoma of AILD (LgX) type. "Burnt-out" germinal centre. Male, 42 years. Supraclavicular node. Giemsa. 256:1

more often, the follicular dendritic cells collect in large, irregularly shaped accu-mulations, which extend far beyond the original B-cell areas and spread out in the tumour tissue, which has a high content of venules. It is difficult to recognize the follicular dendritic cells with conventional stains (Fig. 119), whereas they are easily identified with appropriate immunohistochemical staining (Fig. 120). The follicular dendritic cells may proliferate (they may be Ki-67 positive and may show mitosis)[498] and evidently lose their functional contact with B lymphocytes. We suppose that special lymphokines produced by the lymphoma cells induce proliferation of follicular dendritic cells.[499]

The tumour infiltration is usually not as dense as that of other small cell lymphomas. In many cases areas with lots of cells alternate with other areas that are highly depleted. The spaces between the tumour cells often contain small, amorphous, weakly PAS-positive deposits, which prove to be mostly reticulin fibres and collagenous fibres on electron microscopy.[500]

The infiltrated areas also show a very large number of vessels, mostly epithe-lioid venules, which are frequently branched. A distinctive feature of the epithe-lioid venules is their PAS-positive walls, which vary in thickness (Fig. 121). Elec-tron microscopic studies have shown that the PAS-positive wall consists of thick-ened basement membranes[501] and collagenous fibres.[502] On electron microscopy one can also recognize some fibroblasts and interdigitating cells.[503] In other cases the basement membrane is split into pieces or has disintegrated (or is it insuffi-ciently developed?). Arterioles and arteries are also often surrounded by a broad, hyalinized layer of PAS-positive material or by concentrically arranged, thick bundles of collagenous fibres (Fig. 122).

The tumour cells vary to some extent in cytology (Fig. 123). A majority of the cells are small or medium-sized. They have more or less polymorphic nuclei with small or medium-sized nucleoli and scanty, pale grey to greyish blue cytoplasm. Cells with abundant, "transparent" cytoplasm ("clear cells")[504] are not uncom-mon. These cells are PAS negative and do not contain glycogen. Their nuclei are round or pleomorphic. In addition, there are usually a few large, basophilic blast cells of a varying appearance that is not characteristic of typical immunoblasts. One may also find sporadic multinucleate cells, occasionally with the appearance of Sternberg-Reed cells. Mitotic figures are found in moderate or large numbers.

The tumour cells are often interspersed with many plasma cells (mostly poly-clonal) and plasma cell precursors and with numerous eosinophils. Relatively large numbers of typical B immunoblasts are seen in some cases. A special variant of T-cell lymphoma of AILD (LgX) type shows epithelioid cells arranged in small foci (see p. 186). In a few cases we were able to demonstrate blood basophils in sections routinely prepared with Giemsa staining; this is the equivalent of an increase in basophils in the blood.

---

[498] Feller et al. 1988.
[499] Fliedner et al. 1990.
[500] Knecht and Lennert 1981c.
[501] Knecht and Lennert 1981c.
[502] Schnaidt et al. 1980a; Knecht and Lennert 1981c.
[503] Knecht and Lennert 1981c.
[504] Suchi 1974; Knecht and Lennert 1981c.

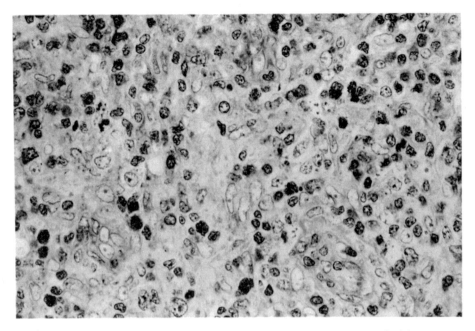

Fig. 119. T-cell lymphoma of AILD (LgX) type. The T cells are interspersed with numerous follicular dendritic cells. The latter are barely recognizable here, but immunohistochemical staining of sections from the same specimen proved their presence. Male, 70 years. Lymph node. Giemsa. 512:1

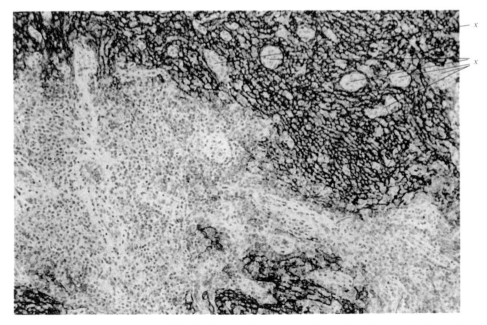

Fig. 120. T-cell lymphoma of AILD (LgX) type. Large, irregularly shaped accumulations of follicular dendritic cells spread over large areas of the node. They also enclose epithelioid venules (*x*). Cryostat section stained with To5 (CD35), APAAP method. 90:1

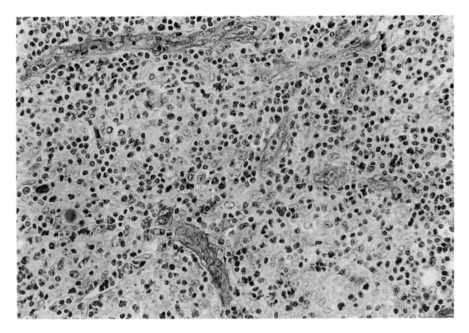

Fig. 121. T-cell lymphoma of AILD (LgX) type. Several venules with thickened walls. Relatively dense, polymorphic infiltrate. Male, 63 years. Inguinal node. Giemsa. 256:1

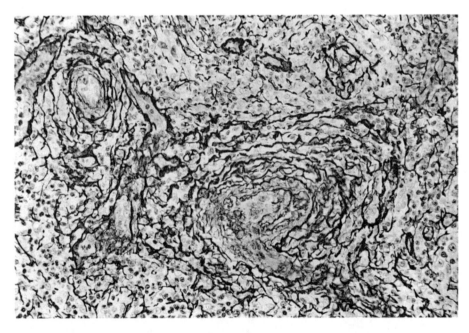

Fig. 122. T-cell lymphoma of AILD (LgX) type. Periarterial fibrosis. Male, 59 years. Gomori. 205:1

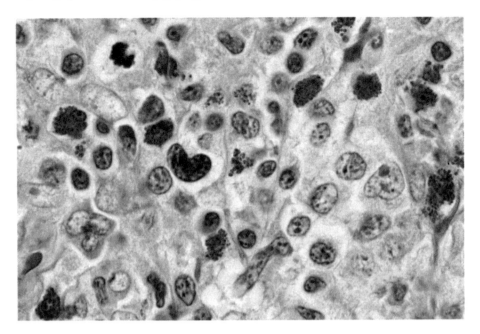

Fig. 123. T-cell lymphoma of AILD (LgX) type. Cells of various sizes with pleomorphic and round nuclei. Eosinophils. One non-characteristic giant cell. Male, 63 years. Giemsa. 1024:1

Depending on the quantity of the various cell types in the infiltrate, we used to distinguish five different types, viz. four with a high content of one cell type (immunoblasts, plasma cells, epithelioid cells or lymphocytes) and a mixed cellularity type without predominance of a particular cell type. This subclassification does not have any significant clinical or prognostic consequences, however, so we no longer bother with it.

Development into a High-Grade Malignant Lymphoma. In some cases, at the onset of the disease the tumour cells are already medium sized and densely packed (at least in places) and they show high mitotic activity, as in a high-grade malignant T-cell lymphoma. We diagnose such cases as a large cell variant of the AILD (LgX) type of T-cell lymphoma.

Sooner or later, approximately 10% of the cases of T-cell lymphoma of AILD (LgX) type develop into a *high-grade malignant T-cell lymphoma*, viz.: pleomorphic, large cell lymphoma; immunoblastic lymphoma; or, most often, large cell anaplastic (CD30+) lymphoma. A somewhat smaller percentage of cases show an increase in monotypic plasma cells and a variable number of B immunoblasts. In the past, such cases would have been classified as *B-immunoblastic lymphoma* (with plasmacytic differentiation).[505] This diagnosis is

---

[505] Lennert et al. 1979.

certainly correct in some cases. In a majority of cases, however, the monotypic immunoblasts (and plasma cells) are still mingled with a large number of neoplastic T cells, without forming cohesive tumour cell clusters. In such cases it is not clear whether a genuine secondary neoplasm has developed, or whether one should assume that the monotypic B-cell proliferation is induced by neoplastic helper T cells.

We have also previously described cases that developed into *Hodgkin's lymphomas*.[506] When we re-examined these cases, however, we discovered that in some the transition was only feigned. In the beginning, a Hodgkin's lymphoma may have an AILD-like appearance, at least partially. In such cases, it is possible to overlook the Hodgkin and Sternberg-Reed cells if only a few of them are present. In only one patient did a second biopsy definitely reveal Hodgkin's lymphoma with a high content of lymphocytes; it differed completely from the first biopsy with the classic picture of the AILD (LgX) type. The simultaneous development of Hodgkin's lymphoma and T-cell lymphoma of AILD (LgX) type in this case was probably coincidental.

Diagnosis. Before we list the distinguishing features of T-cell lymphoma of AILD (LgX) type, we should like to point out once again that we are not able to distinguish between non-neoplastic cases of AILD and T-cell lymphoma of AILD (LgX) type, although other investigators[507] are able to do so. Perhaps this is just a matter of definition of AILD (LgX).

We depend on the following criteria for a diagnosis of the AILD (LgX) type of T-cell lymphoma:

1. When T-cell lymphoma of AILD (LgX) type is suspected, we look at the follicles first. If they do not contain germinal centres and the rest of the picture is compatible with that of the AILD type, we can diagnose the tumour as T-cell lymphoma of AILD (LgX) type. When a few solitary remnants of follicles are found at the periphery, however, or when large germinal centres are seen in parts of an infiltrate of otherwise typical cytology with numerous venules, we cannot completely rule out the possibility of T-cell lymphoma of AILD (LgX) type, but it is unlikely. In such cases, the pathologist must ask for a second biopsy of another enlarged lymph node after a brief interval, to make sure that he is not dealing with a hyperimmune reaction (see Differential Diagnosis). From our follow-up studies we know that a few florid germinal centres occasionally persist at the onset of the disease, but they soon disappear. In our large collection, two of the 26 cases we diagnosed as hyperimmune reaction developed into T-cell lymphoma of AILD (LgX) type.[508]
2. The second important criterion is the high content of epithelioid venules, which are arborized and whose walls contain deposits of PAS-positive material (basement membrane-like substances, hyaline). Such deposits are also found in the adventitia of small and medium-sized arteries.

---

[506] Lennert et al. 1979.
[507] E.g. Frizzera et al. 1989; Knecht 1989.
[508] Knecht et al. 1985.

3. A third, evidently specific but not obligatory feature is the occurrence of large, irregularly shaped accumulations of follicular dendritic cells outside the pre-existent follicles. Often, however, these cells can be recognized clearly only with immunohistochemical stains.
4. The cell density is often lower than that of other small cell lymphomas. The reduced cell density is sometimes merely a focal phenomenon.
5. An admixture of large numbers of plasma cells and plasma cell precursors, together with eosinophils, hardly ever occurs in other T-cell lymphomas.

Differential Diagnosis. Of greatest importance is the distinction between T-cell lymphoma of AILD (LgX) type and *hyperimmune reactions*[509] that show active germinal centres and hyperplastic pulp containing numerous venules. Hence the cytology of the pulp must be studied carefully. In a hyperimmune reaction the pulp does not contain any accumulations of atypical T lymphocytes with pronounced pleomorphism. In all ambiguous cases, very careful clinical observation is necessary, and, if possible, a new biopsy should be performed after a few weeks.

Viral infections, such as rubella and especially EBV infections, may also give a similar impression and thus cause confusion with T-cell lymphoma of AILD (LgX) type.[510] Germinal centres may be lacking or inactive in these conditions, but active germinal centres are seen in some cases. The number of venules is also increased, but they are not hyalinized. The lymph node capsule is infiltrated by lymphoid cells, which cause it to be widened somewhat. The cytology is variegated and includes many B immunoblasts and all kinds of intermediate stages up to small lymphocytes. The T lymphocytes have round or slightly pleomorphic nuclei. "Clear cells" never occur in viral infections. An immunohistochemical analysis with pan-B, pan-T, and *kapppa* and *lambda* antibodies should make it possible to reach a decision in most ambiguous cases. Hyperimmune reactions and viral infections show a relatively large number of (polyclonal) B cells and their functional forms (plasma cells), whereas T-cell lymphoma of AILD (LgX) type exhibits at least focal dominance of the T-cell proliferation. In cases of viral lymphadenitis the usually increased number of small "lymphatic plasma cells" (lymphoplasmacytoid cells) evident with PAP staining is especially useful as a distinguishing sign.

On the basis of immunohistochemical findings, KRUEGER et al.[511] considered the possibility of a connection between the AILD type and rubella. DUMONT et al.[512] demonstrated a herpes-like virus in "AILD" on electron microscopy. SHAMOTO and SUCHI[513] found intracytoplasmic type A particles similar to the Mazon-Pfizer monkey virus in the AILD type.

Occasionally, it is impossible to draw a clear borderline between T-cell lymphoma of AILD (LgX) type and *T-zone lymphoma* (see p. 214), especially when follicles are no longer present.[513a]

---

[509] Knecht and Lennert 1981a,b; Knecht et al. 1985.
[510] Lennert et al. 1981.
[511] 1979; Bergholz et al. 1979.
[512] 1979.
[513] 1979.
[513a] Nakamura and Suchi 1991.

Pleomorphic, small cell T-cell lymphoma shows a higher cell density, a more monotonous-looking T-cell infiltration (no immunoblasts!) and hardly any plasma cells or eosinophils.

In exceptional cases in which an *immunocytoma* shows a marked increase in the number of venules this lymphoma can bear a certain resemblance to T-cell lymphoma of AILD (LgX) type. A false diagnosis is prevented by the greater cell density of the infiltration, which is composed of small lymphocytes that have round nuclei and are interspersed with *monotypic* plasma cells or lymphoplasmacytoid cells.

Prognosis. The available older data[514] probably give a wrong impression. They were collected at a time when the AILD type was still considered to be an abnormal immune reaction. The patients were often treated merely with corticosteroids and received cytostatic drugs much too late, if at all. The results were accordingly poor. Patients treated with corticosteroids alone showed a median survival period of 5.3 months, while with polychemotherapy it was 13.3 months.[515]

A recent prospective study of 53 patients showed complete remission in 29% of the cases treated with prednisone alone.[516] With subsequent chemotherapy (COPLAM/IMVP16) complete remission was achieved in 57% of the cases. Chemotherapy alone led to full remission in only 37%. The remission periods were short, viz. 4.5, 3.5 and 8.5 months, respectively. The mean survival period was almost 24 months. In a new prospective study[516a] the median survival was 15 months. The survival curve showed a plateau (at 40%) after 2 years.

Recently, treatment with low doses of interferon-α_{2a} has been recommended.[517] This agent has been reported to be useful as salvage treatment for patients who are refractory to combination therapy or when the latter is contra-indicated. interferon-α_{2a} may also be useful as adjuvant or maintenance treatment.

A comparison of survival data with the immunophenotype and molecular genetic findings enabled us to distinguish two different groups (I and II; cf. p. 200). Exclusive proliferation of CD4-positive cells was associated with rearrangement of the β- and γ-chain genes of the T-cell receptor. In these cases the mean survival period was 15 ± 13 months. Simultaneous proliferation of CD4-positive and CD8-positive cells was associated with an additional rearrangement of Ig heavy chains. In these cases the mean survival period was 23 ± 8 months. It is not yet possible to confirm these data statistically, however, because the observation period was too short and the number of patients too small (25). The reader may refer to FELLER et al.[518] for further details.

---

[514] Knecht and Lennert 1981b.
[515] Knecht and Lennert 1981b.
[516] Siegert et al. 1989.
[516a] W. Siegert, personal communication.
[517] Trinkler et al. 1989; Siegert et al. 1991.
[518] 1988.

4.1.5 T-Zone Lymphoma

WF: [Some cases of] Malignant lymphoma, diffuse, mixed, small and large cell (F)

Lukes-Collins: T-immunoblastic sarcoma

Definition. We chose the name "T-zone lymphoma" because the tumour develops in T zones and contains all the components of the T zones of lymphoid tissue (analogous to follicular lymphoma, which contains all the components of the B zones), viz. T lymphocytes, interdigitating cells and epithelioid venules. The term "T-zone lymphoma" was also justified by another analogy to follicular centro-blastic-centrocytic lymphoma, which shows neoplastic B regions and non-neo-plastic T regions: the neoplastic T zones are accompanied for some time by non-neoplastic B zones (follicles with or without germinal centres). Eventually, however, the tumour loses its zonal arrangement and shows a completely diffuse pattern, although it is still composed of the same cells. Compared with our earlier definition of T-zone lymphoma,[519] we now consider the tumour cell spectrum to be smaller. Most of the tumour cells are small and monomorphic or slightly pleomorphic. There are *always* some large, transformed cells (T immunoblasts), and "clear cells" are often found. Patients with T-zone lymphoma seldom show a leukaemic blood picture and never have mycosis fungoides-like skin lesions.

Immunology. The tumour cells have the phenotype of mature T cells (CD2+, CD3+, CD5+). The proliferating cells (Ki-67+) simultaneously express CD4. There are also some CD8-positive cells, however, which probably do not belong to the tumour cell clone. In addition, there are a variable number of polyclonal B cells and networks of follicular dendritic cells; either these cells are confined to pre-existent follicles or there are small foci of them distributed among the tumour cells. An increased number of CD1-positive interdigitating cells are often seen within the T-cell infiltrates.

DNA analysis reveals the rearrangement characteristic of other peripheral T-cell lymphomas, viz. TcRγ and TcRβ chain genes, and no rearrangement of Ig heavy chain genes.

Occurrence. T-zone lymphoma as we now define it is a rare disease (approx. 1.0% of the NHL in our collection). Patients range in age from 18 to 82 years, with a peak incidence in the 7th decade of life. The male-to-female ratio is about 1.5:1.

Clinical Picture.[520] The usual presentation is with lymphadenopathy, which develops relatively quickly and tends to become generalized early in the course of the disease. There are some cases, however, in which the tumour is confined to one site for a relatively long period of time. Hepatomegaly and/or splenomegaly and involvement of lungs are frequently observed. Peripheral blood and bone marrow smears occasionally contain a few atypical lymphocytes, but a leukaemic blood

---

[519] Lennert and Mohri 1978; Helbron et al. 1979; Lennert et al. 1981.
[520] Helbron et al. 1979.

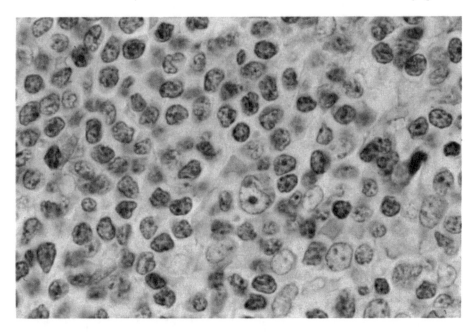

Fig. 124. T-zone lymphoma showing slight pleomorphism. One immunoblast. Male, 76 years. Axillary node. Giemsa. 1024:1

picture has seldom been observed. There is sometimes a marked polyclonal elevation in the serum Ig level. We have observed one patient with severe autoimmune haemolytic anaemia, which required splenectomy (T zones of the spleen were infiltrated). HTLV-1 antibodies are not demonstrable.

Histology. T-zone lymphoma is characterized by a dominant proliferation of T lymphocytes interspersed with a variable number of T immunoblasts and all transitional forms between the two. The nuclei of the lymphocytes are usually monomorphic, but occasionally slightly pleomorphic, and have small nucleoli. Cytoplasm is scanty and appears pale grey with Giemsa staining (Fig. 124). Sometimes there are focal or larger areas in which the lymphocytes show abundant, "transparent" cytoplasm (Fig. 125). These "clear cells" are clearly distinguishable from the other lymphocytes with scanty cytoplasm. The T immunoblasts are usually not as basophilic as B immunoblasts, and they show moderately abundant, grey cytoplasm. The nucleoli of T immunoblasts are also not as basophilic as those of B immunoblasts, but they are central, solitary and large. In addition, there are a few interdigitating cells with crumpled-looking nuclei. Foci of so-called plasmacytoid T cells are seen occasionally. Some eosinophils and a few plasma cells are often present. Occasionally one finds mononuclear and multinucleate giant cells that may resemble Sternberg-Reed cells. Sometimes there is a focal epithelioid cell reaction.

All cases show a markedly increased number of *typical* epithelioid venules. At first, the areas between the neoplastic T zones contain relatively well-preserved (non-neoplastic) follicles with or without germinal centres (Fig. 126). After a

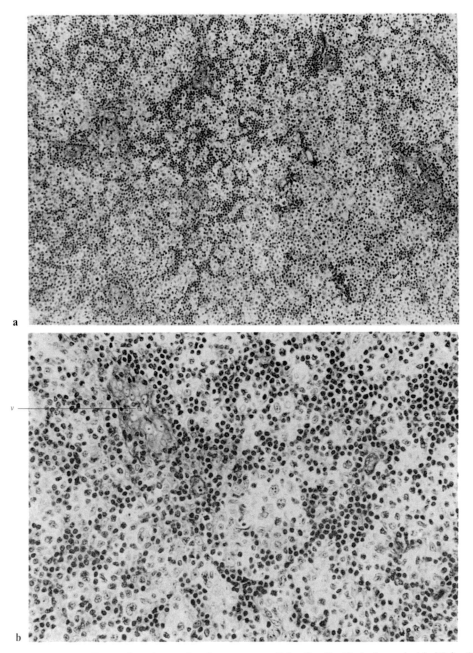

Fig. 125a, b. T-zone lymphoma showing numerous "clear" cells. Typical venule (*v*). Male, 61 years. Inguinal node. Giemsa. **a** 100:1, **b** 256:1

while, however, the follicles begin to disappear, and eventually the whole lymph node is taken over by the T-zone neoplasm.

Cytochemistry. The tumour cells frequently show a granular acid phosphatase reaction. Acid non-specific esterase staining does not reveal a spot-like reaction product, but some of the cells show a granular reaction pattern. A small or moderate number of tumour cells may contain large PAS-positive granules. Occasionally, the cytoplasm of tumour cells has a large number of vacuoles, which are stainable with Sudan red.

Diagnosis. It is easy to make a diagnosis when follicles are still recognizable. They may be hyperplastic, in which case one has to take good care not to make a false diagnosis of centroblastic-centrocytic lymphoma.

The size of the tumour cells is a decisive cytological criterion. A majority of the cells are small (or "intermediate"), and they are interspersed with immunoblasts ("mixed type"). The presence of typical venules and numerous "clear cells" supports a diagnosis of T-zone lymphoma.

Differential Diagnosis. It is occasionally difficult to distinguish T-zone lymphoma from *T-cell lymphoma of AILD (LgX) type* when follicles are no longer recognizable. In the AILD (LgX) type the tumour cells are usually not as densely packed together, and they are more pleomorphic and often larger. The venules have PAS-positive walls and look bizarre, i.e. they are not as well developed as those of T-zone lymphoma. The AILD (LgX) type usually shows a much larger number of eosinophils and plasma cells. On immunohistochemical analysis, a diagnosis of the AILD (LgX) type is supported by the presence of large, irregularly shaped accumulations of follicular dendritic cells, which spread beyond the B-cell areas. Finally, there are also differences in the clinical picture. Patients with T-zone lymphoma do not show the hyperergic phenomena (including exanthema) that are typical of the AILD (LgX) type.

T-zone lymphoma also has to be distinguished from all small cell neoplasms of the T-cell series:

T-CLL shows numerous typical venules—like T-zone lymphoma—but its cytology is more monotonous. The venules usually contain many leukaemic lymphocytes, large numbers of which also migrate through the walls of the venules. There are hardly any blast cells, epithelioid cells or plasma cells. Either the follicles have disappeared, or merely remnants of them are visible. In ambiguous cases, a leukaemic blood picture is an obvious sign of T-CLL.

In *mycosis fungoides* and *Sézary's syndrome* remnants of dermatopathic lymphadenitis are often seen. The nuclei of tumour cells are cerebriform, but this is recognizable only in sections of well-embedded tissue or on electron microscopy. The decisive findings are the clinical ones and the results of histological examination of a skin biopsy.

It is difficult and sometimes impossible to distinguish T-zone lymphoma from *pleomorphic, small cell T-cell lymphoma.* When the neoplasm is associated with follicular hyperplasia, the possibility of pleomorphic, small cell T-cell lymphoma can be excluded. The cytological picture can be relatively monotonous in T-zone

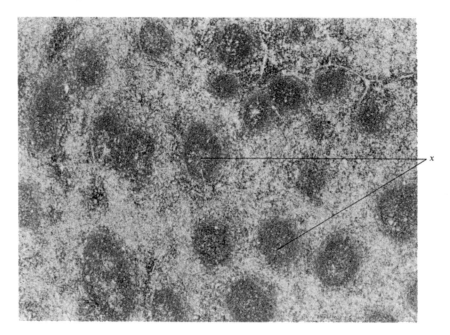

Fig. 126. T-zone lymphoma at a low magnification. The follicles (*x*) are not neoplastic, but simulate a follicular lymphoma. Actually, the pale interfollicular areas (T zones) are neoplastic. Male, 68 years. Submandibular node. Giemsa. 14:1

lymphoma, but the nuclei are more pleomorphic in the small cell variant. Large blast cells hardly ever occur in the pleomorphic, small cell type. There is also no admixture of plasma cells or epithelioid cells. The venules are not as prominent, and they are not as typical as those occurring in T-zone lymphoma.

The possibility of *lymphoepithelioid lymphoma (LeL)* must be considered when foci of epithelioid cells are found in a T-zone lymphoma. Follicles are hardly ever found in LeL, however, and there is no significant increase in the number of venules. There is a certain cytological similarity between these two types of lymphoma (small, and a few large, relatively monomorphic cells).

T-zone lymphoma is misinterpreted most often as a B-cell lymphoma, viz. *immunocytoma*. In early stages of development of immunocytoma, the pulp may be selectively infiltrated and sometimes shows an increase in the number of venules. Seen at a low magnification, the well-preserved or hyperplastic follicles lead to the supposition of T-zone lymphoma. A close look at the tumour cells (admixture of plasma cells or lymphoplasmacytoid cells!) and an immunohisto-chemical analysis of paraffin sections (Ig light chain restriction) save the pathologist from such a misinterpretation.

Finally, we have observed a false diagnosis of T-zone lymphoma made on several lymph node biopsies from children that showed hyperplasia of relatively small cells in the pulp, including T cells of atypical appearance and a small admixture of B cells. The follicles had disappeared almost completely. In one case the lesion was actually caused by a protracted EBV infection. In another case, the patient was recovering from Kawasaki syndrome.

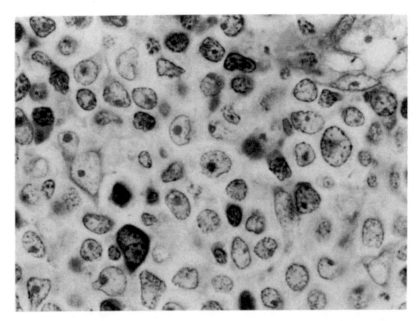

Fig. 127. Same case as Fig. 125, 1 year later. Solitary infiltration of the tonsil by numerous T immunoblasts. Giemsa. 1024:1

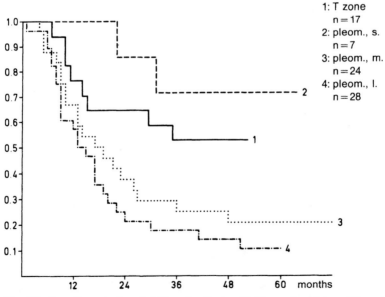

Fig. 128. Overall survival probability of patients with T-zone lymphoma (*T zone*) and pleomorphic T-cell lymphomas of small cell (*pleom., s.*), medium-sized cell (*pleom., m.*) and large cell type (*pleom., l.*). (Based on data from C. von SCHILLING)

Development into a High-Grade Malignant Lymphoma. As the disease progresses, the tumour cells usually become larger and more anaplastic. Eventually, a tumour composed of large, uniform-appearing blast cells (T immunoblasts) may develop (Fig. 127).

Prognosis. Now that we have learned to distinguish T-zone lymphoma from the other peripheral T-cell lymphomas, we find that the prognosis is more favourable than originally assumed.[521] According to data collected by SUCHI et al.,[522] the survival rate of patients with T-zone lymphoma is significantly higher than that of patients with high-grade malignant T-cell lymphomas. Our own most recent survival curves also show a relatively favourable prognosis (Fig. 128).

4.1.6 Pleomorphic, Small Cell T-Cell Lymphoma

WF: Not listed

Lukes-Collins: T-immunoblastic sarcoma

Definition. Pleomorphic, small cell T-cell lymphoma is composed of a relatively monotonous-looking proliferation of small T cells with pleomorphic nuclei, which does not have an admixture of large, basophilic blast cells. A few of the tumour cells with pleomorphic nuclei may be somewhat larger, but they are still of the same appearance as the majority of cells. The tumour can be HTLV-1 positive, especially in Japanese and Caribbean patients, in which case it often shows the clinical picture of *chronic* "adult T-cell lymphoma/leukaemia" (ATLL; cf. p. 223).

Immunology. The tumour cells show the phenotype of mature helper T cells (CD2+, CD3+, CD5+, CD4+). Where they are HTLV-1 positive, the IL-2 receptor (CD25) is also detectable, whereas CD7 is lacking. This combination, i.e. CD25+/CD7−, is not found in HTLV-1-negative T-cell lymphomas, apart from a few exceptional cases. There is clonal rearrangement of the TcRγ and TcRβ-chain genes.

Occurrence. Pleomorphic, small cell T-cell lymphoma can occur early in life. Our youngest patient was 8 years old. Otherwise, it shows the usual peak between the ages of 60 and 80 years. There is a clear male predominance (the male-to-female ratio is approx. 1.8:1), particularly in childhood.

Clinical Picture. Sites of primary manifestation other than lymph nodes in HTLV-1-negative patients are, above all, the *skin* (± lymph node involvement) and, occasionally, the tonsils.

Histology. Despite the pleomorphism of the tumour cell nuclei (Fig. 129), the tumour has a relatively monotonous appearance. The tumour cells are generally

---

[521] Helbron et al. 1979.
[522] 1987; Nakamura and Suchi 1991.

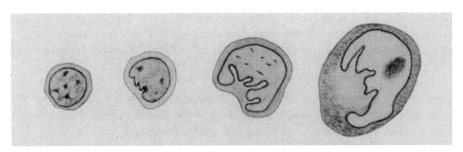

Fig. 129. Various sizes of pleomorphic T cells. *Left to right :* normal lymphocyte; small, medium-sized and large pleomorphic T cell. Drawings based on photomicrographs (320 : 1) of pleomorphic T-cell lymphomas

small and vary only somewhat in size (Fig. 130), but they all show scanty, pale grey cytoplasm. In some cases the cytoplasm is abundant and as clear as water ("clear cells"; Fig. 131). The nuclei are irregularly shaped, with all kinds of forms. They often appear serrated on the concave side, while the convex side looks smooth (cf. Fig. 129). The chromatin is moderately dense. The nucleoli are usually solitary and small. There are practically no other cells interspersed among these cells, with the occasional exception of some eosinophils. The number of mitotic figures is low. Venules are not very conspicuous. Residual follicles may be present in the beginning, but soon disappear. Sometimes there is conspicuous infiltration of small to medium-sized vessels, often with angiodestruction.

Diagnosis. Monotony, the small size of the tumour cells and the irregular shapes of their nuclei are the main criteria for diagnosing pleomorphic, small cell T-cell lymphoma.

Differential Diagnosis. Pleomorphic, small cell T-cell lymphoma must be differentiated first of all from T-zone lymphoma (see p. 214) and centrocytic lymphoma. Centrocytic lymphoma never contains "clear cells". The reticulin fibres are thicker and less abundant. Small vessels often show hyaline deposits in and around their walls. The nuclei are not as pleomorphic as those of the T-cell lymphoma, since they tend to be round or indented and are never serrated. Nevertheless, there are cases of centrocytic lymphoma that cannot be distinguished morphologically from pleomorphic, small cell T-cell lymphoma. Mycosis fungoides may also show certain similarities (see p. 177). Finally, lymphoblastic lymphoma occasionally poses problems in a differential diagnosis (see p. 249).

Prognosis. The life expectancy of patients with pleomorphic, small cell T-cell lymphoma is greater than that of patients with the medium-sized and large cell type. The probability of survival also appears to be somewhat higher than that of patients with T-zone lymphoma (see Fig. 128).

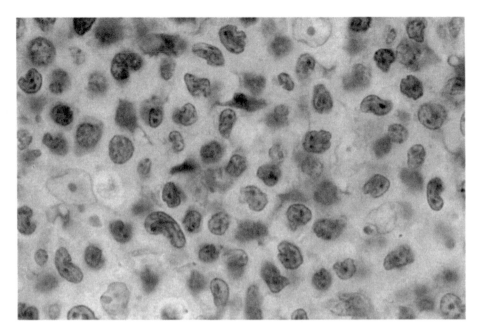

Fig. 130. Pleomorphic, small cell T-cell lymphoma. The tumour cells are interspersed with some large macrophages. Male, 58 years. Cervical node. Giemsa. 1094:1

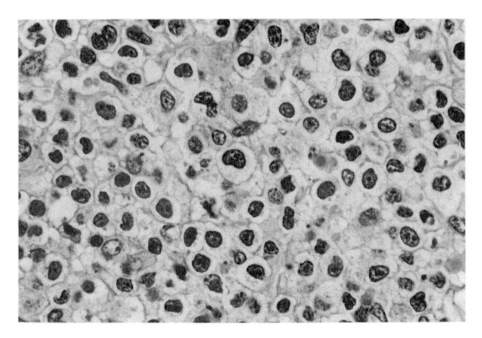

Fig. 131. Pleomorphic, small cell T-cell lymphoma showing "clear" cells. Female, 8 years. Axillary node. H & E. 695:1

4.2 High-Grade Malignant Lymphomas of T-Cell Type

4.2.1 Pleomorphic, Medium-Sized and Large Cell T-Cell Lymphoma

WF: Malignant lymphoma, large cell, immunoblastic, polymorphous (H)

Lukes-Collins: T-immunoblastic sarcoma

Definition. The tumour is composed of medium-sized, of large or of medium-sized and large cells showing a considerable degree of nuclear pleomorphism. The patients can be HTLV-1 positive (in endemic areas). In such virus-positive cases the nuclear *pleo*morphism often tends to show up as "polymorphism"; i.e. the variations in shape among cells of the same type ("pleomorphism") are not as prominent as the presence of various cell types of different sizes, which look like various stages of maturation in a haematological sense ("polymorphism"). Since these cells also show a certain degree of pleomorphism among themselves, we have included the tumours in this category. Our decision to do so was confirmed during the workshop in 1984, when the Japanese experts on ATLL were often, but not always, able to make a histological distinction between virus-positive and virus-negative cases.[523] To avoid mixing up the morphology of HTLV-1-positive and HTLV-1-negative cases, we shall discuss only the HTLV-1-negative European cases in the present section. The endemic pleomorphic T-cell lymphomas caused by HTLV-1 will be described in a separate section (Addendum, p. 223), prepared for the most part by one of the greatest authorities on ATLL, T. SUCHI.

Immunology. Tumour cells characteristically show the phenotype of peripheral T cells (CD2+, CD3+, CD5+, and CD4+ or CD8+). In about 20% of cases there is a partial loss of antigens, which results in an incomplete immunophenotype. Approximately 30% of cases show cells with features of activated cells, viz. expression of IL-2 receptors (CD25) and HLA-DR/DQ or CD30. Cases that are CD25 positive are simultaneously CD7 positive. The lack of the latter antigen, combined with the expression of IL-2 receptors, may be an indication of HTLV-1 positivity. The number of proliferating cells (Ki-67+) also increases as the tumour cells increase in size. Proliferation rates between 15% and 80% are found, with a median of about 60%. Follicular dendritic cells occasionally occur in small, residual foci.

This group of lymphomas shows clonal rearrangement of the TcRγ- and TcRβ-chain genes, as do other types of peripheral T-cell lymphoma.

Occurrence. Pleomorphic, medium-sized and large cell T-cell lymphoma accounts for only about 2.6% of the nodal lymphomas in our collection. It makes up 15.5% of the T-cell lymphomas. The youngest patient in our collection was 13 years old, while the oldest was 87. The age curve reveals a peak incidence in the 8th decade of life. There is a slight predominance of males, with a male-to-female ratio of approximately 1.35:1.

---

[523] Lennert et al. 1985.

Clinical Picture. The tumour is often first diagnosed on a biopsy of an enlarged lymph node. It is not uncommon, however, for the first biopsy to come from the skin, tonsils, soft tissues or stomach. Particular attention should be paid to the so-called *midline granuloma* (see p. 261). The tumour phase of mycosis fungoides shows the picture of pleomorphic, medium-sized and large cell T-cell lymphoma.

Histology. The tumour cells are sometimes predominantly medium-sized (Fig. 132), sometimes predominantly large (Fig. 133); more often, however, there is a mixture of medium-sized and large cells. Typical cases show an extraordinary variety of nuclear configurations. Often the nucleus is convex and smooth on one side, while the opposite side is concave and has many irregular indentations (cf. Fig. 129). The resulting pictures are often very bizarre, occasionally reminding one of jellyfish or embryos. There are also nuclei that could be described as cerebriform.[524] The chromatin is moderately fine or coarse. The nucleoli are large, of varying shape and number, and basophilic. The cytoplasm is moderately abundant and moderately basophilic. Occasionally, a small to moderate number of eosinophils and sporadic mast cells are interspersed among the tumour cells. Now and again one also sees interdigitating cells, which also have bizarre-looking nuclei. These cells show very fine chromatin, however, and the nuclear membrane looks like an outline drawn with a sharp pencil. The cytoplasm is hardly recognizable. At times giant tumour cells are found. The number of mitotic figures is moderately high to high. In a few cases the (medium-sized) nuclei are only slightly pleomorphic. In such cases the nuclei may bear a certain resemblance to those of centroblasts. Angio-invasion and angiodestruction are sometimes prominent.

Diagnosis. Despite the pleomorphism of the nuclei, the appearance of the tumour cells is relatively monotonous (in contrast to those of the HTLV-1-induced tumour in the same category!). The pleomorphism is so characteristic, providing the slides are impeccable, that this type of T-cell lymphoma can even be diagnosed without immunological stainings.

Differential Diagnosis. There is no other type of lymphoma that could be seriously confused with pleomorphic, medium-sized and large cell T-cell lymphoma. Only in exceptional cases showing slight pleomorphism might centroblastic lymphoma be considered in a differential diagnosis. An immunohistochemical analysis quickly provides an answer, however.

It is often but not always possible for an expert to distinguish between virus-positive and virus-negative cases.[525] In virus-positive cases the variation in the size of the nuclei is much more pronounced than the irregularity of the nuclear configuration.

---

[524] Weisenburger et al. 1982.
[525] Lennert et al. 1985.

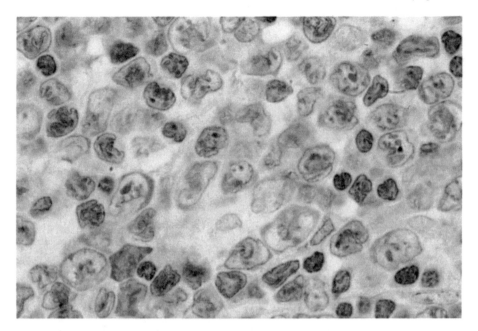

Fig. 132. Pleomorphic, medium-sized cell T-cell lymphoma. The nuclei have bizarre shapes. There are also some large cells. Male, 54 years. Parotid node. Giemsa. 1024 : 1

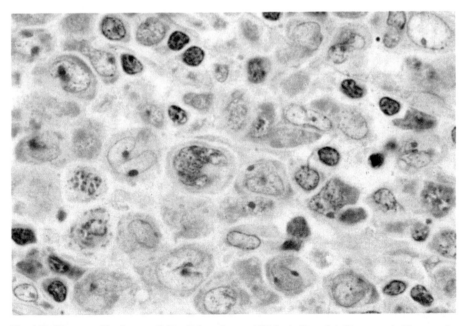

Fig. 133. Pleomorphic, large cell T-cell lymphoma (CD8 +). Female, 42 years. Axillary node. Giemsa. 1024 : 1

Prognosis. The survival rates of our patients with pleomorphic, medium-sized cell T-cell lymphoma were clearly lower than those of the pleomorphic, small cell type and T-zone lymphoma, but somewhat better than that of the pleomorphic, large cell type (Fig. 128). Pleomorphic, medium-sized and large cell T-cell lymphomas hence show the clinical behaviour of high-grade ML.

Addendum: Adult T-Cell Leukaemia/Lymphoma (ATLL)[526]

This particular type of T-cell lymphoma was discovered by TAKATSUKI et al.[527] and found to be endemic in certain parts of southwestern Japan, particularly Kyushu. Shortly thereafter, endemic cases were recognized in the Caribbean basin and in immigrants from this region in England and Holland.[528] Sporadic cases have also been reported in the United States.[529] The lymphoma is caused by the retrovirus HTLV-1.[530]

Epidemiology.[531] A variable proportion (up to 40%) of the inhabitants of the endemic areas are healthy carriers of HTLV-1.[532] These persons are seropositive for the ATLL antigen and have polyclonally integrated viral genomes in their T cells. The virus is transmitted mainly from mother to child or from husband to wife.[533] It has been estimated that one of every 900 male carriers of the virus and one of 2000 female carriers older than 40 years develop ATLL each year.

Immunology. As a rule, the phenotype is that of peripheral helper/inducer T cells (CD3+, CD4+, CD1−, CD8−) with simultaneous expression of the antigens associated with cell activation, viz. HLA-DR and CD25. Only a few cases are of suppressor/cytotoxic subtype (CD8+). A few tumours have shown co-expression of CD4 and CD8, but were CD1 negative.[534] All cases are CD7 negative.

Occurrence. ATLL affects adults; the mean age is 57 years. There is only a slight male preponderance (male-to-female ratio is approx. 1.4:1). This contrasts with most other types of lymphoma in Japan, which affect men much more frequently.

Clinical Picture. ATLL is usually leukaemic or subleukaemic. The neoplastic cells in the peripheral blood have highly lobulated nuclei.[535] Immunologically, they are of helper/inducer type.[536] In some cases, however, the cells suppress B-cell differentiation in vitro.[537]

---

[526] This section was written in collaboration with T. Suchi.
[527] Takatsuki et al. 1976a; Uchiyama et al. 1977.
[528] Catovsky et al. 1982a; Vyth-Dreese and De Vries 1982; Swerdlow et al. 1984.
[529] Grossman et al. 1981; Kadin and Kamoun 1982; Jaffe et al. 1984.
[530] Poiesz et al. 1980; Blattner et al. 1982; Yoshida et al. 1982.
[531] Tajima et al. 1986.
[532] Tajima and Kuroishi 1985.
[533] Tajima et al. 1982; Komuro et al. 1983; Kinoshita et al. 1984; Nakano et al. 1984.
[534] Shamoto et al. 1984.
[535] Hanaoka 1984.
[536] Hattori et al. 1981.
[537] Takatsuki et al. 1982.

Since the bone marrow is usually involved only slightly, anaemia is not a significant symptom. Lymphadenopathy is common and it is often generalized. Hepatomegaly and splenomegaly are also found in many patients. The skin is often affected, with lesions in the form of erythematous patches and papules (histologically, the skin lesions resemble those of mycosis fungoides, since they often show epidermal infiltration and Pautrier's microabscesses!). Hypercalcaemia is associated with ATLL in up to 50% of cases and may result in renal failure. Most patients have hypogammaglobulinaemia, but a few show a polyclonal or even a monoclonal increase in Ig. Cellular immunity is markedly reduced. Due to the considerable reduction in both humoral and cellular immunity, patients are very susceptible to bacterial and viral infections, including opportunistic ones. Hence infections are a common cause of death.

Histology. The nuclei are extremely pleomorphic. They are often even more pleomorphic than those seen in the virus-negative cases (Figs. 134, 135). Particularly striking is the marked variation in the size of the nuclei. The nuclei of medium-sized cells are approximately 6–9 μm in diameter, the large ones about 10–12 μm. The medium-sized cells have dense chromatin. The large cells show round or oval nuclei with a distinct nuclear membrane and from two to five large, basophilic nucleoli. In all cases large cells with nuclei that have multiple indentations on one side ("jellyfish" appearance) are found. The cytoplasm is moderately abundant and grey or blue (basophilic) with Giemsa staining. Many mitotic figures are present.

Giant cells are often found in ATLL (Fig. 135), and two kinds are recognizable, viz. giant cells of the Sternberg-Reed type and those of the cerebriform type. Cells of the first type show large, often lobulated nuclei with a pale nuclear membrane, very fine, weakly stained chromatin and very large, violet, occasionally vacuolated nucleoli. The cytoplasm is abundant and greyish blue with Giemsa staining. Giant cells of the cerebriform type[538] show deep indentations in the nuclear membrane, coarse, basophilic chromatin and two or three large, basophilic nucleoli. This second type appears to be very characteristic of, if not specific to, HTLV-1-positive T-cell lymphomas.[539]

The tumours are generally interspersed with a fair number of macrophages. Plasma cells are rare. Eosinophils, however, are occasionally plentiful. Epithelioid venules may be conspicuous, but generally they are not arborizing.

Prognosis. The prognosis is less favourable than that of the virus-negative pleomorphic, medium-sized and large cell T-cell lymphomas. The median survival time is 4.7 months.[540] This may be due in part to hypercalcaemia. Another reason for the early deaths is the patients' increased susceptibility to bacterial and viral infections. In addition to the rapidly progressive cases of ATLL there is a group of chronic or even smouldering cases that show fewer leukaemic cells in the peripheral blood and a prolonged clinical course. Histologically, such cases correspond to the pleomorphic, small cell type (see p. 217).

---

[538] Kikuchi et al. 1986.
[539] Kikuchi et al. 1986.
[540] Suchi et al. 1987.

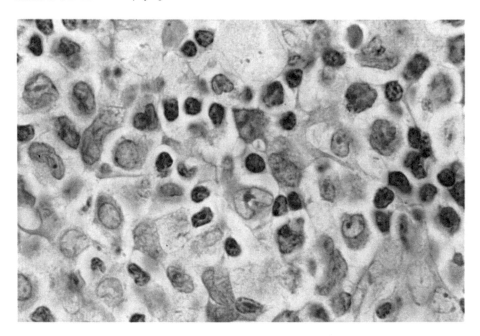

Fig. 134. HTLV-1-positive, Japanese T-cell lymphoma (ATLL). Giemsa. 1024:1

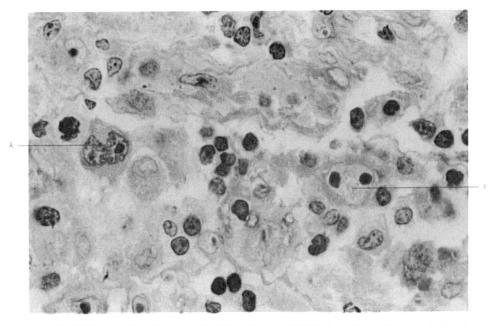

Fig. 135. HTLV-1-positive, Japanese T-cell lymphoma (ATLL). Two giant cells, one of which is of the Sternberg-Reed type (two giant nucleoli, delicate nuclear membrane; *s*). The other giant cell corresponds to the type described by KIKUCHI (markedly pleomorphic, cerebriform nucleus with a thick membrane; nucleoli are somewhat smaller and more basophilic; *k*). Giemsa. 1024:1

4.2.2 Immunoblastic Lymphoma of T-Cell Type

WF: Malignant lymphoma, large cell, immunoblastic, including clear cell (H)

Lukes-Collins: T-immunoblastic sarcoma

Definition. We apply the term "T-immunoblastic lymphoma" to a tumour composed of large cells with round or oval nuclei and one large, solitary nucleolus or several medium-sized nucleoli. The cytoplasm is either markedly basophilic (dark blue), weakly basophilic (grey) or clear as water ("clear cell"). T-immunoblastic lymphoma can be primary, or it can develop secondarily out of various low-grade malignant T-cell lymphomas. HTLV-1-positive cases are found in endemic regions.

Immunology. The cells of this type of lymphoma show the phenotype of peripheral T cells. In most cases the tumour cells express CD4, rarely CD8, but never both. T-immunoblastic lymphoma shows a partial loss of antigens (CD2, CD3, CD5, CD4 or CD8) more often than do low-grade malignant T-cell lymphomas. The number of Ki-67-positive cells is higher than 50%.

As in other types of peripheral T-cell lymphoma, there is rearrangement of the TcRγ- and TcRβ-chain genes.

Occurrence. T-immunoblastic lymphoma is a rare disease. It makes up 1.1% of the cases in our collection, or 6.4% of the T-cell lymphomas. It can occur at any age except for the first decade of life. The youngest patient was 17 years old, the oldest was 83. A peak emerges in the 7th–8th decade.

Clinical Picture. A leukaemic blood picture is frequently seen in the HTLV-1-positive type. This is uncommon in HTLV-1-negative cases. The tumour often develops in lymph nodes and not infrequently in the gastrointestinal tract, including the tonsils; it may also arise in other organs.

Histology. The tumour is composed of fairly uniform, large cells with large (10–12 μm), round or oval nuclei. The chromatin is coarse. Usually, only one large, solitary nucleolus is found, but occasionally there are several medium-sized nucleoli. The cytoplasm varies in appearance such that three variants can be distinguished: (1) It is scanty to moderately abundant and markedly basophilic, i.e. dark blue with Giemsa staining (such cases are usually CD4 +, sometimes HTLV-1 +; Fig. 136). (2) It is moderately abundant and grey (such cases are sometimes CD8 +, sometimes HTLV-1 +; Fig. 137). (3) It is abundant and clear as water (Fig. 138). Giant cells are rare. Sometimes the tumour cells are interspersed with eosinophils, which occasionally occur in large numbers. Mast cells are found now and again. The number of interdigitating cells is small in most cases but may be large in a few cases. Macrophages sometimes occur in large numbers. Clusters of epithelioid cells are seen occasionally. Mitotic activity is high. The venules do not stand out; they have flat endothelial cells and are often incompletely developed.

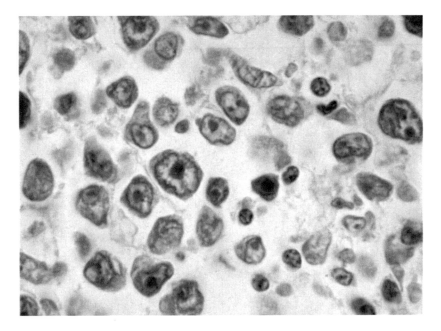

Fig. 136. T-immunoblastic lymphoma with Giemsa staining. Intensely basophilic tumour cells with large, mostly solitary nucleoli. Autopsy specimen, hence the cells are shrunken. Female, 65 years. Abdominal node. 1550 : 1

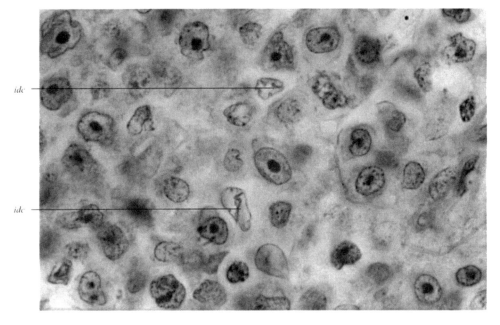

Fig. 137. T-immunoblastic lymphoma showing grey cytoplasm and prominent, solitary nucleoli. Some interdigitating cells (*idc*). Male, 68 years. Cervical node. Giemsa. 1024 : 1

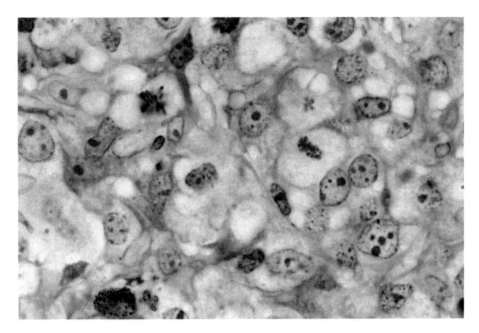

Fig. 138. T-immunoblastic lymphoma of "clear" cell type. Three mitotic figures. At *lower left*, one mast cell. Male, 45 years. Inguinal node. Giemsa. 1024:1

Diagnosis. See Definition.

Differential Diagnosis. T-immunoblastic lymphoma with basophilic cytoplasm is isomorphic with B-immunoblastic lymphoma without plasmacytic differentiation. Immunohistochemical methods are necessary to identify an ambiguous case as a T-immunoblastic lymphoma. T-immunoblastic lymphoma with grey cytoplasm must be distinguished morphologically from large cell anaplastic lymphoma (see p. 242); both types of lymphoma may be CD30 positive. The "clear cell" type does not pose any problems in a differential diagnosis. Otherwise, the differential diagnosis must take into consideration the entire spectrum that we treated in connection with B-immunoblastic lymphoma (see pp. 131 ff.).

Prognosis. The prognosis for most patients with T-immunoblastic lymphoma is apparently unfavourable. This is shown by the survival curves presented by SUCHI et al.[541]

---

[541] 1987.

4.2.3 Large Cell Anaplastic Lymphoma of T-Cell Type (Ki-1 +)

WF: Not listed

Lukes-Collins: T-immunoblastic sarcoma (anaplastic, Ki-1 +)

History and Definition. In a study applying the antibody Ki-1 (CD30) to unclassifiable tumours it was discovered that there is a large cell tumour, often resembling carcinoma, which must be interpreted as ML but which did not fit into any of the categories that had been defined until then.[542] The antibody was developed by fusion with a Hodgkin cell line[543] provided by V. DIEHL and was originally considered to be a valuable marker for Hodgkin and Sternberg-Reed cells. Later, however, STEIN et al.[544] showed that the antibody recognizes an antigen present on activated T and B lymphocytes. Hence Ki-1-positive cells are found in reactive lymph nodes and, with varying degrees of frequency, in a number of ML, particularly of the T-cell type. If all, or all but a few, of the tumour cells react positively there are two possibilities:[545] either the tumour is a large cell anaplastic lymphoma (LCAL), or it is one of the defined high-grade ML of the B-cell or T-cell series (Table 26). If the tumour cannot be placed in one of the other categories of high-grade ML, we call it LCAL, provided the following morphological criteria are fulfilled: the tumour cells are large to giant in size and have abundant, greyish blue cytoplasm (with Giemsa staining) and usually multiple, medium-sized to very large nucleoli. The growth pattern often corresponds to the familiar picture of so-called malignant histiocytosis.[546] Often one suspects a metastasis of an undifferentiated carcinoma or malignant melanoma. With very few exceptions, CD30 can be demonstrated in practically all of the tumour cells with immunohistological stains (BerH2 or HRS-4). What is remarkable is that epithelial membrane antigen (EMA) can also be demonstrated in some cases, but this does not allow one to assume that the tumour is a carcinoma. Since very rare cases of CD30-positive carcinoma do exist and, conversely, exceptional cases of LCAL express cytokeratin (KL1),[546a] it is advisable to take a critical view of a purely immunohistochemical evaluation.[547] Like most of the other antibodies that we use today, Ki-1 (CD30) is not absolutely specific. The diagnostic significance of CD30 expression must be critically assessed in conjunction with other antibody reactions and, above all, with subtle morphological criteria.

The term "large cell anaplastic lymphoma"[548] was introduced because cells of the same morphology do not occur in normal or reactive lymphoid tissue; hence it is not possible to correlate them with a specific cell type, as in other types of NHL. The word "anaplastic" seemed to us to reflect this situation best. We

---

[542] Stein et al. 1985.
[543] Schwab et al. 1982.
[544] 1985.
[545] Lennert and Feller 1985; Engelhard et al. 1986.
[546] Byrne and Rappaport 1973.
[546a] Gustmann et al. 1991.
[547] Pallesen and Hamilton-Dutoit 1988.
[548] Stein et al. 1985; Suchi et al. 1987; Stansfeld et al. 1988.

Table 26. Diagnosis in 95 cases of CD30-positive non-Hodgkin's lymphoma (NHL). (Data from ENGELHARD et al. 1992)

	n			
Large cell anaplastic lymphoma	72			
Primary		52		
Secondary		20		
in T-cell lymphoma			17	
mycosis fungoides				3
lymphoepithelioid lymphoma				1
AILD (LgX) type				3
T-zone lymphoma				5
pleomorphic, medium-sized and				
large cell T-cell lymphoma				5
in Hodgkin's lymphoma			3	
CD30-positive NHL of different morphology	23			
B-cell types		11		
centroblastic			5	
immunoblastic			3	
unclassified			3	
T-cell types		12		
pleomorphic, medium-sized and large cell			10	
immunoblastic			2	

have dropped the original name "Ki-1 lymphoma", which was also used by KADIN et al.,[549] because the decisive feature is the morphology, and not the CD30 expression.

In the United States, for a long time, very little notice was taken of LCAL. Until recently, only KADIN's group had published several papers on LCAL.[550] In the meantime, there have been several other publications.[551] LIEBERMAN et al.[552] have pointed out, justifiably, that LCAL corresponds, at least in part, to the "sinusoidal large cell ('histiocytic') lymphoma" of OSBORNE et al.[553]

Subtypes of CD30-Positive Lymphoma. The cases of ML in which all, or nearly all the tumour cells express CD30 belong to the categories listed in Table 26.[553a]

LCAL may be primary or secondary. The primary type is more frequent (2.6 times) than the secondary type. The secondary type can either occur simultaneously with a peripheral T-cell lymphoma or develop after a certain period of time out of a low-grade malignant T-cell lymphoma or Hodgkin's lymphoma. We refer to a case as a "simultaneous" secondary lymphoma if the LCAL is diagnosed shortly prior to, at the same time as, or up to 3 months after the diagnosis of a low-grade ML or Hodgkin's lymphoma.

---

[549] 1986.

[550] Kadin et al. 1986; Agnarsson and Kadin 1988.

[551] Bitter et al. 1990; Carbone et al. 1990; Ebraim et al. 1990; Kinney et al. 1990; Abbondanzo and Sulak 1991; Dehner 1991; Greer et al. 1991.

[552] 1986.

[553] 1980.

[553a] Cf. Piris et al. 1990.

Secondary LCAL occurred in patients with the following types of lymphoma: mycosis fungoides (three cases), T-zone lymphoma (five cases), LeL (one case), AILD (LgX) type of T-cell lymphoma (three cases), pleomorphic, medium-sized and large cell T-cell lymphoma (i.e. high-grade ML! five cases) and Hodgkin's lymphoma (three cases). The number of LCAL that developed in patients with Hodgkin's lymphoma is underrepresented in Table 26 because our series was preselected.

In the group of CD30-positive NHL of the known categories, T-cell lymphomas were somewhat more frequent than B-cell lymphomas. The B-cell lymphomas were mostly of the centroblastic and immunoblastic types, whereas there were no cases of BL. The T-cell lymphomas were predominantly of the pleomorphic (medium-sized and large cell) type, and there were a few immunoblastic lymphomas. All tumours were high-grade ML. Evidently, lymphoblastic lymphomas are never CD30 positive.

In addition to these completely CD30-positive NHL, the low-grade and high-grade malignant T-cell lymphomas include cases in which a small or fairly large percentage of the tumour cells express CD30. More than half the cases of peripheral T-cell lymphoma show at least a few CD30-positive tumour cells.

Immunology. In the first large-scale study[554] of LCAL (45 cases), 57.8% were definitely of T-cell type, 26.7% were probably of T-cell type, and 15.6% were of B-cell type. Another large series[555] was analysed according to the suggested division of CD30-positive NHL into primary and secondary LCAL and large cell non-anaplastic NHL of different morphology. Immunohistologically, 58% of the LCAL cases were of T-cell type, 10% were of B-cell type, and the rest were either of the "null" type or unclassifiable (Table 27). GRIESSER et al.[556] analysed 16 cases of the "null" type with molecular genetic methods. In 14 cases they found T-cell type rearrangements, sometimes with aberrant Ig_H chain rearrangement. Only two cases did not show rearrangement. The CD30-positive NHL of different morphology ("non-LCAL") included approximately equal proportions of T-cell and B-cell lymphomas. A genotypic analysis of 30 LCAL cases produced results similar to those of immunophenotyping: 16 cases were of T-cell type, six were of B-cell type, and eight cases could not be classified as belonging to either the B-cell or the T-cell system.[557]

Hence we distinguish the following phenotypic subtypes of LCAL:

1. LCAL of T-Cell Type. This type accounts for about two-thirds of the CD30-positive cases of primary and secondary LCAL. The tumour cells show an immunophenotype that is incomplete when compared with that of peripheral T lymphocytes, with predominant expression of CD2, less common expression of CD3 and frequent expression of CD4. CD4 expression, however, may not be

---

[554] Stein et al. 1985.
[555] Engelhard et al. 1992.
[556] 1991.
[557] O'Connor et al. 1987; Feller and Griesser 1989.

Table 27. Immunophenotype of 92 cases of large cell anaplastic lymphoma and Ki-1 (CD30)-positive non-Hodgkin's lymphoma (NHL) of different morphology. (Data from ENGELHARD et al. 1992)

	n	T	B	Null[a]	Unclassified[b]
Large cell anaplastic lymphoma	69	40 (58%)	7 (10%)	16 (23%)	6 (9%)
primary	52	30 (58%)	6 (11%)	11 (21%)	5 (10%)
secondary	17	10 (59%)	1 (6%)	5 (29%)	1 (6%)
Other CD30+ NHL	23	12 (52%)	11 (48%)	–	–

[a] Null = neither T-cell nor B-cell markers in cryostat sections.
[b] Frozen tissue was not available for immunophenotyping.

regarded as a specific feature of T cells. CD25 and HLA class II antigens are frequently expressed, not only in the T-cell type, but also in the B-cell and "null" types.

2. LCAL of B-Cell Type. This type turns out to be relatively rare, after the other categories of CD30-positive NHL have been eliminated. Immunohistochemically, the B-cell antigens CD19 and CD22 and, in exceptional cases, Ig are found.

3. LCAL of "Null" Type. In these cases, only antigens that indicate the state of activation of the cells, such as CD25 and HLA class II, are expressed in addition to CD30.

In a few cases that did not bear either B-cell or T-cell antigens, we found that the tumour cells stained with Ki-M6 (CD68) and Ki-M8. We concluded that LCAL includes a few cases of genuine malignant histiocytosis. STEIN[558] doubts this, because he considers CD30 to be specific to lymphoid cells. This is contradicted, however, by the findings of PALLESEN and HAMILTON-DUTOIT,[559] who have demonstrated the CD30 antigen in a number of embryonic carcinomas and thus in non-lymphoid tumours. Moreover, CD30 has been demonstrated on activated monocytes and myelomonocytic cell lines (THP1).[560] Some CD30-positive cases of genuine malignant histiocytosis have also been reported by CARBONE et al.[561] and BANKS et al.[562]

Furthermore, in all three groups expression of certain antigens is sometimes unexpectedly absent. Leucocyte common antigen (LCA) is expressed in only 30%–40% of the cases, whereas EMA can be demonstrated in one-third of the cases. The CD15 expression that is typical of Sternberg-Reed cells in Hodgkin's lymphomas is hardly ever seen in LCAL. The median percentage of Ki-67-positive cells is approximately 60%.

---

[558] Personal communication 1988.
[559] 1988.
[560] Andreesen et al. 1984; Feller 1989.
[561] 1990.
[562] 1990.

Not all cases of LCAL show expression of CD30. We have seen a few CD30-negative cases (of both B-cell and T-cell types). The existence of such cases justifies our approach: an entity should be defined *first* according to its morphology and then (if necessary) according to immunological reactions.

Cytogenetics and Molecular Genetics. A DNA analysis[563] of our cases demonstrated that the cellular origin of these lymphomas is heterogeneous. In most instances they exhibit a pattern like that of peripheral T-cell lymphomas (TcRγ+, TcRβ+), but in rare cases there is a rearrangement of Ig$_H$ genes. About 20% of cases show Ig$_H$ gene as well as TcR rearrangements, without phenotypical demonstration of B-cell or T-cell antigens. The cellular origin of such cases has not yet been determined. CD30-positive cases of LCAL, especially those of T-cell lineage, are frequently associated with the chromosomal translocation t(2;5)(p23;q35) and less frequently with t(2;13)(p23;q34).[564] Recently, IL-9 expression was demonstrated in LCAL; this antigen is thought to be involved in tumourigenesis or tumour proliferation.[564a]

Clinical Picture.[565] Of the patients listed in Table 26, about two-thirds of those with primary LCAL were in stage I or II at the time of diagnosis, whereas the secondary anaplastic lymphomas (like the CD30-positive NHL of different morphology) were usually detected at a later stage. Most patients with primary LCAL showed initial involvement of lymph nodes (cervical nodes in 15 cases, axillary in seven, mediastinal in six, retroperitoneal in five, iliac in nine and inguinal in seven). Of the sites of extranodal manifestation, skin (five cases) and Waldeyer's ring (four cases) were affected most often. The skin can be infiltrated with or without lymph nodes being involved. Only two patients with primary involvement of the spleen and only one with primary involvement of the stomach were observed. B symptoms were reported in 42% of the patients with primary LCAL and in 65% of those with a secondary lymphoma.

Occurrence. LCAL of the lymph node accounted for 1.3% of our cases of NHL collected in 1983.

We have known for some time[566] that primary LCAL appears most frequently during the first 3 decades of life. The peak occurrence is seen in the 2nd decade. Our youngest patient was 1 year old. We found a second, less steep peak in the 7th decade, however (Fig. 139). Our oldest patient was 73 years old. The male-to-female ratio was 1.65:1.

Secondary LCAL and the CD30-positive NHL of different morphology did not show a peak incidence in the 2nd decade of life, but instead tended to occur more frequently in the 5th decade. The male-to-female ratios also differed from that for primary LCAL, with 3:1 for the secondary type and 0.9:1 for the other types of NHL.

---

[563] Griesser et al. 1986b; Feller and Griesser 1989.
[564] Rimokh et al. 1989; Bitter et al. 1990; Mason et al. 1990; Sainati et al. 1990.
[564a] Merz et al. 1991.
[565] Engelhard et al. 1992.
[566] Lennert et al. 1986.

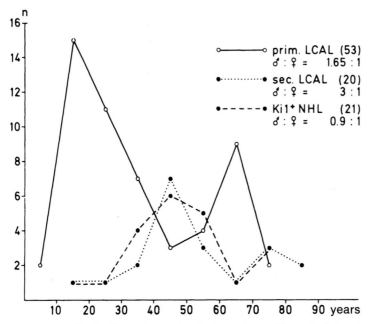

Fig. 139. Age distribution and sex ratio of primary large cell anaplastic lymphoma (*prim. LCAL*), secondary large cell anaplastic lymphoma (*sec. LCAL*) and CD30-positive non-Hodgkin's lymphoma of different morphology (*Ki1⁺ NHL*)

Histology. *Primary* LCAL was previously diagnosed in most cases as other types of neoplasia and not recognized as a specific type of ML. The growth pattern is not uniform, but it usually differs from that of the other large cell NHL.

A diagnosis of LCAL can often be made at a relatively low magnification. One sees large, usually moderately basophilic cells (grey with Giemsa staining) with one of the following characteristic growth patterns:

1. The tumour cells proliferate *in the sinuses* (Fig. 140), causing distension. In early stages of metastatic lymph node infiltration the marginal sinuses are chiefly affected.
2. The tumour cells are intermingled with many large, reactive macrophages. Basophilic and non-basophilic cells show a pattern that was previously considered characteristic of *malignant histiocytosis* (Figs. 141, 142).[567] Other histological features of malignant histiocytosis, as it was previously defined, are also found: The tumour tissue often shows extravasation of erythrocytes (Fig. 144). There may be erythrophagocytosis by the reactive macrophages and, occasionally, even by the tumour cells (Fig. 142). The intrasinusoidal growth pattern (1) also used to be regarded as a typical feature of histiocytosis.
3. The tumour cells form large, solid masses or bands that are reminiscent of the metastases of a carcinoma or melanoma (Fig. 143). The spaces between the

---

[567] Byrne and Rappaport 1973; Rilke et al. 1978b; Collins et al. 1983.

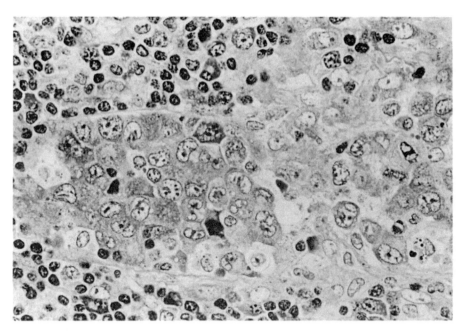

Fig. 140. Large cell anaplastic lymphoma (CD30+). Intrasinusoidal proliferation resembling "malignant histiocytosis" or carcinoma. Male, 69 years. Axillary node. Giemsa. 512:1

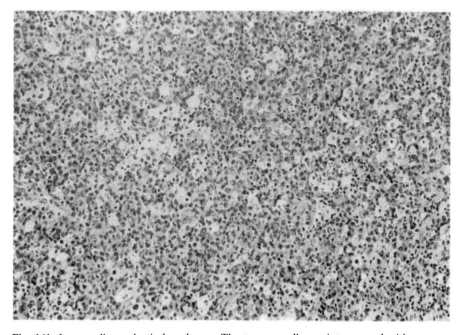

Fig. 141. Large cell anaplastic lymphoma. The tumour cells are interspersed with numerous non-neoplastic macrophages, generating a cribriform appearance. Female, 3 years. Axillary node. H & E. 140:1

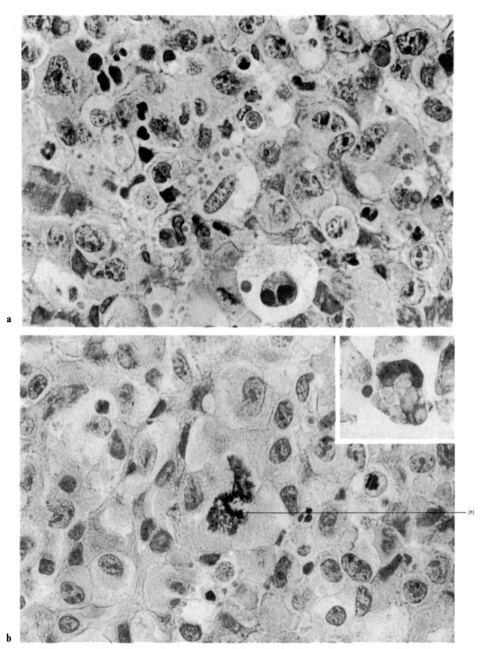

Fig. 142a, b. Large cell anaplastic lymphoma. Note the nuclear structure of the non-neoplastic macrophages—well shown in the *centre* of **a**—which differs from that of the more polymorphic nuclei of the tumour cells. The chromatin is finer, and the nucleoli are smaller that those of the tumour cells. The non-neoplastic macrophages contain tumour cell debris. In the *centre* of **b**, an atypical, polyploid mitosis (*m*). *Inset:* A large tumour cell that has phagocytosed numerous erythrocytes. Same node as Fig. 141. H & E. 875:1

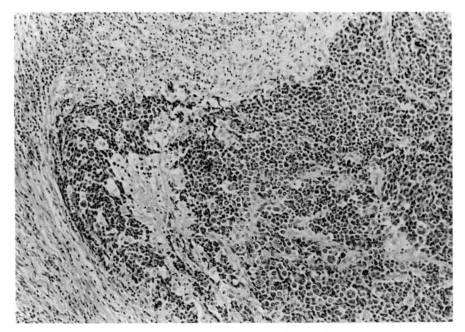

Fig. 143. Large cell anaplastic lymphoma, originally misdiagnosed as metastasis of carcinoma. No primary tumour. Four years later, the neoplasm was identified as large cell anaplastic lymphoma by means of staining with Ki-1 (CD30) antibody. H & E. 100 : 1

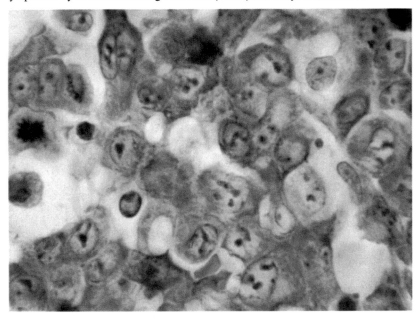

Fig. 144. Large cell anaplastic lymphoma with Giemsa staining. The tumour cells have abundant, basophilic cytoplasm that looks more grey than blue. The nuclei contain a few medium-sized, polymorphic nucleoli. Among the cohesive tumour cells there are some large non-neoplastic macrophages, which are seen better at lower magnification (cf. Fig. 141), and some (extravasated) erythrocytes. Male, 13 years. Subcutaneous tumour mass. 1550 : 1

tumour cell accumulations contain numerous reticulin fibres and small blood vessels, so one is tempted to refer to a tumour stroma. Immunostainings reveal many small T lymphocytes and, frequently, numerous macrophages in the same locations.

Sections stained by silver impregnation often show a marked increase in the number of reticulin fibres. The capsule is often highly fibrous and enlarged. Necrotic areas may be seen, but they are mostly small.

The cytology of LCAL is not completely uniform. The tumour cells range in size from large to giant. Where the appearance resembles histiocytosis one sees multiple, often elongated nucleoli in a nucleus that is generally round or somewhat irregular in shape (Fig. 144). The chromatin is fine to moderately coarse. The cytoplasm is abundant and grey or greyish blue with Giemsa staining. It sometimes shows vacuoles and occasionally a perinuclear pale area. The tumour cells are interspersed with reactive macrophages, which have round nuclei with solitary nucleoli, fine chromatin and very pale cytoplasm that occasionally contains debris of phagocytosis. After chemotherapy the tumour cells may be greatly reduced in size. The tumour may then correspond to a pleomorphic, small cell T-cell lymphoma (Fig. 145).

Where the appearance is closer to that of a carcinoma the tumour cells are usually even larger. In these and in other cases, giant cells may occur that are more basophilic and show very large, solitary or multiple nucleoli. It is practically impossible to distinguish them from Sternberg-Reed cells.

The tumour cells are often interspersed with some (polytypic) plasma cells and eosinophil and neutrophil granulocytes. There may also be a marked increase in the number of eosinophils and neutrophils, in which case one must consider the possibility of Hodgkin's lymphoma, although one cannot make this inference with certainty (the presence of Sternberg-Reed cells in such cases would not, by itself, be proof of a Hodgkin's lymphoma!).

CHAN et al.[568] and CHOTT et al.[569] distinguished two cytological subtypes of LCLA:

Subtype I chiefly consists of polymorphic cells with slightly basophilic cytoplasm. Multinucleate giant cells, occasionally of the Sternberg-Reed type, are frequently found. The nuclei usually show a large, solitary nucleolus.

Subtype II shows relatively monomorphic cells with more or less pronounced basophilia of the cytoplasm. Usually there are only a few giant cells. The nucleoli are quite often multiple and sometimes elongated.

In addition, CHAN et al.[570] have described a sarcomatoid variant that consisted of "interweaving fascicles of plump spindle and oval neoplastic cells" and resembled malignant fibrous histiocytoma. Since the tumour cells not only expressed CD45RO and CD30 but were also LCA positive, the neoplasm was interpreted as LCAL.

---

[568] 1989.

[569] 1990.

[570] 1990.

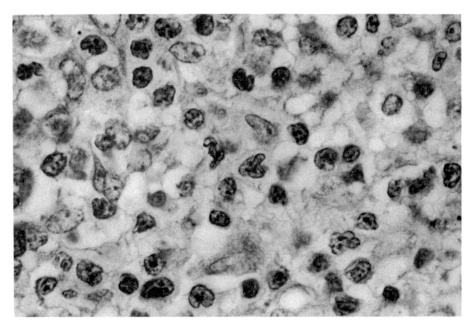

Fig. 145. Same case as Fig. 140. After the patient was treated with chemotherapy the tumour transformed into pleomorphic, small cell T-cell lymphoma. Giemsa. 1024:1

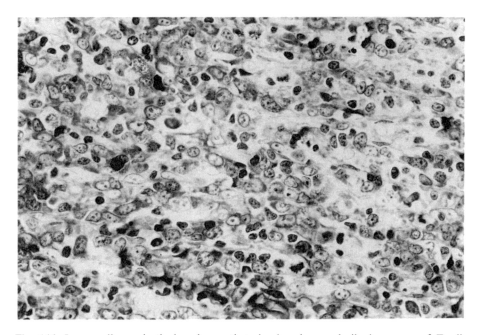

Fig. 146. Large cell anaplastic lymphoma that developed secondarily in a case of T-cell lymphoma of AILD (LgX) type. The secondary tumour has an inhomogeneous appearance. There are narrow bands and groups of large CD30-positive cells among the cells remaining from the T-cell lymphoma of AILD (LgX) type. The large tumour cells express T-cell antigens. Giemsa. 448:1

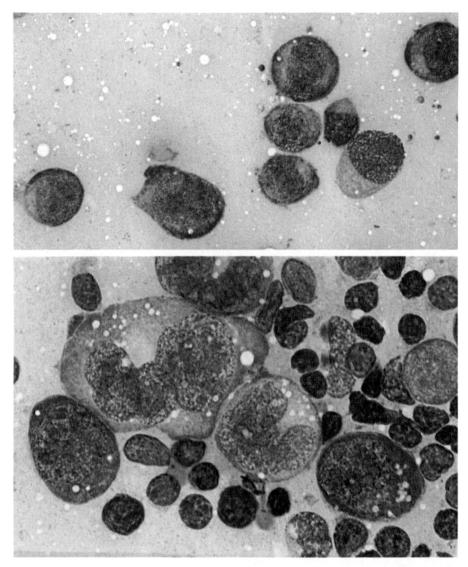

Fig. 147a, b. Large cell anaplastic lymphoma. **a** The cells are large, but there are no giant cells. Same case as Fig. 140. **b** A different case showing large cells and giant cells. Pappenheim. **a** 1024:1, **b** 825:1

Secondary LCAL is often distinctive even at a low magnification, in that it has not developed in a normal lymph node, but instead is surrounded by, and occasionally interspersed with, remnants of the primary low-grade ML or Hodgkin's lymphoma. For example, one finds small to medium-sized, pleomorphic T cells in lieu of the typical small lymphocytes. In another case one might recognize areas containing typical Sternberg-Reed cells, lacunar cells and lymphocytes at the periphery (this would be a case of secondary LCAL in a patient with Hodgkin's

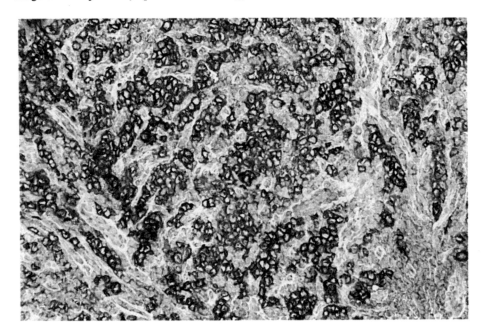

Fig. 148. Large cell anaplastic lymphoma. The tumour cells are arranged in cohesive bands. Male, 14 years. Mediastinal node. Ki-1 staining, APAAP method. 110:1

lymphoma). When the AILD (LgX) type of T-cell lymphoma is the primary neoplasm the CD30-positive cells are sometimes diffusely scattered over the section and do not form large, solid tumour infiltrates (Fig. 146).

Cytology and Cytochemistry. We have previously described the morphology and cytochemistry of lymph node imprints in detail,[571] although at that time we diagnosed the tumour as "malignant histiocytosis" (Fig. 147). We pointed out that the cells are medium-sized to large and basophilic, and that they sometimes show considerable erythrophagocytosis. These cells are intermingled with many reactive macrophages showing signs of phagocytosis. In addition to this type, which resembles histiocytosis, there are cases of LCAL composed of larger cells and showing a pronounced tendency to form giant cells. The giant cells bear a certain similarity to Sternberg-Reed cells. They also have prominent nucleoli, but not of the typical, basophilic, "cut-out" appearance found in classic Hodgkin and Sternberg-Reed cells.

Enzyme cytochemically, the cells show predominantly *focal* non-specific esterase and, more characteristically, focal acid phosphatase reactions.

---

[571] Lennert and Mohri 1978 (p. 460).

Diagnosis. In all large cell tumours in which the cells look grey with Giemsa staining and that are reminiscent of malignant histiocytosis or metastases of poorly differentiated tumours one must consider the possibility of LCAL. By applying the CD30 antibody Ber-H2 or HRS-4 to paraffin sections it is possible to make sure of the diagnosis (Fig. 148). To be even more certain one should use further antibodies, viz. KL1 (keratin), LCA (pan-leucocyte antibody), a pan-T marker and a pan-B marker. Unfortunately, these reactions occasionally overlap. Very sporadically we have seen KL1-positive lymphomas that were simultaneously LCA positive and whose clinical picture (no primary tumour, favourable response to chemotherapy) confirmed the assumption of LCAL.[572] These lymphomas were also proven by detection of TcRcβ rearrangement.[573]

It is sometimes impossible to draw a reliable conclusion about the T-cell or B-cell origin of the tumour cells merely by examining a tissue specimen that has been fixed in formalin.

In ambiguous cases it is very important to weigh the possibility of LCAL so that no time is wasted searching for a primary tumour. In no event should CD30 expression alone be considered automatic proof of LCAL. The cytomorphology must also correspond to that of LCAL. Other high-grade malignant NHL must be distinguished from this type of lymphoma on the basis of their cytological differences.

In order to differentiate between primary and secondary LCAL the pathologist has to pay very careful attention. If a secondary LCAL has developed in the same lymph node as the primary tumour ("simultaneous secondary" LCAL), the pathologist must conscientiously scrutinize the peripheral areas of the LCAL and come to a decision on whether he is dealing with normal or atypical lymphoid tissue. Atypical areas show either a relatively uniform proliferation of atypical T cells or the characteristic picture of Hodgkin's lymphoma. When the primary tumour is Hodgkin's lymphoma, this might be of clinical importance (treatment according to a protocol for Hodgkin's lymphoma?). When the AILD (LgX) type of T-cell lymphoma is the primary neoplasm, irregularly shaped accumulations of follicular dendritic cells can be identified immunohistochemically.

Differential Diagnosis. Other large cell lymphomas that can be classified unmistakably as immunoblastic lymphoma, centroblastic lymphoma or pleomorphic, large cell T-cell lymphoma according to the Kiel classification should not be designated as LCAL, even if 100% of the tumour cells are CD30 positive. In such cases the tumour cells show a characteristic nuclear configuration and a different growth pattern.

Rare cases of large cell ML, particularly of the B-cell series, cannot be assigned to any morphological category. We designate them as unclassified high-grade malignant B-cell lymphomas, even if they are CD30 positive.

We have already mentioned that LCAL must be distinguished from carcinomas (see Diagnosis).

---

[572] Feller 1989.
[573] Gustmann et al. 1991.

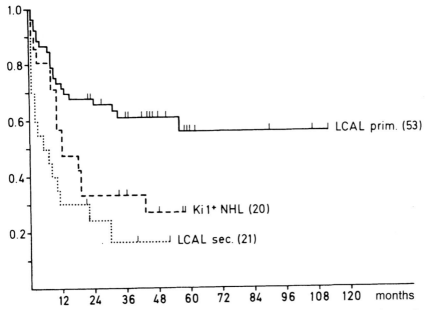

Fig. 149. Overall survival probability of patients with primary (*LCAL prim.*) and secondary large cell anaplastic lymphoma (*LCAL sec.*) and CD30-positive non-Hodgkin's lymphomas of different morphology (*Ki1⁺ NHL*). (Based on data from ENGELHARD et al. 1992)

The distinction between LCAL and malignant histiocytosis, as it used to be defined, is irrelevant: LCAL includes almost all the neoplasms previously called malignant histiocytosis. Nevertheless, there are probably a few cases that still merit the term "malignant histiocytosis".

When LCAL is localized in the skin[574] it must be distinguished from *lymphomatoid papulosis*.[575] This is sometimes impossible, however, or a distinction can be made only with a certain degree of probability. So far, the clinical picture is still of decisive importance. According to KADIN,[576] multiple small lesions with ulceration speak in favour of lymphomatoid papulosis, whereas a few large lesions indicate LCAL. There are, however, borderline and overlapping cases. Not even molecular genetic techniques enable us to make a decision for or against LCAL in such cases, because lymphomatoid papulosis usually shows rearrangement of the TcRβ gene.[577] Even monotonous-looking LCAL infiltrates in the *skin* may show spontaneous regression.

Prognosis.[578] Complete remission is more common and the median survival time is significantly longer in primary LCAL than in secondary cases, irrespective of

---

[574] Feller and Sterry 1989.
[575] Kadin et al. 1985; Slater 1987.
[576] 1990.
[577] Weiss et al. 1986; Kadin et al. 1987.
[578] Nakamura et al. 1991; Engelhard et al. 1992.

whether the LCAL developed simultaneously or subsequently in a case of low-grade ML[579] (Fig. 149). Children appear to respond particularly well to treatment. All 28 children treated in a German-Austrian trial showed complete remission and have not had relapses.[580] Patients with skin involvement, with or without lymphadenopathy, also have a relatively favourable prognosis. The immunological subtype of primary LCAL does not appear to have any influence on survival. According to CHAN et al.[581] and CHOTT et al.,[582] subtype I (slightly basophilic, polymorphic cells) shows a less favourable prognosis than does subtype II (more basophilic, less polymorphic cells). The survival rates of patients with CD30-positive large cell NHL of different morphology are much like that of secondary LCAL. The possible differentiating value of CD30 expression has been described by BELJAARDS et al.[583]

4.2.4 Lymphoblastic Lymphoma of T-Cell Type, Including T-ALL

WF: Malignant lymphoma, lymphoblastic, convoluted cell/non-convoluted cell (I)

Lukes-Collins: Convoluted T

Definition. Lymphoblastic lymphoma of T-cell type is derived from precursor cells of peripheral T lymphocytes. According to their marker profile, they can originate in the bone marrow ("prethymic type") or the thymus ("early" and "late thymus cortex type"). In most cases some of the cells have nuclei with a gyrate (convoluted) outline. This nuclear configuration is not specific, however, since it sometimes occurs in B-lymphoblastic lymphomas as well. Hence the term "convoluted cell type" can no longer pass for a synonym for T-lymphoblastic lymphoma, as originally assumed by LUKES and COLLINS[584] and by the originators of the Kiel classification. The acid phosphatase reaction, however, still plays an important role in the diagnosis. If the reaction is focal, which is true in 80% of the cases, one can be sure that one is dealing with a T-lymphoblastic lymphoma. For the other 20% of cases immunological markers are indispensable. We have not observed a focal acid phosphatase reaction in B-lymphoblastic lymphomas.

Histologically, it is impossible to distinguish a T-lymphoblastic lymphoma, i.e. the genuine tumour variant, from acute lymphoblastic leukaemia of T-cell type (T-ALL). In paediatrics the following clinical distinction is made: for a diagnosis of T-lymphoblastic lymphoma there must be no blast cells demonstrable in the blood and no more than 25% lymphoblasts in the bone marrow.

---

[579] Engelhard et al. 1986.
[580] Bucsky et al. 1989; Heitger et al. 1989.
[581] 1989.
[582] 1990.
[583] 1989; Tashiro et al. 1989.
[584] 1974a,b.

Immunology. A feature that all T-lymphoblastic lymphomas have in common is the expression of the CD7 antigen. Where this is the only antigen expressed, however, one must remember that it can also be demonstrated in about 20% of the immature myelomonocytic neoplasms. Other antigens found in immature T-lymphoblastic lymphomas include CD3 (may be demonstrated in the cytoplasm!), CD2 and CD5. The mature thymus cortex type is characterized by CD1 expression and by simultaneous expression of CD4 and CD8. With increasing maturation into peripheral T cells, either CD4 or CD8 expression is lost. The number of proliferating cells (Ki-67+) corresponds to the figures for B-lymphoblastic lymphoma, with a median of about 45%.

Immunological typing has made it possible to assign all lymphoblastic lymphomas to the B-cell or T-cell series. Blast cell infiltrates that express neither the B cell-associated antigens CD19 and/or CD22 nor the T cell-associated antigen CD7 are of myelomonocytic origin. Even when the T-cell or B-cell nature of the lymphoma is certain, however, one should still search for the expression of myelomonocytic antigens, because it is possible to find antigen coexpression on the same cell or a mixed blast cell infiltration. This would have other therapeutic and prognostic consequences.

According to KNOWLES,[585] about two-thirds of the cases of *T-ALL* express the prothymic phenotype (only CD2+, CD7+), whereas one-third of the cases show the thymus cortex phenotype (CD1+, CD2+, CD3+, CD4+ and CD8+), and only very few cases show the medullary thymus type (CD1−, CD3+, CD4+ or CD8+). In contrast, about two-thirds of the cases of (non-leukaemic) T-lymphoblastic lymphoma must be classified as belonging to the thymus cortex phenotype and one-third to the medullary thymus type. Prothymic phenotypes are almost entirely limited to T-ALL.

Very detailed immunohistochemical investigations allow us to distinguish eight stages of differentiation among the T-lymphoblastic lymphomas and leukaemias.[586] The least mature (prethymic) type expresses CD7 and HLA-DR simultaneously. In the most mature type of T-lymphoblastic lymphoma/leukaemia the partial loss of CD4 or CD8 and CD1 indicates transformation of the cells into peripheral T lymphocytes. A comparison of these phenotypic groups with clinical data revealed that children and adolescents (up to the age of 15 years) predominantly show a more mature cell phenotype (groups 6−8), while in older patients there is a preponderance of the immature differentiation types. It was possible to demonstrate a mediastinal tumour only in differentiation groups 5−7, and not in groups 1−4. Leukaemic blood pictures, however, were chiefly associated with an immature degree of differentiation.[587]

Occurrence. T-lymphoblastic lymphoma accounts for about 3%–4% of all cases of NHL in our collection and occurs mainly in the young. Cases are about equally divided between the first two decades of life; in later life, up to and including the

---

[585] 1988.
[586] Feller et al. 1986b.
[587] Feller et al. 1988.

8th decade, it occurs infrequently. Our youngest patient was 11 months old, the oldest 74 years old. The male-to-female ratio was 2.6 : 1.

Non-leukaemic lymphoblastic lymphoma of T-cell type is much more common than that of the B-cell type. Conversely, ALL of the B-cell type is more than twice as common as that of the T-cell type.

Clinical Picture. In about 80% of the cases T-lymphoblastic lymphoma begins with a ventral mediastinal tumour (generally originating from the thymus), which is often associated with pleural effusions. In addition, lymph nodes in the supraclavicular region or elsewhere may be enlarged. Lymph nodes are sometimes also the first site of visible manifestation of T-lymphoblastic lymphoma. The bone marrow may be free of infiltration at this time, but in 80% of the patients it is sooner or later included in the tumour process, and, as a result, a leukaemic blood picture appears. At this stage various extranodal organs, including the central nervous system, may be involved as well.

In a minority of cases the lymphoblastic proliferation evidently begins in the bone marrow, resulting in development of leukaemia but no mediastinal tumour, or only a small one. This is true above all in patients under 10 years of age, who show predominance of T-ALL of the prethymic immunophenotype.

Histology. The cells are relatively small or medium sized. They are spread apart (not cohesive; Figs. 150–152). The cytoplasm of T lymphoblasts is scanty and only moderately basophilic. In most cases some of the nuclei have a gyrate (convoluted) outline and show only very small, inconspicuous nucleoli and very fine chromatin. According to LUKES and COLLINS,[588] convoluted nuclei usually occur in only a small number of the tumour cells. This means that one has to search for them. We have been unable to find convoluted nuclei in only about 10% of the cases of T-lymphoblastic lymphoma. There is usually high mitotic activity. The tumour cells are occasionally interspersed with eosinophils. A slightly or moderately developed starry-sky pattern (numerous macrophages with phagocytosis of tumour cells) may be evident (Fig. 150). The reticulin fibres are very fine and usually sparse (Fig. 153).

Cytochemistry. A *focal* acid phosphatase reaction ("Golgi type"; Fig. 154) is seen in 80% of the cases. With the method used in our laboratory (no fixation!), the acid non-specific esterase reaction is almost always negative (it is positive only in peripheral T-cell lymphomas). Even with the method used by THIEL et al.[589] (fixation in formalin vapour), the acid non-specific esterase reaction is much weaker than the acid phosphatase reaction in the vast majority of cases of T-lymphoblastic lymphoma, and it is also weaker than the acid non-specific esterase reaction in peripheral T-cell lymphomas. The dipeptidyl peptidase IV (DPPIV) reaction is positive in 40% of the cases, a positive reaction being infallible proof of the T-cell nature of a tumour.[590] In smears PAS staining often discloses large

---

[588] 1974a,b, 1975a,b.
[589] 1978.
[590] Feller 1982; Lennert et al. 1982.

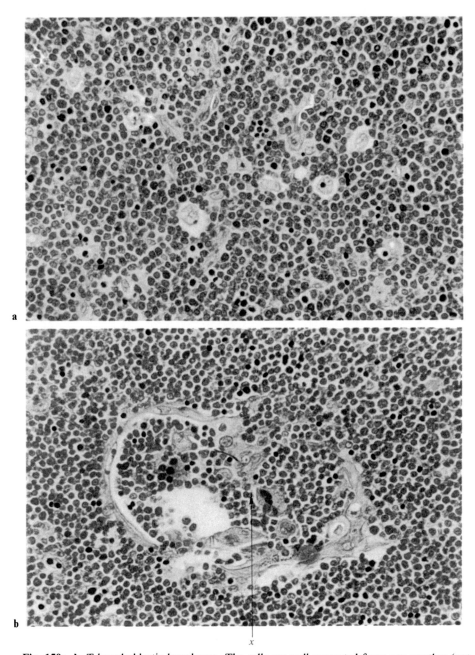

Fig. 150a, b. T-lymphoblastic lymphoma. The cells are well separated from one another (not cohesive) and often pyknotic. Numerous large macrophages with moderate tumour cell phagocytosis. In **b**, a Hassall's corpuscle, infiltrated and partially effaced by tumour cells (*x*). Male, 14 years. Thymic tumour. **a** Giemsa, **b** H & E. 350 : 1

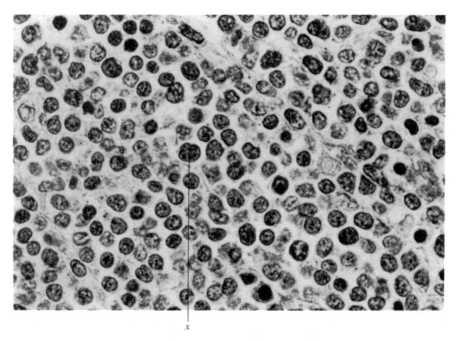

Fig. 151. T-lymphoblastic lymphoma with H & E staining. Some nuclei show "convolutions", for instance in *x*. Chromatin is somewhat coarser, and pyknotic cells and mitotic figures are less prominent than with Giemsa staining (cf. Fig. 152). Tumour cells are not "cohesive". Same case as Fig. 150. 875:1

positive granules (glycogen). Occasionally, a focal PAS reaction can be demonstrated in sections at about the same location in the cells as the acid phosphatase activity (glycoproteins).

Diagnosis. In every case of lymphoblastic lymphoma we try to clarify the nature of the lymphoblasts by applying enzyme cytochemical methods. For such analyses we ask for blood smears in leukaemic cases. In non-leukaemic cases we recommend aspiration of infiltrated organs (e.g. bone marrow or lymph nodes) so that we can apply enzyme cytochemical stains to smears prepared from this material. The best procedure is to have imprints prepared at the time of biopsy. A focal acid phosphatase reaction substantiates the diagnosis (Fig. 154). A positive DPPIV reaction yields the same degree of assurance. If these reactions are negative, however, we recommend investigating immunological markers on smears, imprints or sections of fresh tissue specimens.

Differential Diagnosis. The most important distinction is that between T-lymphoblastic lymphoma and *lymphoblastic lymphoma of B-cell type*. Although the convolutions are usually less pronounced in B-lymphoblastic lymphoma, the nuclear configuration cannot serve as a basis for the decision on whether a lymphoblastic lymphoma is of B-cell or T-cell nature. In contrast, cytochemistry

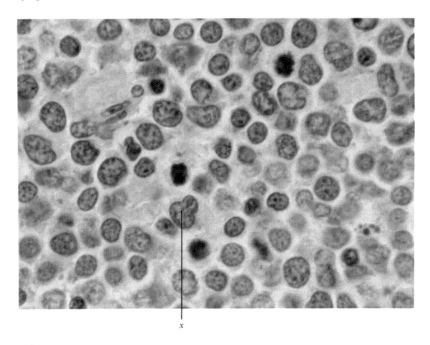

x

Fig. 152. T-lymphoblastic lymphoma with Giemsa staining. The nuclei are somewhat polymorphic and occasionally "convoluted" (*x*). Cytoplasm is hardly visible. Tumour cells are well separated from one another and show multiple, small nucleoli. Several mitotic figures. One pyknotic cell. Same case as Figs. 150 and 151. 1550:1

(acid phosphatase and DPPIV) is useful, as long as the results are positive. If the results are negative, however, we have to rely on investigations of immunological markers in sections of fresh tissue or in fresh smears or imprints.

Centrocytic lymphoma (see p. 101), *pleomorphic, small cell T-cell lymphoma,* and *acute myeloid and myelomonocytic leukaemias* (see p. 101) must also be considered in the differential diagnosis. In pleomorphic, small cell T-cell lymphoma the nuclei are much more pleomorphic and more elongated or irregularly angular. The cytoplasm is somewhat more abundant and less basophilic. The acid phosphatase reaction can be focal or granular; a positive DPPIV reaction is also found in some cases.

Prognosis. About 75% of the children with lymphoblastic lymphoma or ALL of the T-cell type go into lasting complete remission following intensive chemotherapy according to RIEHM's protocol.[591] In adults the prognosis is probably somewhat less favourable.

---

[591] H. Riehm, personal communication 1989; earlier publications by his research group: Müller-Weihrich et al. 1984, 1985; Gadner et al. 1986.

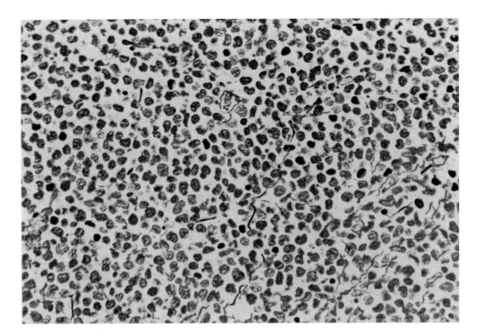

Fig. 153. T-lymphoblastic lymphoma with silver impregnation. Only very few fine reticulin fibres. Tumour cells are not "cohesive". Male, 60 years. Inguinal node. Gomori. 350:1

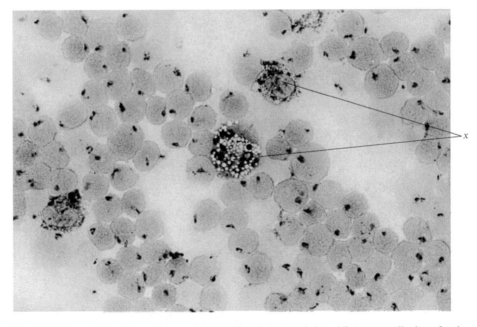

Fig. 154. T-lymphoblastic lymphoma with acid phosphatase staining. All tumour cells show focal activity. Some macrophages (x) with lipid droplets and a strongly positive, diffuse acid phosphatase reaction. Female, 4 years. Patient had a mediastinal tumour. Cerebrospinal fluid. 560:1

Addendum: Unclassified Lymphoblastic Lymphoma

We used to list the unclassified type of lymphoblastic lymphoma as a category of its own. Even today we still use the term for a case of T- or B-lymphoblastic lymphoma when we have no material for investigating cytochemical or immunological markers, since we cannot determine the origin of the tumour cells without them.

4.3 Rare and Ambiguous Types of T-Cell Lymphoma

In the categories of our working classification of T-cell lymphomas[592] we included only those tumour types of which we had seen more than five cases. In so doing, we disregarded definite cases of T-cell lymphoma that, for the time being, did not merit special categories of their own because they were so rare. We have observed, for instance, a case of low-grade malignant T-cell lymphoma consisting of the same cells as LeL, but without epithelioid cells. We do not have any category for this case yet. Likewise, we found two cases of high-grade malignant T-cell lymphoma composed of medium-sized cells that looked somewhat like centroblasts. Should we force them into the pleomorphic, medium-sized cell category, or should we continue to observe them as unclassified high-grade malignant T-cell lymphomas for the time being?

Further, we did not include any types of lymphoma that we had not seen for ourselves or that had not been proven to be separate entities or to be T-cell lymphomas. We have compiled a relatively long list of special types described in the literature. Those we consider important are presented briefly in this chapter.

4.3.1 Hairy Cell Leukaemia of T-Cell Type[593]

Saxon et al.[594] published a case that they considered to be a T-lymphocytic variant of hairy cell leukaemia (HCL). It exhibited the typical morphology of hairy cells on both light and electron microscopy. The hairy cells showed tartrate-resistant acid phosphatase activity, and the patient had massive splenomegaly. In this case Gallo's research group[595] was able to demonstrate HTLV-2 for the first time. Two leucopenic cases of T-CLL resembled HCL and were HTLV-1 or HTLV-2 positive.[596] Other cases of HCL of T-cell type have been described in more or less detail, but they were not always convincing. There have also been reports of cases of HCL of B-cell type in which the cells formed rosettes with sheep erythrocytes in vitro and were accordingly CD2 positive.[597] Other cases

---

[592] Suchi et al. 1987.
[593] Recent critical review: Rosenblatt et al. 1988.
[594] 1978.
[595] Kalyanaraman et al. 1982.
[596] Sohn et al. 1986.
[597] Cawley et al. 1978.

were assumed to contain T/B hybrid cells.[598] Hence the entity "HCL of T-cell
type" does not yet appear to have been sufficiently elucidated.[599] By no means
should the tartrate-resistant acid phosphatase reaction be considered a decisive
criterion, as this reaction is also found in T-CLL and T-PLL.

4.3.2 Large Cell Lymphoma of the Multilobated Cell Type (PINKUS)

PINKUS et al.[600] described a tumour that was composed of large cells with multilobated nuclei. The tumour cells formed rosettes with sheep erythrocytes and were
therefore interpreted as T cells. Three of the four cases were extranodal (skin,
subcutis, bone marrow). Lymph nodes were involved in all cases, but only in one
case was a node the primary site of infiltration. The lymphoma cells showed
relatively fine chromatin and small, inconspicuous nucleoli. The cytoplasm was
abundant and pale. Although the tumour had spread widely, the prognosis appeared to be better than that of other types of T-cell lymphoma. Three of the four
patients were free of disease after 1 1/2 to 5 years.

In a second, retrospective study WEINBERG and PINKUS[601] presented ten more
cases of lymphoma with the same morphology, but they did not provide immunological evidence to back up the diagnoses. They added a case of large cell multilobated lymphoma that could be characterized unequivocally as a B-cell
lymphoma. PALLESEN et al.[602] and VAN DER PUTTE et al.[603] published cases of
multilobated lymphoma of T-cell type of the skin, and BARONI et al.[604] reported
a case in which bones, lymph nodes and subcutaneous tissue were infiltrated.

Almost all the multilobated large cell lymphomas in our collection are B-cell
lymphomas. We have interpreted most of them as centroblastic lymphomas (see
p. 120). Now PINKUS also considers most of the multilobated lymphomas to be
B-cell tumours.[605]

The only case of multilobated T-cell lymphoma that we have been able to
study was presented by O. MIODUSZEWSKA at a meeting of the European
Lymphoma Club (Figs. 155, 156). It was a metastasis in a cervical lymph node.
The 31-year-old patient had multiple skin nodules and died after 3 years of the
disease. Histologically, the lymph node was roughly divided into round nodules
of tumour cells that did not contain reticulin fibres themselves, but were surrounded by fibres and small vessels ("compartmentalization"). There was no
increase in the number of venules. The centre of the nodules occasionally showed
small necrotic areas. The tumour cells were mostly medium sized. Almost all cells

---

[598] Cawley et al. 1978; Jansen et al. 1979.
[599] Swerdlow and Murray 1988.
[600] 1979.
[601] 1981.
[602] 1981.
[603] 1982a,b.
[604] 1987.
[605] Personal communication.

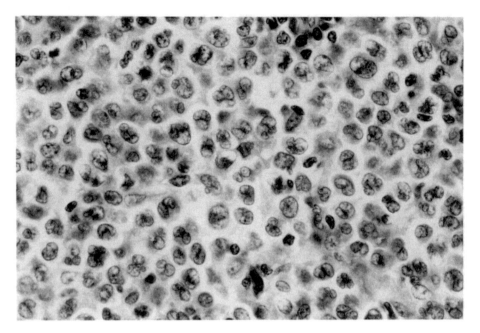

Fig. 155. T-cell lymphoma of multilobated type. Cf. Fig. 66. Male, 31 years. Cervical node. H & E. 700 : 1. (Tissue specimen kindly provided by O. MIODUSZEWSKA, Warsaw, Poland)

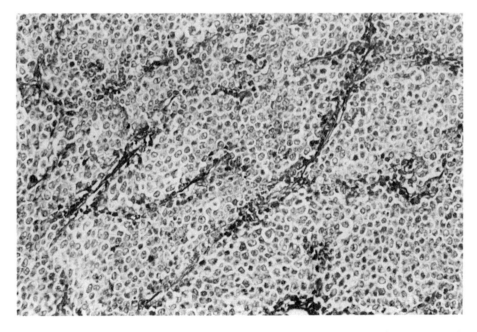

Fig. 156. T-cell lymphoma of multilobated type. Cf. Fig. 67. Same case as Fig. 155. Gomori. 220 : 1

contained multilobated nuclei. Sometimes there was a large nucleolus in a nuclear lobe; otherwise the nucleoli were small or medium sized. The cytoplasm was usually scanty; at times it was moderately abundant, and then it was definitely basophilic. Occasionally there was a central (oxyphilic) pale area in the cytoplasm. In addition to these medium-sized, multilobated cells there were also some large, basophilic cells that resembled immunoblasts. A large number of mitotic figures were found.

4.3.3 Erythrophagocytic Tγ Lymphoma (KADIN)

KADIN et al.[606] described the so-called erythrophagocytic Tγ lymphoma in 1981. It occurred in two men who were both in their thirties. The tumour cells were medium-sized to large blast cells. These cells were peculiar in that they phagocytosed erythrocytes. They corresponded to peripheral T lymphocytes (TdT −!) and were CD8 positive. Unlike a majority of normal CD8-positive lymphocytes, however, they did not show azurophil granules. The patients' blood counts were normal. Polychemotherapy was ineffective.

4.3.4 Malignant Lymphoma of "Plasmacytoid T Cells"

So far, a total of five cases of "ML of plasmacytoid T cells" have been published in the literature.[607] All five cases (see Figs. 157, 158) were associated with, or developed into, a myeloproliferative disorder (myelomonocytic leukaemia in four cases and chronic myeloid leukemia in the fifth case). This indicates that there is a relationship between "plasmacytoid T cells" and the bone marrow. We were also forced to suspect such a connection in a few cases of myeloid leukaemia in which tumour-like masses of "plasmacytoid T cells" appeared in lymph nodes in the blast crisis. Marked infiltration with "plasmacytoid T cells" has also been observed by FACCHETTI et al.[608] in a case of acute leukaemia of "null" type. These authors interpreted the infiltrate as a tumour-associated host reaction (because the cells were CD5 negative). A molecular genetic investigation of our case[609] and that of BEISKE et al.[610] did not reveal rearrangement of the TcRβ gene.

How should we classify these five "ML of plasmacytoid T cells" that developed in cases of myelomonocytic or myeloid leukaemia? Are they truly lymphomas associated with myeloproliferative disorders? This was postulated by FACCHETTI et al.[611] on the basis of CD5 expression, which was also found in the case of BEISKE et al.[612] and our case.[613] The "ML of plasmacytoid T cells" is supposed to be distinguishable from reactive proliferations of "plasmacytoid T

---

[606] 1981; Kadin 1981.
[607] Müller-Hermelink et al. 1983; Prasthofer et al. 1985; Beiske et al. 1986; Facchetti et al. 1990; Harris and Demĺrjian 1991.
[608] 1990.
[609] Müller-Hermelink et al. 1983; Feller et al. 1983b.
[610] 1987.
[611] 1990.
[612] 1986.
[613] Müller-Hermelink et al. 1983.

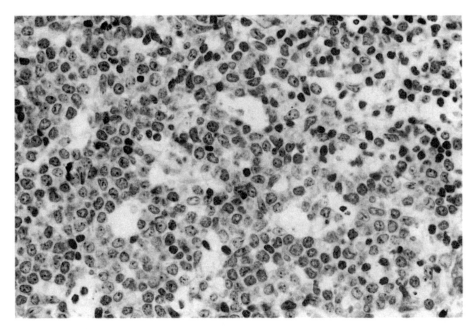

Fig. 157. "Malignant lymphoma of plasmacytoid T cells". At *upper right*, remnants of normal lymphoid tissue. Numerous "starry-sky" macrophages containing disintegrating cells (apoptosis). Giemsa. 440:1. (Case published by MÜLLER-HERMELINK et al. 1983)

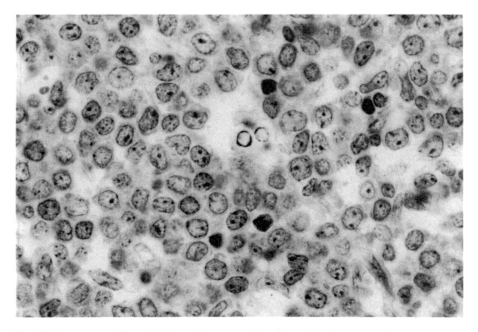

Fig. 158. Same case as Fig. 157. Above the *centre* of the picture there is a macrophage containing disintegrating nuclei. The "plasmacytoid T cells" have a relatively uniform appearance. Some pyknotic nuclei. Giemsa. 875:1

cells" because the latter are CD5 negative. Or do the proliferations of "plasmacy-toid T cells" belong to the myeloproliferative disorders? At present we do not have a final answer.

The "tumour cells" look just like the cells seen in reactive lymph nodes.[614] They are uniformly medium sized and have large, oval nuclei with rather fine chromatin and one small, non-basophilic nucleolus. The cytoplasm is scanty to moderately abundant (much less abundant than that of typical plasma cells!) and grey with Giemsa staining. There are many pyknotic cells, which are phagocy-tosed by macrophages (apoptosis). The lymph node is completely infiltrated by the "tumour cells", so there is hardly any residual lymphoid tissue. The case published by HARRIS and DEMIRJIAN[615] showed infiltration mainly in T regions. This was most obvious in the spleen, where the infiltrates were seen only in T regions, whereas the red pulp showed myeloid infiltration.

Immunohistochemically, the lymphoma cells in our case expressed CD4, CD5 and HLA-DR and showed weak expression of CD10, while they were negative for CD3, CD2, CD8, CIg, B-cell antigens and C3b receptors. The prolif-eration rate was extremely low (2% Ki-67+ cells). In another case, however, we have seen several mitotic figures.

In imprints from our case non-specific esterase staining revealed predomi-nantly negative medium-sized cells. A number of medium-sized cells with oval nuclei struck the eye, however, because they showed a moderately strong or strong, diffuse reaction. They should probably be interpreted as neoplastic mono-cytes and were an indication of the pre-existent myelomonocytic leukaemia.

4.3.5 Lymphohistiocytic Lymphoma

Lymphohistiocytic lymphoma was first presented as a new entity by HAMLIN and STANSFELD at a meeting of the European Lymphoma Club in 1975. Since then we have seen several related cases and have reported on them on a few occasions.[616]

The tumour is composed of CD4-positive lymphocytes, a small to large number of large, CD30-positive blast cells and many lysozyme-positive macrophages. It was these macrophages that first attracted our attention (Fig. 159). With Giemsa staining they are very bright pink to reddish violet; the round nucleus is often eccentric. At a low magnification, these cells give the impression of being plasma cells. Plasma cells, however, are much smaller and have dark blue cytoplasm. The macrophages in the bone marrow and elsewhere occasionally show erythrophagocytosis.

At the meeting in 1975, HAMLIN and STANSFELD already reported that half of their six patients had shown a favourable clinical course, whereas the other half had required chemotherapy and had died of the lymphoma. GALTON, who treated the first of these patients, reported in 1985[617] that the patient had not been treated consistently with chemotherapy and was still alive and well.

---

[614] Vollenweider and Lennert 1983.
[615] 1991.
[616] Lennert et al. 1984; Lennert and Feller 1985.
[617] Discussion of presentation of Lennert and Feller 1985.

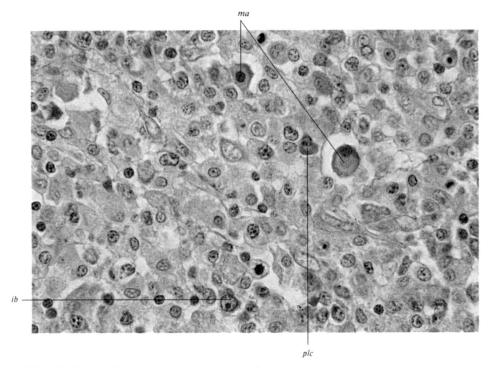

Fig. 159. Lymphohistiocytic lymphoma. Two violet macrophages with pyknotic nuclei (*ma*). Note the much smaller plasma cell (*plc*) and the immunoblast (*ib*). A majority of the cells are small lymphocytes. Giemsa. 560 : 1

Hence we must assume that the morphological picture is actually concealing both a reactive condition, which might be caused by a virus, and a malignant peripheral T-cell lymphoma. Because of the high content of macrophages (showing a distinct morphology!) we call the lymphoma "lympho*histiocytic*". One of our patients showed trisomy 7, an argument (not absolute proof) in favour of interpreting the lesion as a tumour. Signs of proliferation (a positive Ki-67 reaction) were demonstrated only in the lymphoid, chiefly CD30-positive cells, whereas the macrophages were Ki-67 negative. In a recent case, however, we found some mitotic figures in reactive-looking macrophages.

PILERI et al.[618] described 13 cases of lymphohistiocytic T-cell lymphoma, which they placed in the large cell anaplastic lymphoma category because of the frequently high content of CD30-positive large cells. We do not think this global classification is justified, since the T cells were small or medium-sized and CD30 negative, especially in early stages, as evident from several of the photomicrographs published by PILERI et al. Moreover, in later stages the CD30-positive large cells were usually still interspersed with smaller T cells. Lymphohistiocytic T-cell lymphoma may eventually transform into a large cell anaplastic lymphoma, consisting exclusively of CD30-positive large anaplastic cells (sec-

---

[618] 1990.

ondary LCAL). It is remarkable that the patients described by PILERI et al. were relatively young, with a mean age of 14.8 years. The patients presented with systemic symptoms and superficial lymphadenopathy. They responded well to aggressive chemotherapy. It is not possible, however, to determine from the publication whether the cases included non-neoplastic conditions (as mentioned above).

Perhaps there is a relationship between lymphohistiocytic lymphoma and the lesion described by JAFFE et al.[619] as "malignant lymphoma and erythrophagocytosis simulating malignant histiocytosis".

4.3.6 Peripheral T-Cell Lymphoma Associated with Haemophagocytic Syndrome (Histiocytic Medullary Reticulosis of SCOTT and ROBB-SMITH)[620]

In 1939 SCOTT and ROBB-SMITH[621] described a clinicopathological syndrome called "histiocytic medullary reticulosis". This disease has not been included in any lymphoma classification, as bitterly complained by ROBB-SMITH.[622] It has been the fate of all histiocytic or reticulum cell neoplasms to be intentionally left out of new lymphoma classifications, at least for the time being, because too little was known about them at the time. The situation has not improved much. It now seems likely, however, that histiocytic medullary reticulosis is actually not a type of histiocytosis, but rather a lymphoid neoplasm. Hence it should be included in our classification.

FALINI et al.[623] have examined slides from the collection of ROBB-SMITH together with cases of their own. They have provided impressive proof that histiocytic medullary reticulosis is actually a peripheral T-cell lymphoma, which is associated with an exuberant hyperplasia of benign-looking, haemophagocytosing macrophages. The haemophagocytosis leads to severe pancytopenia. Other clinical findings are high fever, loss of weight, prominent hepatosplenomegaly and abnormal liver function tests. Involvement of lymph nodes is only moderate or may even be lacking.

Histologically, lymph nodes show diffuse infiltration by pleomorphic T cells, which may be interspersed with a few T immunoblasts and other large, bizarre-looking cells (Fig. 160). Among the tumour cells there are often large macrophages showing more or less marked haemophagocytosis. This haemophagocytosis is much more pronounced in the spleen and liver than in lymph nodes. Mitotic activity is very high.

The tumour cells were identified by FALINI et al.[624] as T cells. They also showed rearrangement of TcRβ chain genes, indicating monoclonality. Rearrangement of TcRγ or δ was not observed.

---

[619] 1983.
[620] See Robb-Smith 1990 for a historical review.
[621] 1939.
[622] 1990.
[623] 1990.
[624] 1990.

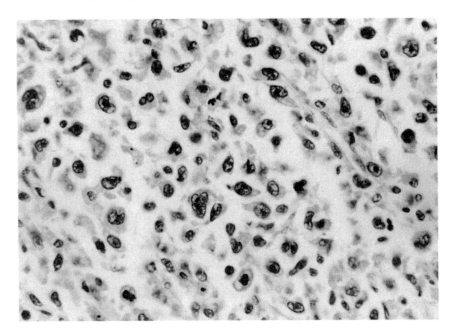

Fig. 160. "Histiocytic medullary reticulosis" (Scott and Robb-Smith). Pleomorphic T-cell lymphoma. Near the *centre*, one giant cell. Lymph node. Van Gieson. 440:1. (Section kindly provided by A. H. T. Robb-Smith)

The clinical course is very rapid (mean survival of 7 weeks[625]). Adults of all ages are affected.

The disease must not be confused with familial haemophagocytic lymphohistiocytosis (Farquhar),[626] which occurs in the first 2 years of life and is often hereditary (autosomally recessive). In this non-neoplastic disorder, *normal*-looking lymphocytes and haemophagocytosing macrophages are widespread in the spleen, liver and bone marrow. Lymph nodes are not enlarged and show severe atrophy of the lymphoid cells, including germinal centres. In contrast to patients with histiocytic medullary reticulosis, those with familial lymphohistiocytosis generally have hyperglyceridemia, hypofibrinogenaemia and a deficit of NK cells and LAK activity. Neurological symptoms are usually observed as well.

Occasionally, the borderline between histiocytic medullary reticulosis and lymphohistiocytic lymphoma may be unclear when the haemophagocytic macrophages take on a plasmacytoid appearance after lysis of the erythrocytes. The distinctions between histiocytic medullary reticulosis and the lymphoma associated with erythrophagocytosis described by Jaffe et al.[627] and infection-as-

---

[625] Falini et al. 1990.
[626] Farquhar et al. 1958; Nézelof and Eliachar 1973; Burgio and Aricó 1989; Aricó 1990; Pileri and Falini 1990.
[627] 1983.

sociated haemophagocytic syndrome in association with a T-cell lymphoma[628] are discussed by FALINI et al.[629] Future studies of larger series of cases should make it possible to assign each case to a certain category.

4.3.7 Signet-Ring Cell Lymphoma of T-Cell Type

GROGAN et al.[630] and WEISS et al.[631] reported three cases of large cell peripheral T-cell lymphoma, which they termed "signet-ring cell lymphoma". A fourth case was recently reported by CROSS et al.[632] The cytoplasm of the tumour cells contained large PAS-positive vacuoles that deformed the nuclei so that they resembled a signet-ring. On electron microscopy, the vacuoles were giant multivesicular bodies. In all four patients the condition began with skin involvement, and all four showed a relatively favourable prognosis. Signet-ring cell lymphoma of B-cell type is discussed on pp. 91 f.

4.3.8 Liebow's Lymphomatoid Granulomatosis, Midline Granuloma and Angiocentric Lymphoma

JAFFE[633] has combined a spectrum of diseases that are supposed to range from benign lymphocytic vasculitis (e.g. in Weber-Christian disease) to malignant lymphomas under the heading "angiocentric immunoproliferative lesions". She considers *lymphomatoid granulomatosis (Liebow)* and *midline granuloma* (also known as polymorphic reticulosis[634]) to be one nosological category, but distinguishes it from "angiocentric lymphoma". Both Liebow's lymphomatoid granulomatosis and midline granuloma are *peripheral T-cell lymphomas* that generally belong to the pleomorphic category (particularly small and medium-sized cell type) and sometimes transform into a T-immunoblastic lymphoma. The vast majority are found in extranodal sites, particularly in the lung, the upper respiratory tract (nasopharynx, paranasal sinuses, palate) and the gastrointestinal tract, but also in the kidney and in the central and peripheral nervous systems.

An angiocentric and angiodestructive growth pattern is characteristic of some types of T-cell lymphoma (Fig. 161). This often results in large areas of necrosis. As far as the naming of these T-cell lymphomas with an angiocentric and angiodestructive growth pattern is concerned, we suggest defining the tumour type as we do all ML, i.e. according to its cytology, and adding that there is an angiocentric $\pm$ angiodestructive growth pattern.

---

[628] Griffin et al. 1978.
[629] 1990.
[630] 1985.
[631] 1985a.
[632] 1989.
[633] 1985; Lipford et al. 1988.
[634] DeRemee et al. 1978.

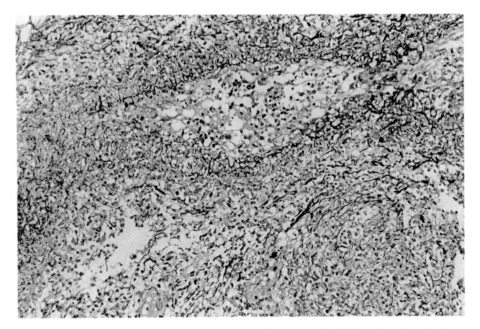

Fig. 161. Pleomorphic, medium-sized cell T-cell lymphoma showing infiltration of a vein ("angiocentric" and "angiodestructive"). Clinically diagnosed as so-called midline granuloma. Male, 41 years. Gomori. 140:1

In many cases *malignant midline granuloma* shows angiocentricity or angio-invasion. Frequently there is a severe inflammatory reaction, which obscures the underlying T-cell proliferation (Fig. 161). In most of our cases immunohisto-chemical analysis revealed expression of antigens of peripheral T-cells (CD2, CD3, CD5 and CD4). Some cases showed CD8 with co-expression of the NK-cell marker CD56. In such cases there was rearrangement of the TcRβ gene, which is evidence of a monoclonal T-cell proliferation. In contrast, Ho et al.[635] of Hong Kong observed cases that did not show rearrangement of the TcRβ gene. These authors reported monoclonal or biclonal EBV genomes in a majority of cases. The patients with midline granuloma were younger, showed a higher male-to-female ratio and had a better overall survival rate than did patients with other types of NHL in the same localization. In some cases the neoplastic T cells carried the EBV genome.[636]

The prognosis appears to be relatively favourable. After radiotherapy most patients with midline granuloma are free of disease, while some patients suffer a relapse.[637] For further clinical data the reader may refer to JAFFE.[638]

[635] 1990a, b.
[636] Harabuchi et al. 1990.
[637] Fauci et al. 1976; DeRemee et al. 1978; Crissman et al. 1982.
[638] 1985.

Addendum: Methods for the Diagnosis of Lymphoma

Preparation of High-Quality Sections [639]

Fixation: 10% buffered formalin.

Processing:

Step	Solution	Hours
1	70% alcohol	1
2	96% alcohol	1
3	96% alcohol	1
4	100% alcohol	1
5	100% alcohol	1
6	100% alcohol	1.5
7	Xylene	1
8	Xylene	1
9	Xylene	1.5
10	Paraplast + ®	1
11	Paraplast + ®	2
12	Paraplast + ®	2

Embedding: Paraplast or Paraplast + ® in an embedding mould.

Cutting: Cut sections with a Jung Hn 40 microtome, knife angle set at 0°. Use a
Feather knife holder and disposable blades (S35).
Cool the block on a coldplate.
Cut the block carefully until the tissue is reached.
Remove four or five sections and dispose of them so as to avoid holes and
cracks.
Continue cutting, moving the knife carefully and steadily, and blowing gently
on the cut surface.

Float the sections on warm water (40°–42 °C). Remove wrinkles and bubbles.

Drying: 2 h at 42 °C
or 5 min at 45°–50 °C and 5 min at 80 °C.

---

[639] The directions for this method were written up by K. MÜLLER.

Re-embedding of Paraffin-Embedded Tissue in JB-4 Resin[640]

1. Dissolve the paraffin block.
2. De-wax the tissue in xylene (12–24 h, depending on the thickness of the specimen).
3. Dehydrate in 100% alcohol (12–24 h).
4. Clarify in methyl benzoate (24 h).
5. Impregnate in catalyzed JB-4 Solution A (12–24 h).
6. Embed in moulding cup trays. Add 1 drop Solution B to 1 ml catalyzed Solution A and stir well. Prepare this mixture immediately before use.

JB-4 Embedding Kit (Polysciences, Warrington, Pennsylvania, USA):

    Solution A: 750 ml
    Catalyst C: 9 g
    Solution B: 50 ml

Giemsa Staining of Paraffin Sections[640]

(Modification of LENNERT 1952, 1961)

1. The de-waxed sections are removed from distilled water and put into the following solution for 1 h:

    80 ml distilled water
    20 ml Giemsa solution (Merck, Darmstadt, Germany)

2. The sections are removed from the Giemsa solution and put into 100 ml distilled water, to which 3–4 drops of undiluted glacial acetic acid have been added. The sections are agitated gently in this solution for a few seconds, slightly differentiated and then immediately put into:

3. 96% ethyl alcohol, in which they are differentiated further until the desired staining is achieved (microscopic control).

4. Differentiation is stopped and, at the same time, dehydration is achieved by dipping in 3 changes of isopropanol for 2 min each and

5. in 3 changes of xylene for 2 min each.

6. Mount with Eukitt (Kindler, Freiburg, Germany).

Results:
    RNA, DNA: blue ("basophilic").
    Acidophilic substances: pink or reddish orange.
    Acid mucopolysaccharides: reddish violet.

---

[640] The directions for this method were written up by K. MÜLLER.

Naphthol AS-D Chloroacetate Esterase in Paraffin Sections

(LEDER 1964; LEDER and STUTTE 1975)

Fixation: formalin or other solution (sufficient fixation is necessary to avoid reactions with other esterases).

Embedding: paraffin (Paraplast) or resin.

Stock solution A ("hexazonium pararosaniline" according to DAVIS and ORNSTEIN 1959):

Mix well:

1 drop of 4% solution of pararosaniline and
1 drop of 4% solution of sodium nitrite.

After about 60 s dilute with:

30 ml veronal acetate buffer, pH 7.62
(if the mixture turns red, then pararosaniline was not sufficiently "hexazotized").

Adjust pH of the mixture to 6.3 with 2 *N* HCl.

Stock solution B:

Dissolve 10 mg naphthol AS-D chloroacetate (Sigma, Munich, Germany) in 1 ml dimethyl formamide.

Stir solution A into solution B, mixing well, and then filter.

Incubate once at room temperature for 30 min or twice for 30 min each, agitating constantly. Then rinse the slides in tap water.

Nuclear staining with haemalum (Merck, Darmstadt, Germany) for 10 min. Then blue in tap water.

Mount with glycerin jelly.

Results:

Enzyme activity is represented by a homogeneous, bright red reaction product. Neutrophil granulocytes, their precursors and mast cells are positive.

Acid Phosphatase in Imprints

(GOLDBERG and BARKA 1962; LEDER 1967; LEDER and STUTTE 1975)

Fixation: none.

Stock solution A ("hexazonium pararosaniline" according to DAVIS and ORNSTEIN 1959):

> Mix well:
>
> 1 drop of 4% solution of pararosaniline and
> 1 drop of 4% solution of sodium nitrite.
>
> After about 60 s dilute with:
>
> 30 ml veronal acetate buffer, pH 7.62
> (if the mixture turns red, then pararosaniline was not sufficiently "hexazotized").
>
> Adjust pH of the mixture to 5.0–5.1 with 2 N HCl.

Stock solution B:

> Dissolve 10 mg naphthol AS-BI phosphate (Sigma, Munich, Germany) in 1 ml dimethyl formamide or 2 ml dimethyl sulfoxide.

Stir solution A into solution B, mixing well, and then filter.

Incubate at room temperature for 4(–10) h. Then rinse the slides in tap water.

Nuclear staining with haemalum (Merck, Darmstadt, Germany) for 10 min. Then blue in tap water.

Mount with glycerin jelly.

Results:

> A red reaction product indicates enzyme activity. One has to distinguish between a focal and a diffuse, granular reaction. As a rule, a focal reaction product corresponds to the Golgi apparatus and is typical of T cells.

Acid Non-specific Esterase in Imprints

(α-naphthyl acetate esterase method of MUELLER et al. 1975)

Fixation: 4 min in buffered (0.1 M sodium cacodylate, pH 7.2) 4% formalin. Dry at room temperature.

Stock solution A:

Dissolve 2 g pararosaniline, acridine-free, C. I. No. 42500 (Chroma, Stuttgart-Untertürkheim, Germany) in
50 ml 2 N HCl. Mix thoroughly.

This solution can be stored in the dark at 4 °C.

Stock solution B:

Freshly prepared 4% aqueous solution of sodium nitrite.

Mix equal parts (1.2 ml each) of solutions A and B until the colour of the mixture becomes amber.

Dissolve substrate (10 mg α-naphthyl acetate; Sigma, St. Louis, Missouri, USA) in 0.4 ml acetone in a second vessel.

Add the mixture of hexazotized pararosaniline and buffer to the substrate. Adjust to pH 5.8 with 2 N NaOH.

Incubate at room temperature for 2 h.

Nuclear staining with haemalum (Merck, Darmstadt, Germany) for 10 min. Then blue in tap water.

Mount with glycerin jelly.

Results:

Enzyme activity is represented by a reddish brown reaction product. Some T lymphocytes show localized, coarse, paranuclear activity. Monocytes and macrophages are diffusely positive.

Peroxidase-Antiperoxidase (PAP) Method for Paraffin Sections

(Modification of method described by TAYLOR and BURNS 1974; MEPHAM et al. 1979)

1. De-wax section in xylene (for about 15–20 min).
2. Dehydrate in alcohol series (100 %–90 %–70 %) for about 3 min each.
3. Inhibit "endogenous" peroxidase (in erythrocytes and granulocytes) by bathing in methanol–H_2O_2 (1 ml H_2O_2/100 ml methanol) for 10–30 min.
4. Rinse in 0.05 M Tris buffer, pH 7.6, for about 10 min.
5. Unmask antigens by bathing in 0.1 % trypsin solution at 37 °C for 15–30 min.
6. Rinse in Tris buffer for about 10 min.
7. Reduce non-specific background activity (e.g. in collagenous fibres) by treating the section with normal sheep or swine serum (SNS), diluted 1 : 5, for about 10 min.
8. Drain off SNS and
9. replace with monospecific polyclonal antiserum (e.g. rabbit antiserum), diluted with Tris buffer, for 30 min.
10. Rinse 3 times in Tris buffer for 10 min each.
11. Apply bivalent anti-rabbit IgG serum, diluted (1 : 50–80) with Tris buffer, for 30 min.
12. Rinse 3 times in Tris buffer for 10 min each.
13. Apply PAP, diluted (1 : 100) with Tris buffer, for 30 min.
14. Rinse 3 times in Tris buffer for 10 min each.
15. Demonstrate peroxidase by staining with
    3,3′-diaminobenzidine (DAB) tetrahydrochloride
    (50 mg DAB/100 ml buffer to which 10 μl of a 10 % H_2O_2 solution is added immediately before use).
16. Rinse in running tap water.
17. Counterstain with haemalum-for about 3–6 min.
18. Blue in lukewarm water for about 5 min.
19. Dehydrate in alcohol series (70 %–90 %–100 %) for 3 min each.
20. Xylene bath for about 5 min.
21. Mount with Eukitt (Kindler, Freiburg, Germany).

Application:
   This method has been widely used for demonstrating cIg in paraffin sections. A reliable demonstration of sIg is not possible. The method is less sensitive than the streptavidin-biotin method (p. 270).

Results:
   A positive reaction for cIg is seen as a dark brown reaction product.

Indirect Immunoperoxidase Method for Cryostat Sections

(STEIN et al. 1982)

1. Dry cryostat section (5 μ) at room temperature, exposed to air. [641]
2. Fix the section with acetone (*pro analysi*) for 10 min.
3. Incubate with monoclonal antibody (diluted 1:3; Tris-NaCl buffer, pH 7.4 + 1% bovine serum albumin) for 30 min.
4. Rinse in buffer.
5. Incubate with secondary antiserum (peroxidase-conjugated rabbit anti-mouse Ig) for 30 min. Dilute (1:2) the antiserum with human serum and buffer.
6. Rinse in buffer.
7. Incubate with tertiary antiserum (peroxidase-conjugated goat anti-rabbit IgG) for 30 min.
8. Rinse in buffer.
9. Demonstrate peroxidase by staining with
   3,3'-diaminobenzidine (DAB) tetrahydrochloride
   (50 mg DAB/100 ml buffer to which 10 μl of a 10% H_2O_2 solution is added immediately before use).
10. Rinse twice in buffer.
11. Counterstain with haemalum for 30 min.
12. Blue in running water.
13. Mount with glycerin jelly.

Application:
This method is widely used for demonstrating surface antigens in cryostat sections or slides prepared from cell suspensions.

---

[641] Suitable monoclonal antibodies can also be applied to paraffin sections.

Streptavidin-Biotin Complex Method for Paraffin Sections[642]

1. De-wax section in xylene (15 min).
2. Dehydrate in alcohol series (100%–90%–70%).
3. Inhibit "endogenous" peroxidase in H_2O_2/absolute methanol for 10 min. Prepare the solution immediately before use.
4. Rinse in running tap water.
5. Warm in 37°C distilled water in a water bath for approx. 5 min.
6. Trypsinize at 37°C and pH 7.8 for 5–16 min in a water bath. Use trypsin T8128 (Sigma, St. Louis, MO, USA) or, if possible, T8253. 100 ml of the trypsin solution should contain 0.1 g trypsin and 0.1 g calcium dichloride dissolved in buffer. The time it takes for the tissue to be digested by trypsin depends on how long the tissue was fixed in formalin.
7. Stop tissue digestion immediately by rinsing in running tap water.
8. Rinse 3 times in buffer for 5 min each.
9. Apply primary antibody and incubate for 30 min.
10. Rinse 3 times in buffer for 5 min each.
11. Apply secondary antibody (E 353 or E 354, Dako, Copenhagen, Denmark), diluted 1 : 200 with human serum (diluted 1 : 20 with PBS), and incubate for 30 min.
12. Rinse 3 times in buffer for 5 min each.
13. Prepare strept-AB complex (using kit K 377, Dako) by mixing 10 ml of A and 10 ml of B with 1000 μl PBS; this corresponds to a dilution of 1 : 100. Pre-incubate the complex for 30 min before use.
14. Apply 100 ml strept-AB complex for 30 min.
15. Rinse 3 times in buffer for 5 min each.
16. Stain with 100 μl diaminobenzidine (DAB) tetrahydrochloride (60 mg DAB [D5905, Sigma] dissolved in 100 ml Tris-HCl buffer, pH 7.6, to which 100 μl of a 30% H_2O_2 solution is added before use) for 5–10 min.
17. Rinse 3 times in buffer for 5 min each.
18. Counterstain with haemalum (Merck, Darmstadt, Germany) for approx. 10 min.
19. Rinse in tap water.
20. Dehydrate in ethanol series (70%–90%–100%).
21. Dehydrate 3 times in xylene for 5 min each.
22. Mount with Eukitt (Kindler, Freiburg, Germany).

Application:

This is a sensitive method for demonstrating cIg and, at least in part, sIg in paraffin sections. It can also be used for cryostat sections, in which case different secondary antibodies (step 11) must be applied. By coupling the strept-AB complex with alkaline phosphatase the reaction product can be developed as described on p. 271 (step 10).

Results:

In paraffin sections the reaction product is either dark brown (cIg) or yellowish brown (sIg). When alkaline phosphatase is used, the reaction product is red.

---

[642] This method was developed by P. G. ISAACSON. The directions were written up by M. TIEMANN.

Alkaline Phosphatase–Anti-Alkaline Phosphatase (APAAP) Method for Cryostat Sections

(CORDELL et al. 1984)

1. Dry cryostat section (5 μm) at room temperature, exposed to air.[643]

2. Fix the section with acetone (*pro analysi*) for 10 min.

3. Incubate with monoclonal antibody (diluted 1:3 with human serum; Tris-NaCl buffer, pH 7.4, + 1% bovine serum albumin) for 30 min.

4. Rinse in buffer.

5. Incubate with secondary antiserum ("bridging antibody", rabbit anti-mouse Ig) for 30 min. Dilute (1:2) the antiserum with human serum and buffer.

6. Rinse in buffer.

7. Incubate with mixture of anti-alkaline phosphatase antibody and alkaline phosphatase (APAAP complex, prepared a few days before use and stored at 4°C) for 30 min.

8. Rinse in buffer.

9. Repeat steps 5–8 twice, but reduce the incubation times to 10 min.

10. Demonstrate alkaline phosphatase by staining with the following mixture:

Solution A:
10 mg naphthol AS-BI phosphate
400 ml dimethyl formamide

Solution B:
1 drop of 5% solution of Astra new fuchsin
3 drops of 4% solution of $NaNO_2$
40 ml propandiol (pH 8.7)

Mix solution A with solution B, filter and shake for 10 min.

11. Counterstain with haemalum for 30 min.

12. Blue in running water.

13. Mount with glycerin jelly.

Application:
This method is suitable for demonstrating antigens in cryostat sections. It can also be used with paraffin sections that have been pretreated in an appropriate manner.

Results:
The reaction product is red.

---

[643] Suitable monoclonal antibodies can also be applied to paraffin sections.

References

Abbondanzo SL, Sulak LE (1991) Ki-1-positive lymphoma developing 10 years after the diagnosis of hairy cell leukemia. Cancer 67:3117–3122

Abe M, Nozawa Y, Wachi E, Tominaga K, Hojo H, Wakasa H (1988) Alkaline phosphatase-positive B cell lymphomas. Eur J Haematol 41:223–229

Addis BJ, Isaacson PG (1986) Large cell lymphoma of the mediastinum: a B-cell tumour of probable thymic origin. Histopathology 10:379–390

Agnarsson BA, Kadin ME (1988) Ki-1 positive large cell lymphoma. A morphologic and immunologic study of 19 cases. Am J Surg Pathol 12:264–274

Aisenberg AC, Wilkes BM, Harris NL, Ault KA, Carey RW (1981) Chronic T-cell lymphocytosis with neutropenia: Report of a case studied with monoclonal antibody. Blood 58:818–822

Aisenberg AC, Krontiris TG, Mak TW, Wilkes BM (1985) Rearrangement of the gene for the beta chain of the T-cell receptor in T-cell chronic lymphocytic leukemia and related disorders. N Engl J Med 313:529–533

Akazaki K, Rappaport H, Berard CW, Bennett JM, Ishikawa E (eds) (1973) Malignant diseases of the hematopoietic system. (GANN monograph on cancer research, vol 15). University of Tokyo Press, Tokyo

Alberti VN, Neiman RS (1984) Lymphoplasmacytic lymphoma. A clinicopathologic study of a previously unrecognized composite variant. Cancer 53:1103–1108

Andreesen R, Osterholz J, Löhr GW, Bross KJ (1984) A Hodgkin cell-specific antigen is expressed on a subset of auto- and alloactivated T (helper) lymphoblasts. Blood 63:1299–1302

Aricò M (1990) Peripheral T-cell lymphoma associated with hemophagocytic syndrome and hemophagocytic lymphohistiocytosis of children: do they share something? [Letter to the Editor] Blood 76:2136

Arseneau JC, Canellos GP, Banks PM, Berard CW, Gralnick HR, DeVita Jr VT (1975) American Burkitt's lymphoma: A clinicopathologic study of 30 cases. I. Clinical factors relating to prolonged survival. Am J Med 58:314–321

Audouin J, Diebold J, Schvartz H, le Tourneau A, Bernadou A, Zittoun R (1988) Malignant lymphoplasmacytic lymphoma with prominent splenomegaly (primary lymphoma of the spleen). J Pathol 155:17–33

Balaton AJ, Vaury P, Videgrain M (1987) Paravertebral malignant rhabdoid tumor in an adult. A case report with immunocytochemical study. Pathol Res Pract 182:713–716

Banks PM (1985) Technical aspects of specimen preparation and special studies. In: Jaffe ES (ed) Surgical pathology of the lymph nodes and related organs. (Major problems in pathology, vol 16) Saunders, Philadelphia, pp 1–21

Banks PM, Arseneau JC, Gralnick HR, Canellos GP, DeVita Jr VT, Berard CW (1975) American Burkitt's lymphoma: A clinicopathologic study of 30 cases. II. Pathologic correlations. Am J Med 58:322–329

Banks PM, Metter J, Allred DC (1990) Anaplastic large cell (Ki-1) lymphoma with histiocytic phenotype simulating carcinoma. Am J Clin Pathol 94:445–452

Banks PM, Chan J, Cleary ML, Delsol G, De Wolf-Peeters C, Gatter K, Grogan TM, Harris NL, Isaacson PG, Jaffe ES, Mason DY, Pileri S, Ralfkiaer E, Stein H, Warnke RA (1992) Mantle cell lymphoma: a proposal for unification of morphologic, immunologic and molecular data. Am J Surg Pathol, submitted

Baroni CD, Pescarmona E, Calogero A, Cassano AM, Pezzella F, Barsotti P, Gallo A, Ruco LP (1987) B- and T-cell non-Hodgkin's lymphomas with large multilobated cells: morphological, phenotypic and clinical heterogeneity. Histopathology 11:1121–1132

Barriga F, Whang-Peng J, Lee E, Morrow C, Jaffe E, Cossman J, Magrath IT (1988) Development of a second clonally discrete Burkitt's lymphoma in a human immunodeficiency virus-positive homosexual patient. Blood 72: 792–795

Bartels H (1980) Prognose der malignen Lymphome der Keimzentren. Habilitationsschrift, Lübeck

Bartels H, Burger A, Common H, Donhuijsen-Ant R, Graubner M, Grupp HJ, Huhn D, Leopold H, Nowicki L, Nürnberger R, Rühl U, Waldner R (Kieler Lymphomgruppe) (1979) Klinik und Prognose des centroblastisch-centrocytischen Lymphoms und des centroblastischen Lymphoms. In: Stacher A, Höcker P (eds) Lymphknotentumoren. Urban and Schwarzenberg, Munich, pp 211–217

Becker H (1978) Maligne Non-Hodgkin-Lymphome: Pathomorphologische Grundlagen. Hautarzt [Suppl III] 29: 21–29

Bednář B (1979) Lymphoepitheloid cell malignant lymphoma (Lennert). Virchows Arch [A] 382: 313–322

Beiske K, Langholm R, Godal T, Marton PF (1986) T-zone lymphoma with predominance of "plasmacytoid T-cells" associated with myelomonocytic leukaemia – a distinct clinicopathological entity. J Pathol 150: 247–255

Beiske K, Munthe-Kaas A, Davies CDL, Marton PF, Godal T (1987) Single cell studies on the immunological marker profile of plasmacytoid T-zone cells. Lab Invest 56: 381–393

Beljaards RC, Meijer CJLM, Scheffer E, Toonstra J, Van Vloten WA, Van der Putte SCJ, Geerts M-L, Willemze R (1989) Prognostic significance of CD30 (Ki-1/Ber-H2) expression in primary cutaneous large-cell lymphomas of T-cell origin. A clinicopathologic and immunohistochemical study in 20 patients. Am J Pathol 135: 1169–1178

Belpomme D, Caillou B, Lelarge N, Botto I, Pujade Lauraine E, Denaro L, Gerard-Marchant R, Davies AJS, Mathé G (1978) Categorization of non-Hodgkin's hematosarcomas (lymphomas) according to T- and B-cell markers: Its value for diagnosis and prognosis. Recent Results Cancer Res 64: 146–157

Benjamin D, Magrath IT, Maguire R, Janus C, Todd HD, Parsons RG (1982) Immunoglobulin secretion by cell lines derived from African and American undifferentiated lymphomas of Burkitt's and non-Burkitt's type. J Immunol 129: 1336–1342

Bennett MH, Millett YL (1969) Nodular sclerotic lymphosarcoma. A possible new clinicopathological entity. Clin Radiol 20: 339–343

Bennett MH, Farrer-Brown G, Henry K, Jelliffe AM (1974) Classification of non-Hodgkin's lymphomas. [Letter to the Editor] Lancet ii: 405–406

Berard CW (1975) Reticuloendothelial system: an overview of neoplasia. In: Rebuck JW, Berard CW, Abell MR (eds) The reticuloendothelial system. (Monographs in pathology no 16) Williams and Wilkins, Baltimore, pp 301–317

Berard CW, Dorfman RF (1974) Histopathology of malignant lymphomas. Clin Hematol 3: 39–76

Berard CW, O'Conor GT, Thomas LB, Torloni H (1969) Histopathological definition of Burkitt's tumour. Bull WHO 40: 601–607

Berard CW, Jaffe ES, Braylan RC, Mann RB, Nanba K (1978) Immunologic aspects and pathology of the malignant lymphomas. Cancer 42: 911–921

Bergholz M, Bartsch H-H, Krueger GRF, Schauer A, Fischer R (1979) Angioimmunoblastische Lymphadenopathie und persistierender Virusinfekt? Erörterung immunhistologischer Befunde an zwei Fällen. Klin Wochenschr 57: 1317–1321

Bitter MA, Franklin WA, Larson RA, McKeithan TW, Rubin CM, Le Beau MM, Stephens JK, Vardiman JW (1990) Morphology in Ki-1 (CD30)-positive non-Hodgkin's lymphoma is correlated with clinical features and the presence of a unique chromosomal abnormality, t(2; 5) (p23; q35). Am J Surg Pathol 124: 305–316

Blattner WA, Kalyanaraman VS, Robert-Guroff M, Lister TA, Galton DAG, Sarin PS, Crawford MH, Catovsky D, Greaves M, Gallo RC (1982) The human type-C retrovirus, HTLV, in Blacks from the Caribbean region, and relationship to adult T-cell leukemia/lymphoma. Int J Cancer 30: 257–264

Bofill M, Janossy G, Janossa M, Burford GD, Seymour GJ, Wernet P, Kelemen E (1985) Human B cell development. II. Subpopulations in the human fetus. J Immunol 134: 1531–1538

Bogomoletz WV, Bernard J, Capron F, Diebold J (1983) T-cell origin of Lennert's lymphoma. Immunohistochemical and immunologic study of one case. Arch Pathol Lab Med 107: 586–588

Bom-van Noorloos AA, van Heerde P, Cleton FJ, Hart AAM, Behrendt H, von dem Borne AEGKr, Melief CJM, Lymphoma Research Group Amsterdam (1980a) Histology, immunological markers and clinical course of non-Hodgkin's lymphomas. In: Bom-van Noorloos AA (ed) Immunological aspects of lymphoid neoplasia. Academisch Proefschrift, Amsterdam, pp 109–126

Bom-van Noorloos AA, Pegels HG, van Oers RHJ, Silberbusch J, Feltkamp-Vroom TM, Goudsmit R, Zeijlemaker WP, von dem Borne AEGKr, Melief CJM (1980b) Proliferation of T/gamma cells with killer-cell activity in two patients with neutropenia and recurrent infections. N Engl J Med 302:933–937

Borisch Chappuis B, Müller H, Stutte J, Hey MM, Hübner K, Müller-Hermelink HK (1990) Identification of EBV-DNA in lymph nodes from patients with lymphadenopathy and lymphomas associated with AIDS. Virchows Arch [B] 58:199–205

Braun-Falco O, Burg G, Schmoeckel C (1978) Klassifikation von malignen Hautlymphomen. Hautarzt 29 [Suppl. III]: 37–45

Brearley RL, Chapman J, Cullen MH, Horton MA, Stansfeld AG, Waters AH (1979) Haematological features of angioimmunoblastic lymphadenopathy with dysproteinaemia. J Clin Pathol 32:356–360

Bremer K, Bartels H, Brittinger G, Burger A, Dühmke E, Gunzer U, König E, Stacher A, Theml H, Waldner R (Kiel Lymphoma Group) (1977) Clinical significance of the Kiel classification of non-Hodgkin's lymphomas (NHL). In: Seno S, Takaku F, Irino S (eds) Topics in hematology (Excerpta Medica International Congress Series No 415), Excerpta Medica, Amsterdam, pp 351–355

Brittinger G, Bartels H, Bremer K, Dühmke E, Gunzer U, König E, Stein H (Kieler Lymphomgruppe) (1976) Klinik der malignen Non-Hodgkin-Lymphome entsprechend der Kiel-Klassifikation: Centrocytisches Lymphom, centroblastisch-centrocytisches Lymphom, lymphoblastisches Lymphom, immunoblastisches Lymphom. In: Löffler H (ed) Maligne Lymphome und monoklonale Gammopathien (Hämatologie und Bluttransfusion Bd 18), Lehmanns, Munich, pp 211–223

Brittinger G, Bartels H, Bremer K, Burger A, Dühmke E, Gunzer U, König E, Stacher A, Stein H, Theml H, Waldner R (Kieler Lymphomgruppe) (1977) Retrospektive Untersuchungen zur klinischen Bedeutung der Kiel-Klassifikation der malignen Non-Hodgkin-Lymphome. Strahlentherapie 153:222–228

Brittinger G, Bartels H, Bremer K, Burger A, Dühmke E, Gunzer U, König E, Schmalhorst U, Stacher A, Stein H, Theml H, Waldner R (Kieler Lymphomgruppe) (1978) Klinische Bedeutung der Kiel-Klassifikation der malignen Non-Hodgkin-Lymphome. Ergebnisse einer retrospektiven Studie. In: Hartwich G (ed) Diagnose und Therapie von Leukämien und malignen Lymphomen. Straube, Erlangen, pp 57–66

Brittinger G, Bartels H, Burger A, Dühmke E, Fülle HH, Gunzer U, Heinz R, Huhn D, Löhr GW, Musshoff K, Nowicki L, Pfoch M, Pralle H, Schmalhorst U (Kieler Lymphomgruppe) (1979a) Grundlagen und bisherige Ergebnisse der prospektiven Studie der Kieler Lymphomgruppe über Non-Hodgkin-Lymphome. In: Stacher A, Höcker P (eds) Lymphknotentumoren. Urban and Schwarzenberg, Munich, pp 193–200

Brittinger G, Bartels H, Fülle HH, Gerhartz H, Gremmel H, Grisar T, Grupp HJ, Gunzer U, Huhn D, Koeppen K-M, Kubanek B, Leopold H, Löffler H, Löhr GW, Nowicki L, Rühl U, Schmidt M, Stacher A, Theml H, Lennert K (Kiel Lymphoma Study Group) (1979b) Principles and present status of a prospective multicentric study on the clinical relevance of the Kiel classification. 5th Meeting Int Soc Haematol, Eur Afr Div, Hamburg, August 26–31

Brittinger G, Bartels H, Common H, Dühmke E, Fülle HH, Gunzer U, Gyenes T, Heinz R, König E, Meusers P, Paukstat M, Pralle H, Theml H, Köpcke W, Thieme C, Zwingers T, Musshoff K, Stacher A, Brücher H, Herrmann F, Ludwig WD, Pribilla W, Burger-Schüler A, Löhr GW, Gremmel H, Oertel J, Gerhartz H, Koeppen K-M, Boll I, Huhn D, Binder T, Schoengen A, Nowicki L, Pees HW, Scheurlen PG, Leopold H, Wannenmacher M, Schmidt M, Löffler H, Michlmayr G, Thiel E, Zettel R, Rühl U, Wilke HJ, Schwarze E-W, Stein H, Feller AC, Lennert K (Kiel Lymphoma Study Group) (1984) Clinical and prognostic relevance of the Kiel classification of non-Hodgkin lymphomas: results of a prospective multicenter study by the Kiel Lymphoma Study Group. Hematol Oncol 2:269–306

Brittinger G, Meusers P, Engelhard M (1986a) Strategien der Behandlung von Non-Hogdkin-Lymphomen. Internist 27:485–497

Brittinger G, Bartels H, Common H, Dühmke E, Engelhard M, Fülle HH, Gunzer U, Gyenes T, Heinz R, König E, Meusers P, Pralle H, Theml H, Zwingers T, Musshoff K, Stacher A, Brücher H, Herrmann F, Ludwig WD, Pribilla W, Burger-Schüler A, Löhr GW, Gremmel H, Oertel J, Gerhartz H, Koeppen K-M, Boll I, Huhn D, Binder T, Schoengen A, Nowicki L, Pees HW, Scheurlen PG, Leopold H, Wannenmacher M, Schmidt M, Löffler H, Michlmayr G, Thiel E, Zettel R, Rühl U, Wilke HJ, Schwarze E-W, Stein H, Feller AC, Lennert K, Kieler Lymphomgruppe (1986b) Klinische und prognostische Relevanz der Kiel-Klassifikation der Non-Hodgkin-Lymphome. Onkologie 9:118–125

Bron D, Stryckmans P (1987) Role of chemotherapy for localized non-Hodgkin's lymphoma? Eur J Cancer Clin Oncol 23:459–463

Brouet JC, Preud'Homme JL, Flandrin G, Chelloul N, Seligmann M (1976) Membrane markers in "histiocytic" lymphomas (reticulum cell sarcomas). J Natl Cancer Inst 56:631–633

Bucsky P, Schwarze E-W, Reiter A, Feickert H-J, Odenwald E, Müller-Weihrich S, Riehm H (1988) Heterogeneity of childhood non-Hodgkin's lymphomas: The BFM experience. Presentation at the 20th Meeting of the International Society of Pediatric Oncology, Trondheim, August 22–26

Bucsky P, Feller AC, Beck JD, Gadner H, Heitger A, Ludwig W-D, Reiter A, Riehm H (1989) Zur Frage der Definition der malignen Histiozytose und des großzelligen anaplastischen (Ki-1) Lymphoms im Kindesalter. Klin Pädiatr 201:233–236

Bucsky P, Feller AC, Reiter A, Beck J, Bertram U, Eschenbach C, Gerein V, Lakomek M, Stollmann B, Tausch W, Urban C, Riehm H (1990) Low grade malignant non-Hodgkin's lymphomas and peripheral pleomorphic T-cell lymphomas in childhood – a BFM Study Group report. Klin Pädiatr 202:258–261

Burgio GR, Aricó M (eds) (1989) Proceedings of the International Workshop on Familial Hemophagocytic Lymphohistiocytosis (FHL), November 24–26, 1988. Pediatr Hematol Oncol 6:199–128

Burke JS, Butler JJ (1976) Malignant lymphoma with a high content of epithelioid histiocytes (Lennert's lymphoma). Am J Clin Pathol 66:1–9

Butler JJ, Cleary KR (1988) Histologic diagnosis and classifications of Hodgkin's disease and non-Hodgkin's lymphoma. In: Fuller LM, Hagemeister FB, Sullivan MP, Velasquez WS (eds) Hodgkin's disease and non-Hodgkin's lymphomas in adults and children. Raven, New York, pp 3–46

Byrne Jr E, Rappaport H (1973) Malignant histiocytosis. In: Akazaki K, Rappaport H, Berard CW, Bennett JM, Ishikawa E (eds) Malignant diseases of the hematopoietic system. (GANN monograph on cancer research no 15) University of Tokyo Press, Tokyo, pp 145–162

Carbone A, Gloghini A, Pinto A, Attadia V, Zagonel V, Volpe R (1989) Monocytoid B-cell lymphoma with bone marrow and peripheral blood involvement at presentation. Am J Clin Pathol 92:228–236

Carbone A, Gloghini A, de Re V, Tamaro P, Boiocchi M, Volpe R (1990) Histopathologic, immunophenotypic, and genotypic analysis of Ki-1 anaplastic large cell lymphomas that express histiocyte-associated antigens. Cancer 66:2547–2556

Cartun RW, Coles FB, Pastuszak WT (1987) Utilization of monoclonal antibody L26 in the identification and confirmation of B-cell lymphomas. A sensitive and specific marker applicable to formalin- and B5-fixed, paraffin-embedded tissues. Am J Pathol 129:415–421

Catovsky D, Greaves MF, Rose M, Galton DAG, Goolden AWG, McCluskey DR, White JM, Lampert I, Bourikas G, Ireland R, Brownell AI, Bridges JM, Blattner WA, Gallo RC (1982a) Adult T-cell lymphoma-leukaemia in Blacks from the West Indies. Lancet i:639–643

Catovsky D, Linch DC, Beverley PCL (1982b) T cell disorders in haematological diseases. Clin Haematol 11:661–695

Catovsky D, Wechsler A, Matutes E, Gomez R, Bourikas G, Cherchi M, Pepys EO, Pepys MB, Kitani T, Hoffbrand AV, Greaves MF (1982c) The membrane phenotype of T-prolymphocytic leukaemia. Scand J Haematol 29:398–404

Cawley JC, Burns GF, Nash TA, Higgy KE, Child JA, Roberts BE (1978) Hairy-cell leukemia with T-cell features. Blood 51:61–69

Cerezo L (1983) B-cell multilobated lymphoma. Cancer 52:2277–2280

Cerilli J, Rynasiewicz JJ, Lemos LB, Rothermel Jr WS (1977) Hodgkin's disease in human renal transplantation. Am J Surg 133:182–184

Chaganti RSK, Jhanwar SC, Koziner B, Arlin Z, Mertelsmann R, Clarkson BD (1983) Specific translocations characterize Burkitt's-like lymphoma of homosexual men with the acquired immunodeficiency syndrome. Blood 61:1269–1272

Chan JKC, Ng CS, Tung S (1986) Multilobated B-cell lymphoma, a variant of centroblastic lymphoma. Report of four cases. Histopathology 10:601–612

Chan JKC, Ng CS, Hui PK (1988) A simple guide to the terminology and application of leucocyte monoclonal antibodies. Histopathology 12:461–480

Chan JKC, Ng CS, Hui PK, Leung TW, Lo ESF, Lau WH, McGuire LJ (1989) Anaplastic large cell Ki-1 lymphoma. Delineation of two morphological types. Histopathology 15:11–34

Chan JKC, Buchanan R, Fletcher CDM (1990) Sarcomatoid variant of anaplastic large-cell Ki-1 lymphoma. Am J Surg Pathol 14:983–988

Cheson BD (1991) New chemotherapeutic agents for non-Hodgkin's lymphomas. In: Armitage JO (ed): Hematology/Oncology Clinics of North America. Non-Hodgkin's Lymphoma. Saunders Company Philadelphia Vol 5, pp 1027–1051

Chirife AM (1979) Immunologic and histologic observations in an unusual lymphoma with epithelioid histiocytes. Cell Mol Biol 24:323–329

Chittal SM, Caverivière P, Voigt J-J, Dumont J, Bénévent B, Fauré P, Bordessoule GD, Delsol G (1987) Follicular lymphoma with abundant PAS-positive extracellular material. Immuno-histochemical and ultrastructural observations. Am J Surg Pathol 11:618–624

Chittal SM, Caverivière P, Schwarting R, Gerdes J, Al Saati T, Rigal-Huguet F, Stein H, Delsol G (1988) Monoclonal antibodies in the diagnosis of Hodgkin's disease. The search for a rational panel. Am J Surg Pathol 12:9–21

Chott A, Kaserer K, Augustin I, Vesely M, Heinz R, Oehlinger W, Hanak H, Radaszkiewicz T (1990) Ki-1-positive large cell lymphoma. A clinicopathologic study of 41 cases. Am J Surg Pathol 14:439–448

Cleary ML, Sklar J (1984) Lymphoproliferative disorders in cardiac transplant recipients are multiclonal lymphomas. Lancet ii:489–493

Cleary ML, Nalesnik MA, Shearer WT, Sklar J (1988) Clonal analysis of transplant-associated lymphoproliferations based on the structure of the genomic termini of the Epstein-Barr virus. Blood 72:349–352

Close P, Lauder I (1990) Mantle zone lymphoma – is it an entity? [Editorial] J Pathol 160:279–281

Close PM, Pringle JH, Ruprai AK, West KP, Lauder I (1990) Zonal distribution of immuno-globulin-synthesizing cells within the germinal centre: an in situ hybridization and immuno-histochemical study. J Pathol 162:209–216

Cogliatti SB, Lennert K, Hansmann M-L, Zwingers TL (1990) Monocytoid B cell lymphoma. Clinical and prognostic features of 21 patients. J Clin Pathol 43:619–625

Cogliatti SB, Schmid U, Schumacher U, Eckert F, Hansmann M-L, Heddrich J, Takahashi H, Lennert K (1991) Primary B-cell gastric lymphoma: a clinicopathological study of 145 patients. Gastroenterology 101:1159–1170

Coleman M, Gerstein G, Topilow A, Lebowicz J, Berhardt B, Chiarieri D, Silver RT, Pasmantier MW (1987) Advances in chemotherapy for large cell lymphoma. Semin Hematol 24 (Suppl 1):8–20

Collins RD (1982) T-neoplasms. Their significance in relation to the classification system of lymphoid neoplasms. Am J Surg Pathol 6:745–754

Collins RD, Leech JH, Waldron JA, Flexner JM, Glick AD (1976) Diagnosis of hematopoietic, mononuclear, and lymphoid cell neoplasms. In: Rose NR, Friedman H (eds) Manual of clinical immunology. American Society for Microbiology, Washington, pp 718–733

Collins RD, Waldron JA, Glick AD (1979) Results of multiparameter studies of T-cell lymphoid neoplasms. Am J Clin Pathol (Suppl) 72:699–707

Collins RD, Bennett B, Glick AD (1983) Neoplasms of the mononuclear phagocyte system. In: Herberman RB, Friedman H (eds) The reticuloendothelial system, vol 5. Plenum, New York, pp 1–33

Common HH, Arnold H, Löhr GW (1980) Diagnostik und Therapie der Lymphogranulomato-sis X (angioimmunoblastische Lymphadenopathie). Verh Dtsch Ges Inn Med 86:484–487

Cooper MD (1979) Early events in B-cell differentiation/maturation. Paper read at Norsk Hydro's Institute for Cancer Research/The Norwegian Cancer Society Symposium "B-Cell Neoplasia in the Perspective of Normal B-Cell Differentiation", Oslo, 14–15 June 1979

Cordell JL, Falini B, Erber WN, Ghosh AK, Abdulaziz Z, MacDonald S, Pulford KAF, Stein H, Mason DY (1984) Immunoenzymatic labeling of monoclonal antibodies using immune complexes of alkaline phosphatase and monoclonal anti-alkaline phosphatase (APAAP complexes). J Histochem Cytochem 32:219-229

Cossman J (1985) Diffuse, aggressive non-Hodgkin's lymphomas. In: Jaffe ES (ed) Surgical pathology of the lymph nodes and related organs. (Major problems in pathology, vol 16) Saunders, Philadelphia, pp 203-217

Coupland RW, Pontifex AH, Salinas FA (1985) Angioimmunoblastic lymphadenopathy with dysproteinemia. Circulating immune complexes and the review of 18 cases. Cancer 55:1902-1906

Cousar JB, McGinn DL, Glick AD, List AF, Collins RD (1987) Report of an unusual lymphoma arising from parafollicular B-lymphocytes (PBLs) or so-called "monocytoid" lymphocytes. Am J Clin Pathol 87:121-128

Crissman JD, Weiss MA, Gluckman J (1982) Midline granuloma syndrome. A clinicopathologic study of 13 patients. Am J Surg Pathol 6:335-346

Cross PA, Eyden BP, Harris M (1989) Signet ring cell lymphoma of T cell type. J Clin Pathol 42:239-245

Davey FR, Elghetany MT, Kurec AS (1990) Immunophenotyping of hematologic neoplasms in paraffin-embedded tissue sections. Am J Clin Pathol 93 (suppl 1):S17-S26

De Almeida PC, Harris NL, Bhan AK (1984) Characterization of immature sinus histiocytes (monocytoid cells) in reactive lymph nodes by use of monoclonal antibodies. Hum Pathol 15:330-335

De Jong D, Voetdijk BMH, van Ommen GJB, Kluin PM (1989) Alterations in immunoglobulin genes reveal the origin and evolution of monotypic and bitypic B cell lymphomas. Am J Pathol 134:1233-1242

Dehner LP (1991) Ki-1 lymphoma. Pediatr Pathol 11:183-189

Delbrück H, Weichert HC, Schmitt G, Firusian N, Wetter O (1978) Der Zusammenhang zwischen Prognose und Kieler Klassifikation der malignen Non-Hodgkin-Lymphome. Eine katamnestische Studie über 201 Patienten. Klin Wochenschr 56:539-543

Dellagi K, Brouet J-C, Seligmann M (1984) Antivimentin autoantibodies in angioimmunoblastic lymphadenopathy. N Engl J Med 310:215-218

Delsol G, Familiades J, Voigt JJ, Gorguet B, Pris J, Laurent G, Fabre J (1977a) Les adénopathies dysimmunitaires et pseudo-lymphomateuses. I. Lymphadénopathies immunoblastiques et plasmocytaires. Ann Anat Pathol (Paris) 22:41-60

Delsol G, Familiades J, Voigt JJ, Gorguet B, Pris J, Lauent G, Fabre J (1977b) Les adénopathies dysimmunitaires et pseudo-lymphomateuses. II. Lymphadénopathies riches en cellules épithélioïdes. Ann Anat Pathol (Paris) 22:61-74

Delsol G, Fabre J, Familiades J, Ohayon E, Kuhlein E, Fedou R, Couret B (1978) Lennert's lymphoma. [Letter to the Editor] Am J Clin Pathol 69:646

Delsol G, Al Saati T, Caverivière P, Voigt JJ, Ancelin E, Rigal-Huguet F (1984) Étude en immunopéroxydase du tissu lymphoïde normal et pathologique. Intérêt des anticorps monoclonaux. Ann Pathol 4:165-183

DeRemee RA, Weiland LH, McDonald TJ (1978) Polymorphic reticulosis, lymphomatoid granulomatosis. Two diseases or one? Mayo Clin Proc 53:634-640

DeVita Jr VT, Hubbard SM, Young RC, Longo DL (1988) The role of chemotherapy in diffuse aggressive lymphomas. Semin Hematol 25 (Suppl 2):2-10

De Waele M, Van Belle S, Gepts W, Thielemans C, Schallier D, Van Camp B (1981) A Lennert lymphoma with a helper-T-cell phenotype. N Engl J Med 305:831-832

Dick FR, Maca RD (1978) The lymph node in chronic lymphocytic leukemia. Cancer 41:283-292

Diebold J, Audouin J (1985) The "Working Formulation of Non-Hodgkin's Lymphoma for Clinical Usage": a critical study. In: Sotto JJ, Vrousos C, Sotto MF, Vincent F (eds) Non-Hodgkin's Lymphomas: New Techniques and Treatments. 4th Cancer Res Workshop, Grenoble 1984. Karger, Basel, pp 13-19

Diebold J, Reynes M, Tricot G, James J-M, Zittoun R, Bilski Pasquier G (1977) Lymphome malin lympho-épithélioïde (lymphome de Lennert). Nouv Presse Méd 6:2145-2151

Diebold J, Tulliez M, Bernadou A, Audouin J, Tricot G, Reynes M, Bilski-Pasquier G (1980) Angiofollicular and plasmacytic polyadenopathy: a pseudotumourous syndrome with dysimmunity. J Clin Pathol 33:1068-1076

Diebold J, Kanavaros P, Audouin J, Bernadou A, Zittoun R (1987) Les lymphomes malins centroblastiques centrocytiques et centroblastiques à prédominance splénique (ou primitifs de la rate). Étude anatomo-clinique de 17 cas. Bull Cancer (Paris) 74:437–453

Diehl V, Schaadt M, Georgii A (1979) Clinical implications of pathological and immunological patterns in non-Hodgkin lymphomas. In: Crowther DG (ed) Leukemia and non-Hodgkin lymphoma (Advances in medical oncology, research and education, vol 7) Pergamon, Oxford, pp 163–177

Dierendonck JH van, Wijsman JH, Keijzer R, Van de Velde CJH, Cornelisse CJ (1991) Cell-cycle-related staining patterns of anti-proliferating cell nuclear antigen monoclonal antibodies. Comparison with BrdUrd labeling and Ki-67 staining. Am J Pathol 138:1165–1172

Dorfman RF (1974) Classification of non-Hodgkin's lymphomas. [Letter to the Editor] Lancet i:1295–1296

Dorfman RF (1975) Lymphadenopathy. [Letter to the Editor] Hum Pathol 6:264

Dorfman RF (1983) The National Cancer Institute sponsored study of the classification of non-Hodgkin's lymphomas. Comment by "expert" pathologists. Hematol Oncol 1:97–98

Dorfman RF, Warnke R (1974) Lymphadenopathy simulating the malignant lymphomas. Hum Pathol 5:519–550

Dühmke E (1976) Zur klinischen Relevanz der histologischen Differenzierung maligner Non-Hodgkin-Lymphome nach der „Kiel-Klassifikation". Eine retrospektive Studie entsprechender Korrelationen bei 228 Fällen aus Schleswig-Holstein. Strahlentherapie 152:129–139

Dumont J, Thiéry JP, Mazabraud A (1979) Adénopathies angio-immunoblastiques: étude ultrastructurale des ganglions. Discussion sur le role éventuel du virus d'Epstein-Barr (EBV). Nouv Rev Fr Hematol 21:257–282

Dura WT, Gladkowska-Dura MJ (1981) Non-Hodgkin's lymphoma in the first two decades. Morphologic and immunocytochemical study. Virchows Arch [A] 390:23–62

Ebraim SA, Ladanyi M, Desai SB, Offit K, Jhanwar SC, Filippa DA, Lieberman PH, Chaganti RS (1990) Immunohistochemical, molecular, and cytogenetic analysis of a consecutive series of 20 peripheral T-cell lymphomas and lymphomas of uncertain lineage, including 12 Ki-1 positive lymphomas. Genes Chromosom Cancer 2:27–35

Editorial (1976) The Lennert lymphoma. Lancet ii:507

Egerter DA, Beckstead JH (1988) Malignant lymphomas in the acquired immunodeficiency syndrome. Additional evidence for a B-cell origin. Arch Pathol Lab Med 112:602–606

Engelhard M, von Schilling C, Diehl V, Pfreundschuh M, Brittinger G, Feller AC, Stein H, Zwingers T, Lennert K (1986) Clinical analysis of Ki1 lymphoma. (Abstract) Blut 53:219

Engelhard M, Meusers P, Bartels H, Binder T, Fülle HH, Görg K, Gunzer U, Havemann K, Kayser W, König E, König HJ, Kuse R, Löffler H, Ludwig W-D, Mainzer K, Martin H, Pralle H, Schoppe WD, Staiger HJ, Theml H, Zurborn KH, Zwingers T, Lennert K, Brittinger G (1989) Zentrozytisches Lymphom: klinisches Bild und Analyse der bisherigen Therapieerfahrungen. In: Thiel E, Wilmanns W, Enghofer E (eds) Non-Hodgkin-Lymphome: Trends in Diagnostik und Therapie. (Onkologisches Kolloquium 3) de Gruyter, Berlin, pp 65–78

Engelhard M, Brittinger G, Heinz R, Theml H, Bartels H, Binder T, Fülle HH, Gerhartz H, Gunzer U, Ludwig F, Ludwig WD, Nowicki L, Oertel J, Pees HW, Pralle H, Rühl U, v. Schilling C, Spann W, Szeimies U, Wetzel HJ, Zwingers T, Feller AC, Stacher A, Stein H, Lennert K (1991) Chronic lymphocytic leukemia (B-CLL) and immunocytoma (LP-IC): Clinical and prognostic relevance of this distinction. Leukemia Lymphoma 5 (Suppl.) 161–173

Engelhard M, Stein H, von Schilling C, Dallenbach F, Zwingers T, Feller AC, Lennert K (1992) Immunomorphological and clinical characterization of CD30 (Ki-1) positive large cell lymphomas: identification of three subgroups with prognostic relevance. submitted for publication

Enzinger FM, Weiss SH (1988) Soft tissue tumors, 2nd edn, Mosby, St. Louis

Ernberg I (1989) Epstein-Barr virus and acquired immunodeficiency syndrome. In: Klein G (ed) Advances in viral oncology, vol 8: tumorigenic DNA viruses. Raven, New York, pp 203–217

Euler HH, von Schilling C, Glass B, Feller AC, Lennert K, Löffler H (1987) Circulating immune complexes (CIC) in angioimmunoblastic lymphadenopathy. (Abstract) Proc Int Conf Malignant Lymphoma 3:P17

Facchetti F, de Wolfe-Peeters C, van den Oord JJ, Desmet VJ (1987) Immunohistochemical visualization of plasmacytoid T cells in paraffin sections. [Letter] Hum Pathol 18:1300

Facchetti F, de Wolf-Peeters C, Mason DY, Pulford K, van den Oord JJ, Desmet VJ (1988) Plasmacytoid T cells. Immunohistochemical evidence for their monocyte/macrophage origin. Am J Pathol 133:15–21

Facchetti F, de Wolf-Peeters C, Kennes C, Rossi G, de Vos R, van den Oord JJ, Desmet VJ (1990) Leukemia-associated lymph nod infiltrates of plasmacytoid monocytes (so-called plasmacytoid T-cells). Evidence for two distinct histological and immunophenotypical patterns. Am J Surg Pathol 14:101–112

Falini B, Pileri S, Martelli MF (1989) Histological and immunohistological analysis of human lymphomas. Crit Rev Oncol/Hematol 9:351–419

Falini B, Pileri S, De Solas I, Martelli MF, Mason DY, Delsol G, Gatter KC, Fagioli M (1990) Peripheral T-cell lymphoma associated with hemophagocytic syndrome. Blood 75:434–444

Farquhar JW, MacGregor AR, Richmond J (1958) Familial haemophagocytic reticulosis. Br Med J 1958/ii:1561–1564

Fauci AS, Johnson RE, Wolff SM (1976) Radiation therapy of midline granuloma. Ann Intern Med 84:140–147

Fellbaum C, Hansmann ML, Parwaresch MR, Lennert K (1988) Monoclonal antibodies Ki-B3 and Leu-M1 discriminate giant cells of infectious mononucleosis and of Hodgkin's disease. Hum Pathol 19:1168–1173

Feller AC (1982) Cytochemical reactivity of Tγ lymphocytes in human lymphatic tissue for dipeptidylaminopeptidase IV. Histochem J 14:889–895

Feller AC (1989) Phänotypische Analyse humaner T-Zell-Lymphome. (Veröffentlichungen aus der Pathologie, Band 131) Fischer, Stuttgart

Feller AC, Griesser H (1989) DNA gene rearrangement studies in Hodgkin's disease and related lymphomas: A contribution to their cellular origin. Recent Results Cancer Res 117:27–34

Feller AC, Sterry W (1989) Large cell anaplastic lymphoma of the skin. Br J Dermatol 121:593–602

Feller AC, Heijnen CJ, Ballieux RE, Parwaresch MR (1982a) Enzymehistochemical staining of Tγ lymphocytes for glycylproline-4-methoxy-beta-naphthylamide-peptidase (DAP IV). Br J Haematol 51:227–234

Feller AC, Parwaresch MR, Bartels H, Lennert K (1982b) Enzymecytochemical heterogeneity of human chronic T-lymphocytic leukemia as demonstrated by reactivity to dipeptidylaminopeptidase IV (DAP IV; EC 3.4.14.4). Leuk Res 6:801–808

Feller AC, Parwaresch MR Lennert K (1983a) Subtyping of chronic lymphocytic leukemia of T-type by dipeptidylaminopeptidase IV (DAP IV), monoclonal antibodies, and Fc-receptors. Cancer 52:1609–1612

Feller AC, Lennert K, Stein H, Bruhn H-D, Wuthe H-H (1983b) Immunohistology and aetiology of histiocytic necrotizing lymphadenitis. Report of three instructive cases. Histopathology 7:825–839

Feller AC, Parwaresch MR, Lennert K (1984) Cytochemical distribution of dipeptidylaminopeptidase IV (DAP IV; EC 3.4.14.5) in T-lymphoblastic lymphoma/leukemia characterized with monoclonal antibodies. Leuk Res 8:397–406

Feller AC, Griesser GH, Mak TW, Lennert K (1986a) Lymphoepithelioid lymphoma (Lennert's lymphoma) is a monoclonal proliferation of helper/inducer T cells. Blood 68:663–667

Feller AC, Parwaresch MR, Stein H, Ziegler A, Herbst H, Lennert K (1986b) Immunophenotyping of T-lymphoblastic lymphoma/leukemia: correlation with normal T-cell maturation. Leuk Res 10:1025–1031

Feller AC, Griesser H, von Schilling C, Wacker HH, Dallenbach F, Bartels H, Kruse R, Mak TW, Lennert K (1988) Clonal gene rearrangement patterns correlate with immunophenotype and clinical parameters in patients with angioimmunoblastic lymphadenopathy. Am J Pathol 133:549–557

Feller AC, Lennert K, Zwingers T (1991) Peripheral T-cell lymphomas [Letter to the Editor] Histopathology 19:481–482

Fellous M, Cartron J-P, Wiels J, Tursz T (1985) A monoclonal antibody against a Burkitt lymphoma associated antigen has an anti-Pk red blood cell specificity. Br J Haematol 60:559–565

Felman P, Bryon PA, Gentilhomme O, Magaud JP, Manel AM, Coiffier B, Lenoir G (1985a) Burkitt's lymphoma: multiparametric analysis of 55 cell lines with special reference to morphometry. In: Cavalli F, Bonadonna G, Rozencweig M (eds) Malignant lymphomas and

Hodgkin's disease: Experimental and therapeutic advances. Proc 2nd Int Conf Malignant Lymphomas, Lugano 1984. Nijhoff, Boston, pp 45–55

Felman P, Bryon P-A, Gentilhomme O, Magaud J-P, Manel A-M, Coiffier B, Lenoir G (1985b) Burkitt's lymphoma. Distinction of subgroups by morphometric analysis of the characteristics of 55 cell lines. Anal Quant Cytol Histol 7:275–282

Fifth International Workshop on Chromosomes in Leukemia-Lymphoma (1987) Correlation of chromosome abnormalities with histologic and immunologic characteristics in non-Hodgkin's lymphoma and adult T cell leukemia-lymphoma. Blood 70:1554–1564

Fischer R (1978) Pathologie der malignen Lymphome unter besonderer Berücksichtigung neuerer Klassifikationen. Med Welt 29:16–20

Fischer R (1986) Aktuelle Fragen zur Histopathologie und Klassifikation der Non-Hodgkin-Lymphome. Internist 27:473–484

Flandrin (1978) Angioimmunoblastic lymphadenopathy: Clinical, biologic, and follow-up study of 14 cases. Recent Results Cancer Res 64:247–262

Flandrin G, Daniel MT, El Yafi G, Chelloul N (1972) Sarcomatoses ganglionnaires diffuses a différenciation plasmocytaire avec anémie hémolytique auto-immune. Actualités Hémat 6:25–41

Fletcher JA, Lynch EA, Kimball VM, Donnelly M, Tantravahi R, Sallan SE (1991) Translocation (9;22) is associated with extremely poor prognosis in intensively treated children with acute lymphoblastic leukemia. Blood 77:435–439

Fliedner A, Parwaresch MR, Feller AC (1990) Induction of antigen expression of follicular dendritic cells in a monoblastic cell line. A contribution to its cellular origin. J Pathol 161:71–77

Forster G, Moeschlin S (1954) Extramedulläres, leukämisches Plasmocytöm mit Dysproteinämie und erworbener hämolytischer Anämie. Schweiz Med Wochenschr 84:1106–1110

French Cooperative Group on Chronic Lymphocytic Leukaemia (1986) Effectiveness of "CHOP" regimen in advanced untreated chronic lymphocytic leukaemia. Lancet i:1346–1349

French Cooperative Group on Chronic Lymphocytic Leukemia (1991) Therapeutic results from the trials managed by the French Cooperative Group on Chronic Lymphocytic Leukemia. Leukemia Lymphoma 5 (Suppl.) 83–88

Frizzera G (1987) The clinico-pathological expressions of Epstein-Barr virus infection in lymphoid tissues. Virchows Arch [B] 53:1–12

Frizzera G, Murphy SB (1979) Follicular (nodular) lymphoma in childhood: A rare clinical-pathological entity. Report of eight cases from four cancer centers. Cancer 44:2218–2235

Frizzera G, Moran EM, Rappaport H (1974) Angio-immunoblastic lymphadenopathy with dysproteinaemia. Lancet i:1070–1073

Frizzera G, Moran EM, Rappaport H (1975) Angio-immunoblastic lymphadenopathy. Diagnosis and clinical course. Am J Med 59:803–818

Frizzera G, Hanto DW, Gajl-Peczalska KJ, Rosai J, McKenna RW, Sibley RK, Holahan KP, Lindquist LL (1981) Polymorphic diffuse B-cell hyperplasias and lymphomas in renal transplant recipients. Cancer Res 41:4262–4279

Frizzera G, Massarelli G, Banks PM, Rosai J (1983) A systemic lymphoproliferative disorder with morphologic features of Castleman's disease. Pathologic findings in 15 patients. Am J Surg Pathol 7:211–231

Frizzera G, Anaya JS, Banks PM (1986) Neoplastic plasma cells in follicular lymphomas. Clinical and pathologic findings in six cases. Virchows Arch [A] 409:149–162

Frizzera G, Kaneko Y, Sakurai M (1989) Angioimmunoblastic lymphadenopathy and related disorders: a retrospective look in search of definitions. Leukemia 3:1–5

Fujita K, Fukuhara S, Nasu K, Yamabe H, Tomono N, Inamoto Y, Shimazaki C, Ohno H, Doi S, Kamesaki H, Ueshima Y, Uchino H (1986) Recurrent chromosome abnormalities in adult T-cell lymphomas of peripheral T-cell origin. Int J Cancer 37:517–524

Gaba AR, Stein RS, Sweet DL, Variakojis D (1978) Multicentric giant lymph node hyperplasia. Am J Clin Pathol 69:86–90

Gadner H, Müller-Weihrich S, Riehm H für die BFM-Studiengruppe (1986) Behandlungsstrategien der malignen Non-Hodgkin-Lymphome im Kindesalter. Onkologie 9:126–130

Galton DAG (1964) Chronic lymphocytic leukaemia: its pathogenesis and relationship to lymphosarcoma. In: Roulet FC (ed) Symposium on lymphoreticular tumours in Africa. Karger, Basel, pp 163–172

Galton DAG, Goldman JM, Wiltshaw E, Catovsky D, Henry K, Goldenberg GJ (1974) Prolymphocytic leukaemia. Br J Haematol 27: 7–23

Garcia CF, Weiss LM, Warnke RA (1986) Small noncleaved cell lymphoma: an immunophenotypic study of 18 cases and comparison with large cell lymphoma. Hum Pathol 17: 454–461

Garwicz S, Landberg T, Lindberg L-G, Åkerman M (1978) Clinico-pathological correlations in the Kiel classification of non-Hodgkin's lymphomata in children. Scand J Haematol 20: 171–180

Geerts M-L (1988) Mycosis fungoides. Een morfologische studie. Proefschrift tot het verkrijgen van de graad van Geaggregeerde voor het Hoger Onderwijs. Rijksuniversiteit, Afd. Huidziekten, Gent

Georgii A, Krmpotic E, Stünkel K, Thiele J, Vykoupil K-F, Diehl V (1979) Verwendung der Kiel-Klassifikation unter gleichzeitigem Einsatz von Zytogenetik, Membranmarkern und Elektronenmikroskopie. In: Stacher A, Höcker P (eds) Lymphknotentumoren. Urban and Schwarzenberg, Munich, pp 82–90

Gérard-Marchant R (1974a) Une nouvelle approche physio-morphologique des lymphomes malins non hodgkiniens. Bull Cancer (Paris) 61: 1–10

Gérard-Marchant R (1974b) Conceptions nosologiques actuelles des lymphomes malins non hodgkiniens. Ann Anat Pathol (Paris) 19: 149–162

Gérard-Marchant R, Hamlin I, Lennert K, Rilke F, Stansfeld AG, van Unnik JAM (1974) Classification of non-Hodgkin's lymphomas. [Letter to the Editor] Lancet ii: 406–408

Gerdes J, Dallenbach F, Lennert K, Lemke H, Stein H (1984) Growth fractions in malignant non-Hodgkin's lymphomas (NHL) as determined in situ with the monoclonal antibody Ki-67. Hematol Oncol 2: 365–371

Glimelius B, Hagberg H, Sundström C (1983) Morphological classification of non-Hodgkin malignant lymphoma. II. Comparison between Rappaport's classification and the Kiel classification. Scand J Haematol 30: 13–24

Gobbi M, Caligaris-Cappio F, Janossy G (1983) Normal equivalent cells of B cell malignancies: analysis with monoclonal antibodies. Br J Haematol 54: 393–403

Gödde-Salz E, Feller AC, Lennert K (1986) Cytogenetic and immunohistochemical analysis of lymphoepithelioid cell lymphoma (Lennert's lymphoma): further substantiation of its T-cell nature. Leuk Res 10: 313–323

Gödde-Salz E, Feller AC, Lennert K (1987) Chromosomal abnormalities in lymphogranulomatosis X (LgrX)/angioimmunoblastic lymphadenopathy (AILD). Leuk Res 11: 181–190

Goldberg AF, Barka T (1962) Acid phosphatase activity in human blood cells. Nature 195: 297

Green I, Jaffe ES, Shevach EM, Edelson RL, Frank MM, Berard CW (1975) Determination of the origin of malignant reticular cells by the use of surface membrane markers. In: Rebuck JW, Berard CW, Abell MR (eds) The reticuloendothelial system. (Monographs in pathology, no 16) Williams and Wilkins, Baltimore, pp 282–300

Greer JP, Kinney MC, Collins RD, Salhany KE, Wolff SN, Hainsworth JD, Flexner JM, Stein RS (1991) Clinical features of 31 patients with Ki-1 anaplastic large-cell lymphoma. J Clin Oncol 9: 539–547

Griesser H, Feller A, Lennert K, Minden M, Mak TW (1986a) Rearrangement of the β chain of the T cell antigen receptor and immunoglobulin genes in lymphoproliferative disorders. J Clin Invest 78: 1179–1184

Griesser H, Feller A, Lennert K, Tweedale M, Messner HA, Zalcberg J, Minden MD, Mak TW (1986b) The structure of the T cell gamma chain gene in lymphoproliferative disorders and lymphoma cell lines. Blood 68: 592–594

Griesser H, Feller AC, Mak TW, Lennert K (1987) Clonal rearrangements of T-cell receptor and immunoglobulin genes and immunophenotypic antigen expression in different subclasses of Hodgkin's disease. Int J Cancer 40: 157–160

Griesser H, Tkachuk D, Reis MD, Mak TW (1989) Gene rearrangements and translocations in lymphoproliferative diseases. Blood 73: 1402–1415

Griesser H, Plendl H, Boie C (1991) Klonale Genrearrangements der α-Kette des T-Zellrezeptors bei lymphoproliferativen Erkrankungen. Verh Dtsch Ges Pathol 75: 408

Griffin JD, Ellman L, Long JC, Dvorak AM (1978) Development of a histiocytic medullary reticulosis-like syndrome during the course of acute lymphocytic leukemia. Am J Med 64:851–858

Grogan TM, Richter LC, Payne CM, Rangel CS (1985) Signet-ring cell lymphoma of T-cell origin. An immunocytochemical and ultrastructural study relating giant vacuole formation to cytoplasmic sequestration of surface membrane. Am J Surg Pathol 9:684–692

Grossman B, Schechter GP, Horton JE, Pierce L, Jaffe E, Wahl L (1981) Hypercalcemia associated with T-cell lymphoma-leukemia. J Clin Pathol 75:149–155

Gustmann C, Altmannsberger M, Osborn M, Griesser H, Feller AC (1991) Cytokeratin expression and vimentin content in large cell anaplastic lymphomas and other non-Hodgkin's lymphomas. Am J Pathol 138:1413–1422

Haas JE, Palmer NF, Weinberg AG, Beckwith JB (1981) Ultrastructure and malignant rhabdoid tumor of the kidney. A distinctive renal tumor of children. Hum Pathol 12:646–657

Habeshaw JA, Catley PF, Stansfeld AG, Brearley RL (1979) Surface phenotyping, histology and the nature of non-Hodgkin lymphoma in 157 patients. Br J Cancer 40:11–34

Hall PA, D'Ardenne AJ, Richards MA, Stansfeld AG (1987) Lymphoplasmacytoid lymphoma: an immunohistological study. J Pathol 153:213–223

Hall PA, Donaghy M, Cotter FE, Stansfeld AG, Levison DA (1989) An immunohistological and genotypic study of the plasma cell form of Castleman's disease. Histopathology 14:333–346

Hall PA, Levison DA, Woods AL, Yu CC-W, Kellock DB, Watkins JA, Barnes DM, Gillett CE, Camplejohn R, Dover R, Waseem NH, Lane DP (1990) Proliferating cell nuclear antigen (PCNA) immunolocalization in paraffin sections: an index of cell proliferation with evidence of deregulated expression in some neoplasms. J Pathol 162:285–294

Hamilton-Dutoit SJ, Pallesen G (1989) B cell associated monoclonal antibody L26 may occasionally label T cell lymphomas. Acta Pathol Microbiol Immunol Scand [A] 97:1033–1036

Hamilton-Dutoit SJ, Pallesen G, Karkov J, Skinhoj P, Franzmann MB, Pedersen C (1989) Identification of EBV-DNA in tumour cells of AIDS-related lymphomas by in-situ hybridisation. Lancet i:554–555

Hamilton-Dutoit SJ, Pallesen G, Franzmann MB, Karkov J, Black F, Skinhoj P, Pedersen C (1991) AIDS-related lymphoma. Histopathology, immunophenotype, and association with Epstein-Barr virus as demonstrated by in situ nucleic acid hybridization. Am J Pathol 138:149–163

Hanaoka M (1984) Adult T cell leukemia and Sézary syndrome. Leuk Rev Int 2:17–44

Hanaoka M, Shirakawa S, Yodoi J, Uchiyama T, Takatsuki K (1979) Adult T cell leukemia. Histological features of the lymphoid tissues. In: Müller-Ruchholtz W, Müller-Hermelink HK (eds) Function and structure of the immune system. (Advances in experimental medicine and biology, vol 144) Plenum, New York, pp 613–621

Hanaoka M, Takatsuki K, Shimoyama M (eds) (1982) Adult T cell leukemia and related diseases. (GANN monograph on cancer research, no 28) Japan Scientific Societies Press, Tokyo and Plenum, New York

Hansen MM, Andersen E, Birgens H, Christensen BE, Christensen TG, Geisler C, Meldgaard K, Pedersen D (1991) CHOP versus chlorambucil + prednisolone in chronic lymphocytic leukemia. Leukemia Lymphoma 5 (Suppl.) 97–100

Hanson CA, Frizzera G, Patton DF, Peterson BA, McClain KL, Gajl-Peczalska KJ, Kersey JH (1988) Clonal rearrangement for immunoglobulin and T-cell receptor genes in systemic Castleman's disease. Association with Epstein-Barr virus. Am J Pathol 131:84–91

Hanto DW, Frizzera G, Purtilo DT, Sakamoto K, Sullivan JL, Saemundsen AK, Klein G, Simmons RL, Najarian JS (1981) Clinical spectrum of lymphoproliferative disorders in renal transplant recipients and evidence for the role of Epstein-Barr virus. Cancer Res 41:4253–4261

Hanto DW, Gajl-Peczalska KJ, Frizzera G, Arthur DC, Balfour HH, McClain K, Simmons RL, Najarian JS (1983) Epstein-Barr virus (EBV) induced polyclonal and monoclonal B-cell lymphoproliferative diseases occurring after renal transplantation. Clinical, pathologic, and virologic findings and implications for therapy. Ann Surg 198:356–369

Harabuchi Y, Yamanaka N, Kataura A, Imai S, Kinoshita T, Mizuno F, Osato T (1990) Epstein-Barr virus in nasal T-cell lymphomas in patients with lethal midline granuloma. Lancet 335:128–130

Harris M, Eyden B, Read G (1981) Signet ring cell lymphoma. A rare variant of follicular lymphoma. J Clin Pathol 34:884–895

Harris NL, Bhan AK (1985a) Mantle zone lymphoma. A pattern produced by lymphomas of more than one cell type. Am J Surg Pathol 9:872–882

Harris NL, Bhan AK (1985b) B-cell neoplasms of the lymphocytic, lymphoplasmacytoid, and plasma cell types: immunologic analysis and clinical correlation. Hum Pathol 16:829–837

Harris NL, Demirjian Z (1991) Plasmacytoid T-zone cell proliferation in a patient with chronic myelomonocytic leukemia. Histologic and immunohistologic characterization. Am J Surg Pathol 15:87–95

Harris NL, Nadler LM, Bhan AK (1984) Immunohistologic characterization of two malignant lymphomas of germinal center type (centroblastic/centrocytic and centrocytic) with mono- clonal antibodies. Follicular and diffuse lymphomas of small-cleaved-cell type are related but distinct entities. Am J Pathol 117:262–272

Hastrup N, Ralfkiaer E, Pallesen G (1989) Aberrant phenotypes in peripheral T cell lymphomas. J Clin Pathol 42:398–402

Hastrup N, Hamilton-Dutoid S, Ralfkiaer E, Pallesen G (1991) Peripheral T-cell lymphomas: an evaluation or reproducibility of the updated Kiel classification. Histopathology 18:99–105

Hattori T, Uchiyama T, Toibana T, Takatsuki K, Uchino H (1981) Surface phenotype of Japanese adult T-cell leukemia cells characterized by monoclonal antibodies. Blood 58:644– 647

Hayes D, Robertson JH (1979) Malignant lymphoma with a high content of epithelioid histio- cytes. J Clin Pathol 32:675–680

Heimann R, Vannineuse A, De Sloover C, Dor P (1978) Malignant lymphomas and undifferen- tiated small cell carcinoma of the thyroid: a clinicopathological review in the light of the Kiel classification for malignant lymphomas. Histopathology 2:201–213

Heinz R, Stacher A, Theml H, Pralle H, Bremer K, Brunswicker F, Burkert M, Common H, Fülle HH, Grüneisen A, Hermann F, Leopold H, Liffers R, Nowicki L, Nürnberger R, Rengshausen H, Rühl U, Schoengen A, Schmidt M, Wirthmüller R, Schwarze E-W (Kiel Lymphoma Study Group) (1979) Immunocytic lymphoma, a clinical entity distinct from chronic lymphocytic leukemia. 5th Meeting. Intern. Soc. Haematol., European and African Division, Hamburg, August 26–31, 1979

Heitger A, Gadner H, Bucsky P, Feller AC, Ritter J, Riehm H (1989) Das großzellige anaplasti- sche Lymphom im Kindesalter – Klinische Erfahrungen bei einer histologisch neu definierten Entität. Klin Pädiatr 201:237–241

Helbron D, Brittinger G, Lennert K (1979) T-Zonen-Lymphom. Klinisches Bild, Therapie und Prognose. Blut 39:117–131

Henry K (1979) Reactive and proliferative disorders of the alimentary tract. VIIth Eur. Congr. Pathol., Valencia, Spain, September 17–21, 1979

Hill W, Burkhardt R (1984) "Epitheloid cell lymphogranulomatosis" in the bone marrow. In: Lennert K, Hübner K (eds) Pathology of the bone marrow. Fischer, Stuttgart, pp 351–354

Ho FCS, Choy D, Loke SL, Kung ITM, Fu KH, Liang R, Todd D, Khoo RKK (1990a) Polymorphic reticulosis and conventional lymphomas of the nose and upper aerodigestive tract: a clinicopathologic study of 70 cases, and immunophenotypic studies of 16 cases. Hum Pathol 21:1041–1050

Ho FCS, Srivastava G, Loke SL, Fu KH, Leung BPY, Liang R, Choy D (1990b) Presence of Epstein-Barr virus DNA in nasal lymphomas of B and 'T' cell type. Hematol Oncol 8:271– 281

Ho JHC, Lau WH, Kwan HC, Chan CL, Au GKH, Saw D, de Thé G (1981) Diagnostic and prognostic serological markers in nasopharyngeal carcinoma (NPC). In: Grundmann E, Krueger GRF, Ablashi DV (eds) Nasopharyngeal carcinoma. Cancer campaign, vol 5, Fischer, Stuttgart, pp 219–224

Hofmann WJ, Momburg F, Möller P, Otto HF (1988) Intra- and extrathymic B cells in physi- ologic and pathologic conditions. Immunohistochemical study on normal thymus and lymphofollicular hyperplasia of the thymus. Virchows Arch [A] 412:431–442

Hoppe RT, Wood GS, Abel EA (1990) Mycosis fungoides and the Sézary syndrome: pathology, staging, and treatment. Curr Probl Cancer 14:295–371

Horny H-P, Feller AC, Horst H-A, Lennert K (1987) Immunocytology of plasmacytoid T cells: Marker analysis indicates a unique phenotype of this enigmatic cell. Hum Pathol 18:28–32

Hossfeld DK, Höffken K, Schmidt CG, Diedrichs H (1976) Chromosome abnormalities in angioimmunoblastic lymphadenopathy. Lancet i:198

Hsu S-M, Raine L, Fanger H (1981) Use of avidin-biotin-peroxidase complex (ABC) in immunoperoxidase techniques: a comparison between ABC and unlabeled antibody (PAP) procedures. J Histochem Cytochem 29:577–580

Hu E, Weiss LM, Warnke R, Sklar J (1987) Non-Hodgkin's lymphoma containing both B and T cell clones. Blood 70:287–292

Hui PK, Feller AC, Pileri S, Gobbi M, Lennert K (1987) New aggressive variant of suppressor/cytotoxic T-CLL. Am J Clin Pathol 87:55–59

Hui PK, Feller AC, Lennert K (1988) High-grade non-Hodgkin's lymphoma of B-cell type. I. Histopathology. Histopathology 12:127–143

Humphrey JH (1981) Tolerogenic or immunogenic activity of hapten-conjugated polysaccharides correlated with cellular localization. Eur J Immunol 11:212–220

Ioachim HL, Cooper MC, Hellman GC (1985) Lymphomas in men at high risk for acquired immune deficiency syndrome (AIDS). A study of 21 cases. Cancer 56:2831–2842

Isaacson P (1979) Middle East lymphoma and α-chain disease. An immunohistochemical study. Am J Surg Pathol 3:431–441

Isaacson PG (1989) Castleman's disease. (Commentary) Histopathology 14:429–432

Isaacson PG, Spencer J (1987) Malignant lymphoma of mucosa-associated lymphoid tissue. Histopathology 11:445–462

Isaacson P, Wright DH (1984) Extranodal malignant lymphoma arising from mucosa-associated lymphoid tissue. Cancer 53:2515–2524

Isobe T, Ikeda Y, Ohta H (1979) Comparison of sizes and shapes of tumor cells in plasma cell leukemia and plasma cell myeloma. Blood 53:1028–1030

Iversen OH, Iversen U, Ziegler JL, Bluming AZ (1974) Cell kinetics in Burkitt lymphoma. Eur J Cancer 10:155–163

Jackson Jr H, Parker Jr F (1947) Hodgkin's Disease and Allied Disorders. Oxford University Press, New York

Jacobs RH, Vokes EE, Golomb HM (1985) Second malignancies in hairy cell leukemia. Cancer 56:1462–1467

Jacobson JO, Aisenberg AC, Lamarre L, Willett CG, Linggood RM, Miketic LM, Harris NL (1988) Mediastinal large cell lymphoma. An uncommon subset of adult lymphoma curable with combined modality therapy. Cancer 62:1893–1898

Jaffe ES (1985) Post-thymic lymphoid neoplasia. In: Jaffe ES (eds) Surgical pathology of the lymph nodes and related organs. (Major problems in pathology, vol 16) Saunders, Philadelphia, pp 218–248

Jaffe ES (1988) The morphologic spectrum of T-cell lymphoma. (Abstract) Am J Surg Pathol 12:158–159

Jaffe ES, Costa J, Fauci AS, Cossman J, Tsokos M (1983) Malignant lymphoma and erythrophagocytosis simulating malignant histiocytosis. Am J Med 75:741–749

Jaffe ES, Blattner WA, Blayney DW, Bunn Jr PA, Cossman J, Robert-Guroff M, Gallo RC (1984) The pathologic spectrum of adult T-cell leukemia/lymphoma in the United States. Am J Surg Pathol 8:263–275

Jaffe ES, Bookman MA, Longo DL (1987) Lymphocytic lymphoma of intermediate differentiation – mantle zone lymphoma: a distinct subtype of B-cell lymphoma. Hum Pathol 18:877–880

Jansen J, Schuit HRE, Schreuder GMT, Muller HP, Meijer CJLM (1979) Distinct subtype within the spectrum of hairy cell leukemia. Blood 54:459–467

Jennette JC, Reddick RL, Saunders AW, Wilkman AS (1982) Diffuse T-cell lymphoma preceded by nodular lymphoma. J Clin Pathol 78:242–248

Jones DB, Wright DH, Paul F, Smith JL (1986) Phenotypic heterogeneity displayed by T-non Hodgkin's lymphoma (T-NHL) cells dispersed from diagnostic lymph node biopsies. Hematol Oncol 4:219–226

Jones EL (1983) Antibody probes in diagnosis and classification of lymphomas. J Pathol 141:259–286

Jones SE, Fuks Z, Bull M, Kadin ME, Dorfman RF, Kaplan HS, Rosenberg SA, Kim H (1973) Non-Hodgkin's lymphomas. IV. Clinicopathologic correlation in 405 cases. Cancer 31:806–823

Jones SE, Miller TP, Connors JM (1989) Long-term follow-up and analysis for prognostic factors for patients with limited-stage diffuse large-cell lymphoma treated with initial chemotherapy with or without adjuvant radiotherapy. J Clin Oncol 7:1186–1191

Kadin ME (1981) T gamma cells: A missing link between malignant histiocytosis and T cell leukemia-lymphoma? Hum Pathol 12:771–772

Kadin ME (1990) Lymphomatoid papulosis and Ki-1$^+$ large cell lymphomas of the skin: pathology, immunology, natural history, and relevance to Hodgkin's disease. In: Hanaoka M, Kadin ME, Mikata A, Watanabe S (eds) Lymphoid malignancy: immunocytology and cytogenetics. Field and Wood, Philadelphia, pp 189–195

Kadin ME, Kamoun M (1982) Nonendemic adult T-cell leukemia/lymphoma. Hum Pathol 13:691–693

Kadin ME, Kamoun M, Lamberg J (1981) Erythrophagocytic Tγ lymphoma. A clinicopathologic entity resembling malignant histiocytosis. N Engl J Med 304:648–653

Kadin M, Nasu K, Sako D, Said J, Vonderheit E (1985) Lymphomatoid papulosis. A cutaneous proliferation of activated helper T cells expressing Hodgkin's disease-associated antigens. Am J Pathol 119:315–325

Kadin ME, Sako D, Berliner N, Franklin W, Woda B, Borowitz M, Ireland K, Schweid A, Herzog P, Lange B, Dorfman R (1986) Childhood Ki-1 lymphoma presenting with skin lesions and peripheral lymphadenopathy. Blood 68:1042–1049

Kadin ME, Vonderheid EC, Sako D, Clayton LK, Olbricht S (1987) Clonal composition of T cells in lymphomatoid papulosis. Am J Pathol 126:13–17

Kaiserling E (1977) Non-Hodgkin-Lymphome. Ultrastruktur und Cytogenese (Veröffentlichungen aus der Pathologie, Heft 105). Fischer, Stuttgart

Kaiserling E (1978) Ultrastructure of non-Hodgkin's lymphomas. In: Lennert K et al. (eds) Malignant lymphomas other than Hodgkin's disease (Handbuch der speziellen pathologischen Anatomie und Histologie, vol 1, part 3 B) Springer, Berlin Heidelberg New York, pp 471–528

Kaiserling E, Patsouris E, Müller-Hermelink HK, Wichterich D, Lennert K (1989) Bacterial lymphadenitis with the picture of a lymphoepithelioid cell lymphoma (Lennert's lymphoma). Histopathology 14:161–178

Kalter SP, Riggs SA, Cabanillas F, Butler JJ, Hagemeister FB, Mansell PW, Newell GR, Velasquez WS, Salvador P, Barlogie B, Rios A, Hersh EM (1985) Aggressive non-Hodgkin's lymphomas in immunocompromised homosexual males. Blood 66:655–659

Kalyanaraman VS, Sarngadharan MG, Miyoshi I, Blayney D, Golde D, Gallo RC (1982) A new subtype of human T-cell leukemia virus (HTLV-II) associated with a T-cell variant of hairy cell leukemia. Science 218:571–573

Kamel OW, LeBrun DP, Davis RE, Berry GJ, Warnke RA (1991) Growth fraction estimation of malignant lymphomas in formalin-fixed paraffin-embedded tissue using anti-PCNA/Cyclin 19A2. Correlation with Ki-67 labeling. Am J Pathol 138:1471–1477

Kaneko Y, Larson RA, Variakojis D, Haren JM, Rowley JD (1982) Nonrandom chromosome abnormalities in angioimmunoblastic lymphadenopathy. Blood 60:877–887

Kaneko Y, Maseki N, Sakurai M, Takayama S, Nanba K, Kikuchi M, Frizzera G (1988) Characteristic karyotypic pattern in T-cell lymphoproliferative disorders with reactive "angioimmunoblastic lymphadenopathy with dysproteinemia-type" features. Blood 72:413–421

Kansu E, Hauptman SP (1979) Suppressor cell population in Sézary syndrome. Clin Immunol Immunopathol 12:341–350

Karpinski A, Krueger GRF, Wustrow J, Haas W, Ablashi DV, Pearson GR (1981) Epstein-Barr virus antibody titers in various histological types of carcinoma in the nasopharynx. In: Grundmann E, Krueger GRF, Ablashi DV (eds) Nasopharyngeal carcinoma. Cancer campaign, vol 5, Fischer, Stuttgart, pp 95–99

Keating MJ, Kantarjian H, O'Brien S, Robertson L, Huh Y (1991) New agents and strategies in CLL treatment. Leukemia Lymphoma 5 (Suppl.) 139–142

Kelényi G (1978) Die Klassifikation der Non-Hodgkin-Lymphome: Tatsachen und Perspektiven. Folia Haematol (Leipz) 105:585–605

Kelly DR, Nathwani BN, Griffith RC, Shuster JJ, Sullivan MP, Hvizdala E, Murphy SB, Berard CW (1987) A morphologic study of childhood lymphoma of the undifferentiated type. The Pediatric Oncology Group experience. Cancer 59:1132–1137

Kerl H, Kresbach H (1979) Lymphoreticuläre Hyperplasien und Neoplasien der Haut. In: Schnyder UW (ed) Histopathologie der Haut, 2nd edn, part 2: Stoffwechselkrankheiten und Tumoren. (Spezielle pathologische Anatomie, vol 7, part 2) Springer, Berlin Heidelberg New York, pp 351–480

Keuning FJ, Bos WH (1967) Regeneration patterns of lymphoid follicles in the rabbit spleen after sublethal X-irradiation. In: Cottier H, Odartchenko N, Schindler R, Congdon CC (eds) Germinal centers in immune responses. Springer, Berlin Heidelberg New York, pp 250–258

Keuning FJ, van der Meer J, Nieuwenhuis P, Oudendijk P (1963) The histophysiology of the antibody response. II. Antibody responses and splenic plasma cell reactions in sublethally x-irradiated rabbits. Lab Invest 12:156–170

Kikuchi M, Mitsui T, Matsui N, Sato E, Tokunaga M, Hasui K, Ichimaru M, Kinoshita K, Kamihira S (1979) T-cell malignancies in adults: histopathological studies of lymph nodes in 110 patients. Jpn J Clin Oncol 9 (Suppl):407–422

Kikuchi M, Mitsui T, Takeshita M, Okamura H, Naitoh H, Eimoto T (1986) Virus associated adult T-cell leukemia (ATL) in Japan: clinical, histological and immunological studies. Hematol Oncol 4:67–81

Kim H, Dorfman RF (1974) Morphological studies of 84 untreated patients subjected to laparotomy for the staging of non-Hodgkin's lymphomas. Cancer 33:657–674

Kim H, Dorfman RF, Rappaport H (1978a) Signet ring cell lymphoma. A rare morphologic and functional expression of nodular (follicular) lymphoma. Am J Surg Pathol 2:119–132

Kim H, Jacobs C, Warnke RA, Dorfman RF (1978b) Malignant lymphoma with a high content of epithelioid histiocytes. A distinct clinicopathologic entity and a form of so-called "Lennert's lymphoma". Cancer 41:620–635

Kim H, Nathwani BN, Rappaport H (1980) So-called "Lennert's lymphoma". Is it a clinicopathologic entity? Cancer 45:1379–1399

Kimby E, Mellstedt H for the Lymphoma Group of Central Sweden (1991) Chlorambucil/Prednisone versus CHOP in symptomatic chronic lymphocytic leukemia of B-cell type. A randomized trial. Leukemia Lymphoma 5 (Suppl.) 93–96

Kinney MC, Glick AD, Stein H, Collins RD (1990) Comparison of anaplastic large cell Ki-1 lymphomas and microvillous lymphomas in their immunologic and ultrastructural features. Am J Surg Pathol 14:1047–1060

Kinney MC, Greer JP, Glick AD, Salhany KE, Collins RD (1991) Anaplastic large-cell Ki-1 malignant lymphomas. Recognition, biological and clinical implications. Pathol Annu 26/I: 1–24

Kinoshita K, Hino S, Amagasaki T, Ikeda S, Yamada Y, Suzuyama J, Momita S, Toriya K, Kamihira S, Ichimaru M (1984) Demonstration of adult T-cell leukemia virus antigen in milk from three seropositive mothers. Gann 75:103–105

Kittas C, Hansmann M-L, Borisch B, Feller AC, Lennert K (1985) The blood microvasculature in T-cell lymphomas. A morphological, ultrastructural and immunohistochemical study. Virchows Arch [A] 405:439–452

Kjeldsberg CR, Kim H (1981) Polykaryocytes resembling Warthin-Finkeldey giant cells in reactive and neoplastic lymphoid disorders. Hum Pathol 12:267–272

Klajman A, Yaretzky A, Schneider M, Holoshitz Y, Shneur A, Griffel B (1981) Angioimmunoblastic lymphadenopathy with paraproteinemia: A T- and B-cell disorder. Cancer 48:2433–2437

Klein G, Klein E (1985) Evolution of tumours and the impact of molecular oncology. Nature 315:190–195

Klein MA, Jaffe R, Neiman RS (1977) "Lennert's lymphoma" with transformation to malignant lymphoma, histiocytic type (immunoblastic sarcoma). Am J Clin Pathol 68:601–605

Knapp W, Rieber P, Dörken B, Schmidt RE, Stein H, v. dem Borne AEGKr (1989) Towards a better definition of human leucocyte surface molecules. Immunol Today 10:253–258

Knecht H (1989) Angioimmunoblastic lymphadenopathy: ten years' experience and state of current knowledge. Semin Hematol 26:208–215

Knecht H, Lennert K (1981a) Vorgeschichte und klinisches Bild der Lymphogranulomatosis X (einschließlich [angio]immunoblastischer Lymphadenopathie). Schweiz Med Wochenschr 111:1108–1121

Knecht H, Lennert K (1981 b) Verlauf, Therapie und maligne Transformation der Lymphogranulomatosis X (einschließlich [angio]immunoblastischer Lymphadenopathie). Schweiz Med Wochenschr 111:1122–1130

Knecht H, Lennert K (1981 c) Ultrastructural findings in lymphogranulomatosis X ([angio]immunoblastic lymphadenopathy). Virchows Arch [B] 37:29–47

Knecht H, Schwarze E-W, Lennert K (1985) Histological, immunological and autopsy findings in lymphogranulomatosis X (including angio-immunoblastic lymphadenopathy). Virchows Arch [A] 406:105–124

Knecht H, Odermatt BF, Hayoz D, Kühn L, Bachmann F (1989) Polyclonal rearrangements of the T-cell receptor β-chain in fatal angioimmunoblastic lymphadenopathy. Br J Haematol 73:491–496

Knowles II DM (1985) Lymphoid cell markers. Their distribution and usefulness in the immunophenotypic analysis of lymphoid neoplasms. Am J Surg Pathol 9 [Suppl]:85–108

Knowles DM (1988) Phenotypic markers and gene rearrangement analysis in T-cell neoplasia. (abstract) Am J Surg Pathol 12:160–163

Knowles II DM, Dodson LD, Raab R, Mittler RS, Talle MA, Goldstein G (1983) The application of monoclonal antibodies to the characterization and diagnosis of lymphoid neoplasms: a review of recent studies. Diagn Immunol 1:142–149

Knowles II DM, Dodson L, Burke JS, Wang JM, Bonetti F, Pelicci P-G, Flug F, Dalla-Favera R, Wang CY (1985) SIg⁻E⁻ ("null-cell") non-Hodgkin's lymphomas. Multiparametric determination of their B- or T-cell lineage. Am J Pathol 120:356–370

Kojima M, Sakuma H, Mori N (1983) Histopathological features of plasma cell dyscrasia with polyneuropathy and endocrine disturbances, with special reference to germinal center lesions. Jpn J Clin Oncol 13:557–576

Komuro A, Hayami M, Fujii M, Miyahara S, Hirayama M (1983) Vertical transmission of adult T-cell leukaemia virus. [Letter to the Editor] Lancet i:240

König E, Bartels H, Burger-Schüler A, Common H, Dühmke E, Engelhard M, Fülle HH, Gunzer U, Koeppen K-M, Leopold H, Nowicki L, Oertel J, Paetzmann S, Rühl U, Schmidt M, Schoengen A, Scholle H, Stacher A, Wolf-Hornung B, Schwarze EW (Kiel Lymphoma Study Group) (1979 a) Germinal center cell lymphomas: Prognostic significance of their histopathological differentiation. 5th Meeting Intern Soc Haematol, European and African Division, Hamburg, August 26–31, 1979

König E, Schmalhorst U, Bartels H, Brunswicker F, Common H, Graubner M, Heinz R, Leopold H, Mende S, Nowicki L, Nürnberger R, Theml H, Zitzelsberger G (Kieler Lymphomgruppe (1979 b) Klinik und Prognose des centrocytischen Lymphoms. In: Stacher A, Höcker P (eds) Lymphknotentumoren. Urban and Schwarzenberg, Munich, pp 207–210

Kövary PM, Niedorf H, Sommer G, Breu H, Kamanabroo P, Büchner T, Macher E (1977) Paraproteinaemia in Sézary syndrome. Dermatologica 154:138–146

Krueger GRF, Bergholz M, Bartsch H-H, Fischer R, Schauer A (1979) Rubella virus antigen in lymphocytes of patients with angioimmunoblastic lymphadenopathy (AIL). J Cancer Res Clin Oncol 95:87–91

Krüger GRF, Grisar T, Lennert K, Schwarze E-W, Brittinger G (Kiel Lymphoma Study Group) (1981) Histopathological correlation of the Kiel with the original Rappaport classification of malignant non-Hodgkin lymphomas. Blut 43:167–181

Krueger GRF, Medina JR, Klein HO, Konrads A, Zach J, Rister M, Janik G, Evers KG, Hirano T, Kitamura H, Bedoya VA (1983) A new Working Formulation of non-Hodgkin's lymphomas. A retrospective study of the new NCI classification proposal in comparison to the Rappaport and Kiel classifications. Cancer 52:833–840

Kruschwitz M, Fritzsche G, Schwarting R, Micklem K, Mason DY, Falini B, Stein H (1991) Ber-ACT8: new monoclonal antibody to the mucosa lymphocyte antigen. J Clin Pathol 44:636–645

Lamarre L, Jacobson JO, Aisenberg AC, Harris NL (1989) Primary large cell lymphoma of the mediastinum. A histologic and immunophenotypic study of 29 cases. Am J Surg Pathol 13:730–739

Leahu S, Niculescu R (1987) Special types of malignant lymphomas limited to intrathoracic sites. Arch Anat Cytol Pathol 35:95–99

Leder L-D (1964) Über die selektive fermentcytochemische Darstellung von neutrophilen myeloischen Zellen und Gewebsmastzellen im Paraffinschnitt. Klin Wochenschr 42:553

Leder L-D (1967) Die fermentcytochemische Erkennung normaler und neoplastischer Erythro-poesezellen in Schnitt und Ausstrich. Blut 15: 289–293

Leder L-D, Stutte HJ (1975) Seminar für hämatologisch-zytochemische Techniken. Verh Dtsch Ges Pathol 59: 503–509

Leibetseder F, Thurner J (1973) Angiofollikuläre Lymphknotenhyperplasie (Zwiebelschalen-lymphom). Med Klin 68: 817–820

Lennert K (1952) Zur histologischen Diagnose der Lymphogranulomatose. Habilitationsschrift, Frankfurt/M

Lennert K (1953a) Histologische Studie zur Lymphogranulomatose. I. Die Cytologie der Lymphogranulomzellen. Frankf Z Pathol 64: 209–234

Lennert K (1953b) Studien zur Histologie der Lymphogranulomatose. II. Die diagnostische Bedeutung der einzelnen Zellelemente. Frankf Z Pathol 64: 343–356

Lennert K (1958) Die Frühveränderungen der Lymphogranulomatose. Frankf Z Pathol 69: 103–122

Lennert K (1961) Lymphknoten. Diagnostik in Schnitt und Ausstrich. Cytologie und Lymphadenitis (Handbuch der speziellen pathologischen Anatomie und Histologie, vol 1, part 3 A) Springer, Berlin Göttingen Heidelberg

Lennert K (1967) Classification of malignant lymphomas (European concept). In: Rüttimann A (ed) Progress in lymphology. Thieme, Stuttgart, pp 103–109

Lennert K (1969) Pathologisch-anatomische Klassifikation der malignen Lymphome. Strahlen-therapie [Sonderbd] 69: 1–7

Lennert K (1973) Pathologisch-histologische Klassifizierung der malignen Lymphome. In: Stacher A (ed) Leukämien und maligne Lymphome. Urban and Schwarzenberg, Munich, pp 181–194

Lennert K (1976) Klassifikation und Morphologie der Non-Hodgkin-Lymphome. In: Löffler H (ed) Maligne Lymphome und monoklonale Gammopathien (Hämatologie und Bluttransfu-sion, Vol 18) Lehmanns, Munich, pp 145–166

Lennert K, in collaboration with Mohri N, Stein H, Kaiserling E, Müller-Hermelink HK (1978) Malignant lymphomas other than Hodgkin's disease (Handbuch der speziellen pathologi-schen Anatomie und Histologie, vol 1, part 3 B) Springer, Berlin Heidelberg New York

Lennert K (1981) Histopathologie der Non-Hodgkin-Lymphome (nach der Kiel-Klassifikation). In Zusammenarbeit mit H. Stein. Springer, Berlin Heidelberg New York

Lennert K (1983) The National Cancer Institute sponsored study of the classifications of non-Hodgkin's lymphomas. Comments by "expert" pathologists. Hematol Oncol 1: 95–96

Lennert K, Feller AC (1985) Morphology and immunohistology of T cell lymphomas. In: Quaglino D, Hayhoe FGJ (eds) The cytobiology of leukaemias and lymphomas. (Serono Symposia Publications, vol 20). Raven, New York, pp 81–90

Lennert K, Hansmann ML (1987) Progressive transformation of germinal centers: clinical significance and lymphocytic predominance Hodgkin's disease – the Kiel experience. (ab-stract) Am J Surg Pathol 11: 149–150

Lennert K, Mestdagh J (1968) Lymphogranulomatosen mit konstant hohem Epitheloidzellge-halt. Virchows Arch [A] 344: 1–20

Lennert K, Mohri N (1978) Histopathology and diagnosis of non-Hodgkin's lymphomas. In: Lennert K et al (eds) Malignant lymphomas other than Hodgkin's disease (Handbuch der speziellen pathologischen Anatomie und Histologie, vol I/3 B) Springer, Berlin Heidelberg New York, pp 111–469

Lennert K, Remmele W (1958) Karyometrische Untersuchungen an Lymphknotenzellen des Menschen. II. Mitt. Reticulum- und Endothelzellen. Acta Haematol (Basel) 20: 301–317

Lennert K, Löffler H, Leder L-D (1961) Fermenthistochemische Untersuchungen des Lymph-knotens. I. Mitt. Alkalische Phosphatase in Schnitt und Ausstrich. Virchows Arch [A] 334: 399–418

Lennert K, Mohri N, Stein H, Kaiserling E (1975) The histopathology of malignant lymphoma. Br J Haematol 31 [Suppl]: 193–203

Lennert K, Kaiserling E, Mazzanti T (1978) Diagnosis and differential diagnosis of lymphoep-ithelial carcinoma in lymph nodes: Histological, cytological and electron-microscopic find-ings. In: De-Thé G, Ito Y (eds) Nasopharyngeal carcinoma: etiology and control (IARC scientific publications, vol 20) Intern Agency for Research on Cancer, Lyon, pp 51–64

Lennert K, Knecht H, Burkert M (1979) Vorstadien maligner Lymphome. Verh Dtsch Ges Pathol 63:170–196

Lennert K, Schwarze E-W, Krüger G (1981) Lymphknotenveränderungen durch Virusinfektionen. Verh Dtsch Ges Pathol 65:151–171

Lennert K, Stein H, Feller AC, Gerdes J (1982) Morphology, cytochemistry and immunohistology of T cell lymphomas. In: Vitetta ES (ed) B and T cell tumors. (UCLA symposia on molecular and cellular biology Vol XXIV) Academic, New York, pp 9–28

Lennert K, Collins RD, Lukes RJ (1983) Concordance of the Kiel and Lukes-Collins classifications of non-Hodgkin's lymphomas. Histopathology 7:549–559

Lennert K, Feller AC, Radzun HJ (1984) Malignant histiocytosis/histiocytic sarcoma and related neoplasms. Recent Adv RES Res 24:1–16

Lennert K, Kikuchi M, Sato E, Suchi T, Stansfeld AG, Feller AC, Hansmann M-L, Müller-Hermelink HK, Gödde-Salz E (1985) HTLV-positive and -negative T-cell lymphomas. Morphological and immunohistochemical differences between European and HTLV-positive Japanese T-cell lymphomas. Int J Cancer 35:65–72

Lennert K, Feller AC, Gödde-Salz E (1986) Morphologie, Immunhistochemie und Genetik peripherer T-Zellen-Lymphome. Onkologie 9:97–107

Lennert K, Tamm I, Wacker H-H (1991) Histopathology and immunocytochemistry of lymph node biopsies in chronic lymphocytic leukemia and immunocytoma. Leuk Lymphoma (Suppl) 157–160

Lenoir GM, Bornkamm GW (1987) Burkitt's lymphoma, a human cancer model for the study of the multistep development of cancer: proposal for a new scenario. In: Klein G (ed) Advances in viral oncology, vol 7: analysis of multistep scenarios in the natural history of human or animal cancer. Raven, New York, pp 173–206

Leonard RCF, Cuzick J, MacLennan ICM, Vanhegan RI, Mackie PH, McCormick CV, Oxford Lymphoma Group (1983) Prognostic factors in non-Hodgkin's lymphoma: the importance of symptomatic stage as an adjunct to the Kiel histopathological classification. Br J Cancer 47:91–102

Leong AS-Y (1983) A critique of some contemporary classifications of non-Hodgkin's lymphoma. Which one should we now use? Pathology 15:437–442

Levine A (1981) Clinical manifestations of T-cell lymphomas. 2nd Int Lymphoma Conf, Athens, April 5–10

Levine AM, Meyer PR, Begandy MK, Parker JW, Taylor CR, Irwin L, Lukes RJ (1984) Development of B-cell lymphoma in homosexual men. Clinical and immunologic findings. Ann Intern Med 100:7–13

Levine PH, Cho BR, Connelly RR, Berard CW, O'Conor GT, Dorfman RF, Easton JM, DeVita VT (1975) The American Burkitt lymphoma registry: A progress report. Ann Intern Med 83:31–36

Levine PH, Connelly RR, McKay FW (1985) Burkitt's lymphoma in the USA: cases reported to the American Burkitt Lymphoma Registry compared with population-based incidence and mortality data. In: Lenoir GM, O'Conor GT, Olweny CLM (eds) Burkitt's lymphoma: a human cancer model. (IARC scientific publications, no 60) International Agency for Research on Cancer, Lyon, pp 217–224

Levitt LJ, Aisenberg AC, Harris NL, Linggood RM, Poppema S (1982) Primary non-Hodgkin's lymphoma of the mediastinum. Cancer 50:2486–2492

Li G, Hansmann M-L, Zwingers T, Lennert K (1990) Primary lymphomas of the lung: morphological, immunohistochemical and clinical features. Histopathology 16:519–531

Liao KT, Rosai J, Daneshbod K (1972) Malignant histiocytosis with cutaneous involvement and eosinophilia. Am J Clin Pathol 57:438–448

Lichtenstein AK, Levine A, Taylor CR, Boswell W, Rossman S, Feinstein DI, Lukes RJ (1980) Primary mediastinal lymphoma in adults. Am J Med 68:509–514

Lieberman PH, Filippa DA, Straus DJ, Thaler HT, Cirrincione C, Clarkson BD (1986) Evaluation of malignant lymphomas using three classifications and the Working Formulation. 482 cases with median follow-up of 11.9 years. Am J Med 81:365–380

Lipford EH, Smith HR, Pittaluga S, Jaffe ES, Steinberg AD, Cossman J (1987) Clonality of angioimmunoblastic lymphadenopathy and implications for its evolution to malignant lymphoma. J Clin Invest 79:637–642

Lipford Jr EH, Margolick JB, Longo DL, Fauci AS, Jaffe ES (1988) Angiocentric immunoproliferative lesions: A clinicopathologic spectrum of post-thymic T-cell proliferations. Blood
72:1674–1681

Lippman SM, Volk JR, Spier CM, Grogan TM (1988) Clonal ambiguity of human immunodeficiency virus-associated lymphomas. Similarity to posttransplant lymphomas. Arch
Pathol Lab Med 112:128–132

Liu Y-J, Johnson GD, Gordon J, MacLennan ICM (1992) Germinal centres in T-cell-dependent
antibody responses. Immunol Today 13:17–21

Lojda Z (1977) Studies on glycyl-proline naphthylamidase. I. Lymphocytes. Histochemistry
54:299–309

Longo DL, Glatstein E, Duffey PL, Ihde DC, Hubbard SM, Fisher RI, Jaffe ES, Gilliom M,
Young RC, DeVita Jr VT (1989) Treatment of localized aggressive lymphomas with combination chemotherapy followed by involved-field radiation therapy. J Clin Oncol 7:1295–1302

Lopes Cardozo P (1976) Atlas of Clinical Cytology. Verlag Chemie, Weinheim

Loughran Jr TP, Hammond WP (1986) Adult-onset cyclic neutropenia is a benign neoplasm
associated with clonal proliferation of large granular lymphocytes. J Exp Med 164:2089–2094

Loughran Jr TP, Starkebaum G, Ruscetti FW (1988) Similar rearrangements of T-cell receptor
β gene in cell lines and uncultured cells from patients with large granular lymphocyte
leukemia. Blood 72:613–615

Lukes RJ (1979) The immunologic approach to the pathology of malignant lymphomas. Am J
Clin Pathol 72:657–669

Lukes RJ (1983) The National Cancer Institute sponsored study of the classifications of non-
Hodgkin's lymphomas. Comments by "expert" pathologists. Hematol Oncol 1:96–97

Lukes RJ, Collins RD (1974a) A functional approach to the classification of malignant
lymphoma. Recent Results Cancer Res 46:18–30

Lukes RJ, Collins RD (1974b) Immunologic characterization of human malignant lymphomas.
Cancer 34:1488–1503

Lukes RJ, Collins RD (1975a) New approaches to the classification of the lymphomata. Br J
Cancer 31 [Suppl II]:1–28

Lukes RJ, Collins RD (1975b) A functional classification of malignant lymphomas. In: Rebuck
JW, Berard CW, Abell MR (eds) The reticuloendothelial system (Monographs in pathology,
no 16) Williams and Wilkins, Baltimore, pp 213–242

Lukes RJ, Tindle BH (1973) Immunoblastic lymphadenopathy: Presented at the Pathology Panel
for Clinical Trials, NCI, January 26–28, 1973

Lukes RJ, Tindle BH (1975) Immunoblastic lymphadenopathy. A hyperimmune entity resembling Hodgkin's disease. N Engl J Med 292:1–8

Lukes RJ, Tindle BH (1978) Immunoblastic lymphadenopathy: A prelymphomatous state of
immunoblastic sarcoma. Recent Results Cancer Res 64:241–246

Lukes RJ, Butler JJ, Hicks EB (1966) Natural history of Hodgkin's disease as related to its
pathologic picture. Cancer 19:317–344

Lukes RJ, Parker JW, Taylor CR, Tindle BH, Cramer AD, Lincoln TL (1978a) Immunologic
approach to non-Hodgkin lymphomas and related leukemias. Analysis of the results of
multiparameter studies of 425 cases. Semin Hematol 15:322–351

Lukes RJ, Taylor CR, Parker JW, Lincoln TL, Pattengale PK, Tindle BH (1978b) A morphologic and immunologic surface marker study of 299 cases of non-Hodgkin lymphomas and
related leukemias. Am J Pathol 90:461–486

Machado JC, Leimig T, Sales Rodrigues ML (1978) Ocorrencia dos linfomas malignos nao
Hodgkin segundo a classificaçao de Lennert (Kiel) em Sao Paulo-Brasil. Rev Bras Cancerol
28:11–17

MacLennan I (1991) The centre of hypermutation. Nature 354:352–353

MacLennan ICM, Gray D (1986) Antigen-driven selection of virgin and memory B cells.
Immunol Rev 91:61–85

MacLennan ICM, Gray D, Kumararatne DS, Bazin H (1982) The lymphocytes of splenic
marginal zones. A distinct B-cell lineage. Immunol Today 3:305–307

MacLennan ICM, Oldfield S, Liu Y-J, Lane PJL (1989a) Regulation of B-cell populations. Curr
Top Pathol 79:37–57

MacLennan ICM, Liu Y-J, Joshua DE, Gray D (1989b) The production and selection of memory B cells in follicles. In: Melchers F et al. (eds) Progress in immunology, vol VII (Proc 7th Int Congr Immunol, Berlin 1989). Springer, Berlin Heidelberg New York, pp 443–447

Magrath I, Benjamin D, Papadopoulos N (1983) Serum monoclonal immunoglobulin bands in undifferentiated lymphomas of Burkitt and non-Burkitt types. Blood 61:726–731

Malik STA, Amess J, D'Ardenne AJ, Lister TA (1989) Hairy cell leukemia – mediastinal involvement. A report of two cases and review of the literature. Hematol Oncol 7:303–306

Mandard AM, Tanguy A, Vernhes JC, Abbatucci JS, Mandard JC (1977) Lymphomes malins non hodgkiniens. Étude rétrospective de 64 cas classés selon les nomenclatures de Kiel et Rappaport. Bull Cancer (Paris) 64:347–364

Mann RB (1985) Follicular lymphoma and lymphocytic lymphoma of intermediate differentiation. In: Jaffe ES (ed) Surgical pathology of the lymph nodes and related organs. (Major problems in pathology, vol 16) Saunders, Philadelphia, pp 165–202

Mann RB, Jaffe ES, Braylan RC, Nanba K, Frank MM, Ziegler JL, Berard CW (1976) Non-endemic Burkitt's lymphoma. A B-cell tumor related to germinal centers. N Engl J Med 295:685–691

Mann RB, Jaffe ES, Berard CW (1979) Malignant lymphomas – A conceptual understanding of morphologic diversity. Am J Pathol 94:104–192

Mason DY, Gatter KC (1987) The role of immunocytochemistry in diagnostic pathology. J Clin Pathol 40:1042–1054

Mason DY, Bastard C, Rimokh R, Dastugue N, Huret J-L, Kristoffersson U, Magaud J-P, Nezelof C, Tilly H, Vannier J-P, Hemet J, Warnke R (1990) CD30-positive large cell lymphomas ('Ki-1 lymphoma') are associated with a chromosomal translocation involving 5q35. Br J Haematol 74:161–168

Mathé G, Rappaport H, O'Conor GT, Torloni H (1976) Histological and cytological typing of neoplastic diseases of haematopoietic and lymphoid tissues (International Histological Classification of Tumors No 14) World Health Organization, Geneva

Matsuzaki H, Yamaguchi K, Kagimoto T, Nakai R, Takatsuki K, Oyama W (1985) Monoclonal gammopathies in adult T-cell leukemia. Cancer 56:1380–1383

Matthews MJ (1985) Surgical pathology of mycosis fungoides and Sézary syndrome. In: Jaffe ES (ed) Surgical pathology of the lymph nodes and related organs. (Major problems in pathology, vol 16) Saunders, Philadelphia, pp 329–356

Matutes E, Garcia Talavera J, O'Brien M, Catovsky D (1986) The morphological spectrum of T-prolymphocytic leukaemia. Br J Haematol 64:111–124

McKenna RW, Parkin J, Kersey JH, Gajl-Peczalska KJ, Peterson L, Brunning RD (1977) Chronic lymphoproliferative disorder with unusual clinical, morphologic, ultrastructural and membrane surface marker characteristics. Am J Med 62:588–596

McKenna RW, Parkin J, Brunning RD (1979) Morphologic and ultrastructural characteristics of T-cell acute lymphoblastic leukemia. Cancer 44:1290–1297

Medeiros J, Van Krieken JH, Jaffe ES, Raffeld M (1990) Association of bcl-1 rearrangements with lymphocytic lymphoma of intermediate differentiation. Blood 76:2086–2090

Menestrina F, Chilosi M, Bonetti F, Lestani M, Scarpa A, Novelli P, Doglioni C, Todeschini G, Ambrosetti A, Fiore-Donati L (1986) Mediastinal large-cell lymphoma of B-type, with sclerosis: histopathological and immunohistochemical study of eight cases. Histopathology 10:589–600

Mentlein R, Heymann E, Scholz W, Feller AC, Flad H-D (1984) Dipeptidyl peptidase IV as a new surface marker for a subpopulation of human T-lymphocytes. Cell Immunol 89:11–19

Mepham BL, Frater W, Mitchell BS (1979) The use of proteolytic enzymes to improve immunoglobulin staining by the PAP technique. Histochem J 11:345–357

Merz H, Houssiau FA, Orscheschek K, Renauld JC, Fliedner A, Herin M, Noël H, Kadin M, Mueller-Hermelink HK, Van Snick J, Feller AC (1991) Interleukin-9 expression in human malignant lymphomas: unique association with Hodgkin's disease and large cell anaplastic lymphoma. Blood 78:1311–1317

Meugé C, Hoerni B, de Mascarel A, Durand M, Richaud P, Hoerni-Simon G, Chauvergne J, Lagarde C (1978) Non-Hodgkin malignant lymphomas. Clinico-pathologic correlations with the Kiel classification. Retrospective analysis of a series of 274 cases. Eur J Cancer 14:587–592

Meusers P, Bartels H, Brittinger G, Common H, Dühmke E, Fülle HH, Gunzer U, Heinz R, König E, Musshoff K, Pralle H, Schmalhorst U, Theml H, Krüger GRF, Lennert K (1979) Heterogeneity of diffuse "histiocytic" lymphoma according to the Kiel classification. [Letter to the Editor] N Engl J Med 301:384

Meusers P, Engelhard M, Bartels H, Binder T, Fülle HH, Görg K, Gunzer U, Havemann K, Kayser W, König E, König HJ, Kuse R, Löffler H, Luwig W-D, Mainzer K, Martin H, Pralle H, Schoppe WD, Staiger HJ, Theml H, Zurborn KH, Zwingers T, Lennert K, Brittinger G (1989) Multicentre randomized therapeutic trial for advanced centrocytic lymphoma: Anthracycline does not improve the prognosis. Hematol Oncol 7:365–380

Miliauskas JR, Berard CW, Young RC, Garvin AJ, Edwards BK, DeVita Jr VT (1982) Undifferentiated non-Hodgkin's lymphomas (Burkitt's and non-Burkitt's types). The relevance of making this histologic distinction. Cancer 50:2115–2121

Miller JB, Variakojis D, Bitran JD, Sweet Jr DL, Golomb HM, Ultmann JE (1978) Diffuse histiocytic lymphoma with sclerosis: a clinicopathologic entity with frequent occurrence of superior venacaval obstruction. Blood 52 (Suppl 1):263

Miller R, Spicer SS, Kurtz SM (1979) Histiocytic lymphoma in a patient with Lennert's lymphoma. Report of a case with unusual cytoplasmic inclusions. Arch Pathol Lab Med 103:279–283

Mitrou PS, Queisser W, Lennert K, Sandritter W (1969) Kombinierte autoradiographisch-cytophotometrische Untersuchungen von Keimzentrumszellen der menschlichen Tonsille. Virchows Arch [B] 3:156–170

Moir DH (1983) War of the words: Classification of the non-Hodgkin's lymphomas. Pathology 15:359–360

Moldenhauer G, Mielke B, Dörken B, Schwartz-Albiez R, Möller P (1990) Identity of HML-1 antigen on intestinal intraepithelial T cells and of B-ly7 antigen on hairy cell leukaemia. Scand J Immunol 32:77–82

Molenaar WM, Bartels H, Koudstaal J (1984) Histological, epidemiological and clinical aspects of centroblastic-centrocytic lymphomas subdivided according to the "working formulation". Br J Cancer 49:263–268

Monfardini S, Vaccher E, Foà R, Tirelli U, Italian Cooperative Group on AIDS-Related Tumors (GICAT) (1990) AIDS-associated non-Hodgkin's lymphoma in Italy: intravenous drug users versus homosexual men. Ann Oncol 1:203–211

Möller P, Lämmler B, Herrmann B, Otto HF, Moldenhauer G, Momburg F (1986) The primary mediastinal clear cell lymphoma of B-cell type has variable defects in MHC antigen expression. Immunology 59:411–417

Möller P, Moldenhauer G, Momburg F, Lämmler B, Eberlein-Gonska M, Kiesel S, Dörken B (1987) Mediastinal lymphoma of clear cell type is a tumor corresponding to terminal steps of B cell differentiation. Blood 69:1087–1095

Möller P, Mielke B, Moldenhauer G (1990) Monoclonal antibody HML-1, a marker for intraepithelial T cells and lymphomas derived thereof, also recognizes hairy cell leukemia and some B-cell lymphomas. Am J Pathol 136:509–512

Mori Y, Lennert K (1969) Electron microscopic atlas of lymph node cytology and pathology. Springer, Berlin Heidelberg New York

Mueller J, Brun del Re G, Buerki H, Keller H-U, Hess MW, Cottier H (1975) Nonspecific esterase activity: A criterion for differentiation of T and B lymphocytes in mouse lymph nodes. Eur J Immunol 5:270–274

Müller-Hermelink HK, Lennert K (1978) The cytologic, histologic, and functional bases for a modern classification of lymphomas. In: Lennert K et al. (ed) Malignant lymphomas other than Hodgkin's disease (Handbuch der speziellen pathologischen Anatomie und Histologie, vol 1 part 3 B) Springer, Berlin Heidelberg New York, pp 1–71

Müller-Hermelink HK, Stein H, Steinmann G, Lennert K (1983) Malignant lymphoma of plasmacytoid T-cells. Morphologic and immunologic studies characterizing a special type of T-cell. Am J Surg Pathol 7:849–862

Müller-Weihrich S, Beck J, Henze G, Jobke A, Kornhuber B, Lampert F, Ludwig R, Prindull G, Schellong G, Spaar HJ, Stollmann B, Treuner J, Wahlen W, Weinel P, Riehm H (1984) BFM-Studie 1981/83 zur Behandlung hochmaligner Non-Hodgkin-Lymphome bei Kindern:

Ergebnisse einer nach histologisch-immunologischem Typ und Ausbreitungsstadium strate-fizierten Therapie. Klin Pädiatr 196:135–142

Müller-Weihrich S, Henze G, Odenwald E, Riehm H (1985) BFM trials for childhood non-Hodgkin's lymphomas. In: Cavalli F, Bonadonna G, Rozencweig M (eds) Malignant lymphomas and Hodgkin's disease: experimental and therapeutic advances. Proc 2nd Int Conf Malignant Lymphomas, Lugano 1984. Nijhoff, Boston, pp 633–642

Musshoff K (1979) Die Strahlentherapie der Non-Hodgkin-Lymphome. Indikation und Probleme. In: Stacher A, Höcker P (eds) Lymphknotentumoren. Urban and Schwarzenberg, Munich, pp 157–165

Musshoff K (1987) Maligne Systemerkrankungen. In: Scherer E (ed) Strahlentherapie – Radiologische Onkologie. 3rd edn. Springer, Berlin Heidelberg New York, pp 1080–1332

Musshoff K, Schmidt-Vollmer H, Lennert K, Sandritter W (1976) Preliminary clinical findings on the Kiel classification of malignant lymphomas. Z Krebsforsch 87:229–238

Myhre MJ, Isaacson PG (1987) Primary B-cell gastric lymphoma. A reassessment of its histogenesis. J Pathol 152:1–11

Nakamura S, Suchi T (1991) A clinicopathologic study of node-based, low-grade, peripheral T-cell lymphoma. Angioimmunoblastic lymphoma, T-zone lymphoma, and lymphoepithelioid lymphoma. Cancer 67:2565–2578

Nakamura S, Takagi N, Kojima M, Motoori T, Kitoh K, Osada H, Suzuki H, Ogura M, Kurita S, Oyama A, Ueda R, Takahashi T, Suchi T (1991) Clinicopathologic study of large cell anaplastic lymphoma (Ki-1-positive large cell lymphoma) among the Japanese. Cancer 68:118–129

Nakano S, Ando Y, Ichijo M, Moriyama I, Saito S, Sugamura K, Hinuma Y (1984) Search for possible routes of vertical and horizontal transmission of adult T-cell leukemia virus. Gann 75:1044–1045

Nanba K, Jaffe ES, Braylan RC, Soban EJ, Berard CW (1977) Alkaline phosphatase-positive malignant lymphoma. A subtype of B-cell lymphomas. Am J Clin Pathol 68:535–542

Nanba K, Sasaki N, Dohy H, Takahashi M (1987a) Malignant lymphomas with marked epithelioid cell reactions: a summary of clinicopathological, enzyme histochemical, immunohistochemical and electron microscopic study of 17 cases. Recent Adv RES Res 23:171–178

Nanba K, Yamamoto H, Kamada N, Kikuchi M, Suchi T, Frizzera G, Berard CW, Shimamura K, Kaneko Y, Sakurai M (1987b) Agreement rates and American-Japanese pathologists' comparability of a modified Working Formulation for non-Hodgkin's lymphomas. An analysis of the cases collected for the Fifth International Workshop on Chromosomes in Leukemia-Lymphoma. Cancer 59:1463–1469

Nathwani BN (1987) Classifying non-Hodgkin's lymphomas. In: Berard CW, Dorfman RF, Kaufman N (eds) Malignant lymphoma. (Monographs in pathology no 29) Williams and Wilkins, Baltimore, pp 18–80

Nathwani BN, Kim H, Rappaport H (1976) Malignant lymphoma, lymphoblastic. Cancer 38:964–983

Nathwani BN, Rappaport H, Moran EM, Pangalis GA, Kim H (1978) Evolution of immunoblastic lymphoma in angioimmunoblastic lymphadenopathy. Recent Results Cancer Res 64:235–240

Nathwani BN, Winberg CD, Diamond LW, Bearman RM, Kim H (1981) Morphologic criteria for the differentiation of follicular lymphoma from florid reactive follicular hyperplasia: a study of 80 cases. Cancer 48:1794–1806

Newland JR, Linke RP, Lennert K (1986) Amyloid deposits in lymph nodes: A morphologic and immunohistochemical study. Hum Pathol 17:1245–1249

Nézelof C, Eliachar E (1973) La lymphohistiocytose familiale. Revue générale à propos de trois observations. Liens éventuels avec les syndromes secondaires. Nouv Rev Fr Hematol 13:319–338

Ng CS, Chan JKC (1987) Monocytoid B-cell lymphoma. Hum Pathol 18:1069–1071

Ngan B-Y, Nourse J, Cleary ML (1989) Detection of chromosomal translocation t(14;18) within the minor cluster region of bcl-2 by polymerase chain reaction and direct genomic sequencing of the enzymatically amplified DNA in follicular lymphomas. Blood 73:1759–1762

Nieuwenhuis P, Lennert K (1980) Histophysiology of normal lymphoid tissue and immune reactions. In: Van den Tweel JG (ed) Malignant lymphoproliferative diseases (Boerhaave series for postgraduate medical education vol 17) Leiden University Press, The Hague, pp 3–12

Nizze H, Cogliatti SB, von Schilling C, Feller AC, Lennert K (1991) Monocytoid B-cell lymphoma: morphological variants and relationship to low-grade B-cell lymphoma of the mucosa-associated lymphoid tissue. Histopathology 18:403–414

Noël H, Helbron D, Lennert K (1979) Die epitheloidzellige Lymphogranulomatose (sogenanntes „Lennert's lymphoma"). In: Stacher A, Höcker P (eds) Lymphknotentumoren. Urban and Schwarzenberg, Munich, pp 40–45

Noël H, Helbron D, Lennert K (1980) Epithelioid cellular lymphogranulomatosis (lymphoepithelioid cell lymphoma). Histologic and clinical observations. In: Van den Tweel JG (ed) Malignant lymphoproliferative diseases (Boerhaave series for postgraduate medical education vol 17) Leiden University Press, The Hague, pp 433–445

The Non-Hodgkin's Lymphoma Pathologic Classification Project (1982) National Cancer Institute sponsored study of classifications of non-Hodgkin's lymphomas. Summary and description of a Working Formulation for clinical usage. Cancer 49:2112–2135

Norton AJ, Isaacson PG (1987) Detailed phenotypic analysis of B-cell lymphoma using a panel of antibodies reactive in routinely fixed wax-embedded tissue. J Pathol 128:225–240

Norton AJ, Isaacson PG (1989a) Lymphoma phenotyping in formalin-fixed and paraffin wax-embedded tissues. I. Range of antibodies and staining patterns. Histopathology 14:437–446

Norton AJ, Isaacson PG (1989b) Lymphoma phenotyping in formalin-fixed and paraffin wax-embedded tissues: II. Profiles of reactivity in the various tumour types. Histopathology 14:557–579

O'Connor NTJ (1987) Genotypic analysis of lymph node biopsies. J Pathol 151:185–190

O'Connor NTJ, Wainscoat JS, Weatherall DJ, Gatter KC, Feller AC, Isaacson P, Jones D, Lennert K, Pallesen G, Ramsey A, Stein H, Wright DH, Mason DY (1985) Rearrangement of the T-cell-receptor β-chain gene in the diagnosis of lymphoproliferative disorders. Lancet i:1295–1297

O'Connor NTJ, Feller AC, Wainscoat JS, Gatter KC, Pallesen G, Stein H, Lennert K, Mason DY (1986a) T-cell origin of Lennert's lymphoma. Br J Haematol 64:521–528

O'Connor NTJ, Crick JA, Wainscoat JS, Gatter KC, Stein H, Falini B, Mason DY (1986b) Evidence for monoclonal T lymphocyte proliferation in angioimmunoblastic lymphadenopathy. J Clin Pathol 39:1229–1232

O'Connor NTJ, Stein H, Gatter KC, Wainscoat JS, Crick J, Al Saati T, Falini B, Delsol G, Mason DY (1987) Genotypic analysis of large cell lymphomas which express the Ki-1 antigen. Histopathology 11:733–740

Orell SR, Skinner JM (1982) The typing of non-Hodgkin's lymphomas using fine needle aspiration cytology. Pathology 14:389–394

Osborne BM, Butler JJ, Mackay B (1980) Sinusoidal large cell ("histiocytic") lymphoma. Cancer 46:2484–2491

Osborne BM, Mackay B, Butler JJ, Ordonez NG (1983) Large cell lymphoma with microvillus-like projections: and ultrastructural study. Am J Clin Pathol 79:443–450

Osborne BM, Butler JJ, Pugh WC (1990) The value of immunophenotyping on paraffin sections in the identification of T-cell rich B-cell large-cell lymphomas: lineage confirmed by J_H rearrangement. Am J Surg Pathol 14:933–938

Ott MM, Müller-Hermelink HK, Schmitt B, Feller AC (1991) Chromosomal translocation detected by bcl-1 and bcl-2 rearrangement in low grade B-cell lymphomas of a European population. Histopathology 19:163–167

Oviatt DL, Cousar JB, Flexner JM, Kurtin PJ, Collins RD, Stein RS (1983) Malignant lymphoma of follicular center cell origin in humans. IV. Small transformed (noncleaved) cell lymphoma of the non-Burkitt's type. Cancer 52:1196–1201

Pallesen G (1983) Burkitt's lymphoma: diagnostic and taxonomic aspects. In: Molander DW (ed) Diseases of the lymphatic system. Diagnosis and therapy. Springer, Berlin Heidelberg New York, pp 89–102

Pallesen G (1988) Immunophenotypic markers for characterizing malignant lymphoma, malignant histiocytosis and tumors derived from accessory cells. Cancer Rev 8:1–65

Pallesen G, Hamilton-Dutoit SJ (1988) Ki-1 (CD30) antigen is regularly expressed by tumor cells of embryonal carcinoma. Am J Pathol 133:446–450

Pallesen G, Hamilton-Dutoit SJ (1989) Monoclonal antibody (HML-1) labelling of T-cell lymphomas. Lancet i: 223

Pallesen G, Zeuthen J (1987) Distribution of the Burkitt's lymphoma-associated antigen (BLA) in normal human tissue and malignant lymphoma as defined by immunohistological staining with monoclonal antibody 38.13. J Cancer Res Clin Oncol 113: 78–86

Pallesen G, Madsen M, Hastrup J (1981) Large-cell T-lymphoma with hypersegmented nuclei. Scand J Haematol 26: 72–79

Pallesen G, Beverley PCL, Lane EB, Madsen M, Mason DY, Stein H (1984) Nature of non-B, non-T lymphomas: an immunohistological study on frozen tissues using monoclonal antibodies. J Clin Pathol 37: 911–918

Palutke M, Varadachari C, Weise RW, Husain M, Tabaczka P (1978) Lennert's lymphoma, a T-cell neoplasm. [Letter to the Editor] Am J Clin Pathol 69: 643–646

Palutke M, Tabaczka, P, Weise RW, Axelrod A, Palacas C, Margolis H, Khilanani P, Ratanatharathorn V, Piligian J, Pollard R, Husain M (1980) T-cell lymphomas of large cell type. A variety of malignant lymphomas: "histiocytic" and mixed lymphocytic-"histiocytic". Cancer 46: 87–101

Pangalis GA, Nathwani BN, Rappaport H (1977) Malignant lymphoma, well differentiated lymphocytic. Its relationship with chronic lymphocytic leukemia and macroglobulinemia of Waldenström. Cancer 39: 999–1010

Papadimitriou CS, Schwarze EW (1983) Extramedullary non-gastrointestinal plasmocytoma. An immunohistochemical study of sixteen cases. Pathol Res Pract 176: 306–312

Papadimitriou CS, Müller-Hermelink U, Lennert K (1979) Histologic and immunohistochemical findings in the differential diagnosis of chronic lymphocytic leukemia of B-cell type and lymphoplasmacytic/lymphoplasmacytoid lymphoma. Virchows Arch [A] 384: 149–158

Paryani SB, Hoppe RT, Cox RS, Colby TV, Rosenberg SA, Kaplan HS (1983) Analysis of non-Hodgkin's lymphomas with nodular and favorable histologies, stages I and II. Cancer 52: 2300–2307

Patsouris E, Noël H, Lennert K (1988) Histological and immunohistological findings in lymphoepithelioid cell lymphoma (Lennert's lymphoma). Am J Surg Pathol 12: 341–350

Patsouris E, Noël H, Lennert K (1989a) Angioimmunoblastic lymphadenopathy-type of T-cell lymphoma with a high content of epithelioid cells. Histopathology and comparison with lymphoepithelioid cell lymphoma. Am J Surg Pathol 13: 262–275

Patsouris E, Noël H, Lennert K (1989b) Cytohistologic and immunohistochemical findings in Hodgkin's disease, mixed cellularity type, with a high content of epithelioid cells. Am J Surg Pathol 13: 1014–1022

Patsouris E, Noël H, Lennert K (1990) Lymphoplasmacytic/lymphoplasmacytoid immunocytoma with a high content of epithelioid cells. Histologic and immunohistochemical findings. Am J Surg Pathol 14: 660–670

Payne CM, Grogan TM, Cromey DW, Bjore Jr CG, Kerrigan DP (1987) An ultrastructural morphometric and immunophenotypic evaluation of Burkitt's and Burkitt's-like lymphomas. Lab Invest 57: 200–218

Pelicci P-G, Knowles II DM, Dalla Favera R (1985) Lymphoid tumors displaying rearrangements of both immunoglobulin and T cell receptor genes. J Exp Med 162: 1015–1024

Pelicci P-G, Knowles II DM, Arlin ZA, Wieczorek R, Luciw P, Dina D, Basilico C, Dalla-Favera R (1986) Multiple monoclonal B cell expansions and c-myc oncogene rearrangements in acquired immune deficiency syndrome-related lymphoproliferative disorders. Implications for lymphomagenesis. J Exp Med 164: 2049–2076

Penn I, Starzl TE (1972) Malignant tumors arising de novo in immunosuppressed organ transplant recipients. Transplantation 14: 407–417

Percy C, O'Conor G, Ries LG, Jaffe ES (1984) Non-Hodgkin's lymphomas. Application of the International Classification of Diseases for Oncology (ICD-O) to the Working Formulation. Cancer 54: 1435–1438

Perrone T, Frizzera G, Rosai J (1986) Mediastinal diffuse large-cell lymphoma with sclerosis. A clinicopathologic study of 60 cases. Am J Surg Pathol 10: 176–191

Peters JPJ, Rademakers LHPM, Roelofs JMM, de Jong D, van Unnik JAM (1984) Distribution of dendritic reticulum cells in follicular lymphoma and reactive hyperplasia. Light microscopic identification and general morphology. Virchows Arch [B] 46: 215–228

Pezzella F, Gatter KC, Mason DY, Bastard C, Duval C, Krajewski A, Turner GE, Ross FM, Clark H, Jones DB, Leroux D, Le Marc'Hadour F (1990a) Bcl-2 protein expression in follicular lymphomas in absence of 14;18 translocation. Lancet 336:1510–1511

Pezzella F, Tse AGD, Cordell JL, Pulford KAF, Gatter KC, Mason DY (1990b) Expression of the bcl-2 oncogene protein is not specific for the 14;18 chromosomal translocation. Am J Pathol 137:225–232

Picker LJ, Weiss LM, Medeiros LJ, Wood GS, Warnke RA (1987) Immunophenotypic criteria for the diagnosis of non-Hodgkin's lymphoma. Am J Pathol 128:181–201

Pileri S (1985) Linfomi maligni non-Hodgkin. Dalla tecnica alla diagnostica. Con la collaborazione di Rivano MT et al. Società Editirice Esculapio, Bologna

Pileri S, Falini B (1990) Peripheral T-cell lymphoma associated with hemophagocytic syndrome and hemophagocytic lymphohistiocytosis of children: do they share something? [Letter to the Editor, Response] Blood 76:2163–2164

Pileri S, Brandi G, Rivano MT, Govoni E, Martinelli G (1982) Report of a case of non-Hodgkin's lymphoma of large multilobated cell type with B-cell origin. Tumori 68:543–548

Pileri S, Rivano MT, Gobbi M, Taruscio D, Lennert K (1985) Neoplastic and reactive follicles within B-cell malignant lymphomas. A morphological and immunological study of 30 cases. Hematol Oncol 3:243–260

Pileri S, Falini B, Delsol G, Stein H, Baglioni P, Poggi S, Martelli MF, Rivano MT, Mason DY, Stansfeld AG (1990) Lymphohistiocytic T-cell lymphoma (anaplastic large cell lymphoma CD30+/Ki-1+ with a high content of reactive histiocytes). Histopathology 16:383–391

Pinkus GS, Said JW, Hargreaves HK (1979) Malignant lymphoma, T cell type: A distinct morphologic variant with large multilobated nuclei. Report of four cases. Am J Clin Pathol 72:540–550

Piris MA, Rivas C, Morente M, Oliva H, Rubio C (1986) Immature sinus histiocytosis: a monocytoid B-lymphoid reaction. J Pathol 148:159–167

Piris MA, Rivas C, Morente M, Cruz MA, Rubio C, Oliva H (1988) Monocytoid B-cell lymphoma, a tumour related to the marginal zone. Histopathology 12:383–392

Piris M, Brown DC, Gatter KC, Mason DY (1990) CD30 expression in non-Hodgkin's lymphoma. Histopathology 17:211–218

Plank L, Beseda A, Plank J (1983) Farebny Atlas Malígnych Lymfómov. Vydavatel'stvo Osveta, Martin

Plank L, Lennert K, Hansmann M-L, Meusers P, Brittinger G, Zwingers T (1991) Centrocytic malignant lymphoma. A histological, histomorphometrical, and immunohistological study of 62 biopsy cases with relation to the prognosis. In preparation

Poiesz BJ, Ruscetti FW, Gazdar AF, Bunn PA, Minna JD, Gallo RC (1980) Detection and isolation of type C retrovirus particles from fresh and cultured lymphocytes of a patient with cutaneous T-cell lymphoma. Proc Natl Acad Sci USA 77:7415–7419

Poppema S (1984) Plastic embedment in routine pathology. In: Lennert K, Hübner K (eds) Pathology of the bone marrow. Fischer, Stuttgart, pp 15–17

Poppema S, Halie R, Elema JD (1978) Alkaline phosphatase positive lymphoma, functional and morphological aspects. Z Immunitaetsforsch 154:351–352

Poppema S, Kaiserling E, Lennert K (1979) Nodular paragranuloma and progressively transformed germinal centers. Ultrastructural and immunohistologic findings. Virchows Arch [B] 31:211–225

Poppema S, Hollema H, Visser L, Vos H (1987) Monoclonal antibodies (MT1, MT2, MB1, MB2, MB3) reactive with leukocyte subsets in paraffin-embedded tissue sections. Am J Pathol 127:418–429

Porwit-Ksiazek A, Mioduszewska O (1983) Clinical significance of histologic (Kiel) classification combined with immunologic definition of malignant lymphoma. Neoplasma 30:173–180

Prasthofer EF, Grizzle WE, Prchal JT, Grossi CE (1985) Plasmacytoid T-cell lymphoma associated with chronic myeloproliferative disorder. Am J Surg Pathol 9:380–387

Pringle JH, Ruprai AK, Primrose L, Keyte J, Potter L, Close P, Lauder I (1990) In situ hybridization of immunoglobulin light chain mRNA in paraffin sections using biotinylated or hapten-labelled oligonucleotide probes. J Pathol 162:197–207

Pugh WC, Manning JT, Butler JJ (1988) Paraimmunoblastic variant of small lymphocytic lymphoma/leukemia. Am J Surg Pathol 12:907–917

Pui C-H, Frankel LS, Carroll AJ, Raimondi SC, Shuster JJ, Head DR, Crist WM, Land VJ, Pullen DJ, Steuber CP, Behm FG, Borowitz MJ (1991) Clinical characteristics and treatment outcome of childhood acute lymphoblastic leukemia with the t(4;11) (q21;q23): a collaborative study of 40 cases. Blood 77:440–447

Radaszkiewicz T, Lennert K (1975) Lymphogranulomatosis X. Klinisches Bild, Therapie und Prognose. Dtsch Med Wochenschr 100:1157–1163

Radaszkiewicz T, Hansmann M-L, Lennert K (1989) Monoclonality and polyclonality of plasma cells in Castleman's disease of the plasma cell variant. Histopathology 14:11–24

Radzun HJ, Hansmann ML, Heidebrecht HJ, Bödewadt-Radzun S, Wacker HH, Kreipe H, Lumbeck H, Hernandez C, Kuhn C, Parwaresch MR (1991) Detection of a monocyte/macrophage differentiation antigen in routinely processed paraffin-embedded tissues by monoclonal antibody Ki-M1P. Lab Invest 65:306–315

Rai KR, Sawitzky A, Cronkite EP, Chanana AD, Levy RN, Pasternack BS (1975) Clinical staging of chronic lymphocytic leukemia. Blood 46:219–234

Ramsay AD, Smith WJ, Isaacson PG (1988) T-cell-rich B-cell lymphoma. Am J Surg Pathol 12:433–443

Raphael M, Gentilhomme O, Tulliez M, Byron P-A, Diebold J, French Study Group of Pathology for Human Immunodeficiency Virus-Associated Tumors (1991) Histopathologic features of high-grade non-Hodgkin's lymphomas in acquired immunodeficiency syndrome. Arch Pathol Lab Med 115:15–20

Rappaport H (1966) Tumors of the hematopoietic system. Atlas of tumor pathology, sect 3, fasc 8. Armed Forces Institute of Pathology, Washington

Rappaport H, Winter WJ, Hicks EB (1956) Follicular lymphoma. A re-evaluation of its position in the scheme of malignant lymphoma, based on a survey of 253 cases. Cancer 9:792–821

Reinherz EL, Schlossman SF (1981) Derivation of human T-cell leukemias. Cancer Res 41:4767–4770

Rennke H, Lennert K (1973) Käsig-tuberkuloide Reaktion bei Lymphknotenmetastasen lymphoepithelialer Carcinome (Schmincke-Tumoren). Virchows Arch [A] 358:241–247

Rice L, Shenkenberg T, Lynch EC, Wheeler TM (1982) Granulomatous infections complicating hairy cell leukemia. Cancer 49:1924–1928

Richards MA, Stansfeld AG (1988) Updated Kiel classification. [Letter] Lancet i:937

Rilke F, Lennert K (1981) Bezug der Kiel-Klassifikation zu anderen neuen Lymphom-Klassifikationen und besonders zur „Working Formulation". In: Lennert K (1981) Histopathologie der Non-Hodgkin-Lymphome (nach der Kiel-Klassifikation). In Zusammenarbeit mit H. Stein. Springer, Berlin Heidelberg New York, pp 112–118

Rilke F, Pilotti S, Carbone A, Lombardi L (1978a) Morphology of lymphatic cells and of their derived tumours. J Clin Pathol 31:1009–1056

Rilke F, Carbone A, Musumeci R, Pilotti S, de Lena M, Bonadonna G (1978b) Malignant histiocytosis: a clinicopathologic study of 18 consecutive cases. Tumori 64:211–227

Rilke F, Giardini R, Lombardi L, Pilotti S, Clemente C (1980) Malignant lymphomas – Histopathological diagnoses and their conceptual bases. In: Fenoglio CM, Wolff M (eds) Progress in surgical pathology, vol II. Masson, New York, pp 145–185

Rimokh R, Magaud J-P, Berger F, Samarut J, Coiffier B, Germain D, Mason DY (1989) A translocation involving a specific breakpoint (q35) on chromosome 5 is characteristic of anaplastic large cell lymphoma ('Ki-1 lymphoma'). Br J Haematol 71:31–36

Rivas C, Oliva H (1980) Linfomas no-Hodgkin. Salvat Editores, Barcelona

Robb-Smith AHT (1975) The interrelationship of lymphoreticular hyperplasia and neoplasia. Excerpta Medica Int Congr Series 384:165–171

Robb-Smith AHT (1976) Lennert lymphoma. [Letter to the Editor] Lancet ii:970

Robb-Smith AHT (1982) U.S. National Cancer Institute Working Formulation of non-Hodgkin's lymphomas of clinical use. Lancet ii:432–434

Robb-Smith AHT (1990) Before our time: half a century of histiocytic medullary reticulosis: a T-cell teaser? Histopathology 17:279–283

Robb-Smith AHT, Taylor CR (1981) Lymph node biopsy. A diagnostic atlas with 300 photomicrographs in full colour. Miller Heyden, London

Rohatiner AZS, Lister TA (1991) Myeloablative therapy for follicular lymphoma. In: Armitage JO (ed): Hematology/Oncology Clinics of North America. Non-Hodgkin's Lymphoma. Saunders Company Philadelphia, vol 5, pp 1003–1012

Rooney CM, Gregory CD, Rowe M, Finerty S, Edwards C, Rupani H, Rickinson AB (1986) Endemic Burkitt's lymphoma: phenotypic analysis of tumor biopsy cells and of derived tumor cell lines. JNCI 77: 681–687

Rosenberg SA (1983) The National Cancer Institute sponsored study of the classifications of non-Hodgkin's lymphomas. Comment by the principal investigator. Hematol Oncol 1: 93–94

Rosenberg SA (1985) The low-grade non-Hodgkin's lymphomas: Challenges and opportunities. J Clin Oncol 3: 299–310

Rosenblatt JD, Chen ISY, Wachsman W (1988) Infection with HTLV-I and HTLV-II: evolving concepts. Semin Hematol 25: 230–246

Rowe M, Rooney CM, Rickinson AB, Lenoir GM, Rupani H, Moss DJ, Stein H, Epstein MA (1985) Distinctions between endemic and sporadic forms of Epstein-Barr virus-positive Burkitt's lymphoma. Int J Cancer 35: 435–441

Rowley JD (1984) Biological implications of consistent chromosome rearrangements in leukemia and lymphoma. Cancer Res 44: 3159–3168

Sacks EL, Donaldson SS, Gordon J, Dorfman RF (1978) Epithelioid granulomas associated with Hodgkin's disease. Clinical correlations in 55 previously untreated patients. Cancer 41: 562–567

Sainati L, Montaldi A, Stella M, Putti MC, Zanesco L, Basso G (1990) A novel variant translocation t(2; 13) (p23; q34) in Ki-1 large cell anaplastic lymphoma. Br J Haematol 75: 621–622

Sandritter W, Grimm H (1977) Non-Hodgkin-Lymphome. Eine Übersicht. Med Welt 28: 1533–1538

Saxon A, Stevens RH, Golde DW (1978) T-lymphocyte variant of hairy-cell leukemia. Ann Intern Med 88: 323–326

Scarpa A, Bonetti F, Zamboni G, Menestrina F, Chilosi M (1989) T-cell-rich B-cell lymphoma. [Letter to the Editor] Am J Surg Pathol 13: 335–337

Scheffer E, Meijer CJLM, Van Vloten WA (1980) Dermatopathic lymphadenopathy and lymph node involvement in mycosis fungoides. Cancer 45: 137–148

Scheurlen PG, Hellriegel KP (1971) „Epitheloidzellige Lymphogranulomatose" mit Gammopathie und Chromosomenaberrationen. Klin Wochenschr 49: 597–604

Schilling C von, Feller AC, Johansen P, Lennert K (1987) Sinusoidal B-cell lymphoma is the malignant lymphoma of so-called immature sinus histiocytosis. The Third International Conference on Malignant Lymphoma, Lugano 1987: Abstract 64

Schlegelberger B, Feller AC, Gödde-Salz E, Grote W, Lennert K (1990) Stepwise development of chromosomal abnormalities in angioimmunoblastic lymphadenopathy. Cancer Genet Cytogenet 50: 15–29

Schmalhorst U, Bartels H, Boll I, Burger-Schüler A, Common H, Fülle HH, Graubner M, Heinz R, Huhn D, Leopold H, Meusers P, Nowicki L, Nürnberger R, Oertel J, Rühl U, Sieber G, Schmidt M, Schoengen A, Strassner A, Schwarze EW (Kiel Lymphoma Study Group) (1979) Clinical and prognostic heterogeneity of high-grade malignant lymphomas. 5th Meeting Intern Soc Haematol, European and African Division, Hamburg, August 26–31, 1979

Schmid U, Helbron D, Lennert K (1982) Development of malignant lymphoma in myoepithelial sialadenitis (Sjögren's syndrome). Virchows Arch [A] 395: 11–43

Schmid U, Karow J, Lennert K (1985) Follicular malignant non-Hodgkin's lymphoma with pronounced plasmacytic differentiation: a plasmacytoma-like lymphoma. Virchows Arch [A] 405: 473–481

Schmidt D, Harms D, Zieger G (1982) Malignant rhabdoid tumor of the kidney. Histopathology, ultrastructure and comments on differential diagnosis. Virchows Arch [A] 398: 101–108

Schmidt D, Leuschner I, Harms D, Sprenger E, Schäfer H-J (1989) Malignant rhabdoid tumor. A morphological and flow cytometric study. Pathol Res Pract 184: 202–210

Schnaidt U, Thiele J, Georgii A (1980a) Angioimmunoblastic lymphadenopathy. Fine structure of the lymph nodes by correlation of light and electron microscopical findings. Virchows Arch [A] 389: 381–395

Schnaidt U, Vykoupil KF, Thiele J, Georgii A (1980b) Angioimmunoblastic lymphadenopathy. Histopathology of bone marrow involvement. Virchows Arch [A] 389: 369–380

Schneider DR, Taylor CR, Parker JW, Cramer AC, Meyer PR, Lukes RJ (1985) Immunoblastic sarcoma of T- and B-cell types: morphologic description and comparison. Hum Pathol 16:885–900

Schoengen A, Dietrich M, Kubanek B, Haferkamp O, Heimpel H (1976) Immunoblastische Lymphadenopathie mit pseudoleukämischem Blutbild. Blut 32:29–36

Schwab U, Stein H, Gerdes J, Lemke H, Kirchner H, Schaadt M, Diehl V (1982) Production of a monoclonal antibody specific for Hodgkin and Sternberg-Reed cells of Hodgkin's disease and a subset of normal lymphoid cells. Nature 299:65–67

Schwalbe P, Arndt D, Müller-Hermelink HK (1978) Untersuchungen mit Gewebsextrakten maligner menschlicher Lymphome im Leukozyten-Migrations-Test. Acta Biol Med Germ 37:1105–1112

Schwarting R, Stein H, Wang CY (1985) The monoclonal antibodies αS-HCL 1 (αLeu-14) and αS-HCL 3 (αLeu-M5) allow the diagnosis of hairy cell leukemia. Blood 65:974–983

Schwarting R, Dienemann D, Kruschwitz M, Fritsche G, Stein H (1990) Specificities of monoclonal antibodies B-ly7 and HML-1 are identical. [Letter to the Editor] Blood 75:320

Schwarze E-W (1979) Alkalische Phosphatase-positive Non-Hodgkin-Lymphome – Eine cytochemische Studie. Verh Dtsch Ges Pathol 63:488

Schwarze E-W (1986) Non-Hodgkin-Lymphome. Cytologie und Cytochemie. (Veröffentlichungen aus der Pathologie, vol 123) Fischer, Stuttgart

Schwarze E-W, Gödde-Salz E, Lennert K (1982) Zytogenetische Befunde bei Morbus Hodgkin, Lymphogranulomatosis X und T-Zonen-Lymphom. Verh Dtsch Ges Pathol 66:127–133

Scott RB, Robb-Smith AHT (1939) Histiocytic medullary reticulosis. Lancet ii:194–198

Second MIC Cooperative Study Group (1988) Morphologic, immunologic and cytogenetic (MIC) working classification of the acute myeloid leukaemias. Br J Haematol 68:487–494

Semenzato G, Pandolfi F, Chisesi T, de Rossi G, Pizzolo G, Zambello R, Trentin L, Agostini C, Dini E, Vespignani M, Cafaro A, Pasqualetti D, Giubellino MC, Migone N, Foa R (1987) The lymphoproliferative disease of granular lymphocytes. A heterogeneous disorder ranging from indolent to aggressive conditions. Cancer 60:2971–2978

Seo IS, Min KW, Brodhecker C, Mirkin LD (1988) Malignant renal rhabdoid tumour. Immunohistochemical and ultrastructural studies. Histopathology 13:657–666

Shamoto M, Suchi T (1979) Intracytoplasmic type A virus-like particles in angioimmunoblastic lymphadenopathy. Cancer 44:1641–1643

Shamoto M, Kito K, Akatsuka H, Suchi T (1984) Immunoelectron microscopic studies on peripheral T-cell lymphomas using monoclonal antibodies. Virchows Arch [B] 47:281–290

Sheibani K, Winberg C, Burke J, Rappaport H (1984) Monocytoid cells in reactive follicular hyperplasia with and without multifocal histiocytic reactions: An immunohistochemical study of 21 cases including suspected cases of toxoplasmic lymphadenitis. Lab Invest 50:53 A–54 A

Sheibani K, Sohn CC, Burke JS, Winberg CD, Wu AM, Rappaport H (1986) Monocytoid B-cell lymphoma: a novel B-cell neoplasm. Am J Pathol 124:310–318

Sheibani K, Burke JS, Swartz WG, Nademanee A, Winberg CD (1988) Monocytoid B-cell lymphoma. Clinicopathologic study of 21 cases of a unique type of low-grade lymphoma. Cancer 62:1531–1538

Shimoyama M, Minato K, Saito H, Takenaka T, Watanabe S, Nagatani T, Naruto M (1979) Immunoblastic lymphadenopathy (IBL)-like T-cell lymphoma. Jpn J Clin Oncol 9 (Suppl):347–356

Shimoyama M, Tobinai K, Minato K, Watanabe S (1987) Immunoblastic lymphadenopathy (IBL)-like T cell lymphoma. Recent Adv RES Res 23:161–170

Shtern RD (1980) Pathology of the non-Hodgkin's malignant lymphomas (based on the Kiel classification). [russ] Arch Patologii 42:71–80

Sibley R, Rosai J, Froehlich W (1980) A case for the panel: anemone cell tumor. Ultrastruct Pathol 1:449–453

Sibley R, Rosai J, Froehlich W (1985) Anemone cell tumor: comments by the panel. Ultrastruct Pathol 8:369–373

Siegert W, Schwerdtfeger R, Hartmann R, Agthe A, Huhn D, Tiemann M, Lennert K (1989) Lymphogranulomatosis X – a multicenter evaluation of a standardized treatment. (Abstract) Blood 74 (Suppl 1):280 a

Siegert W, Nerl C, Meuthen I, Zahn T, Brack N, Lennert K, Huhn D (1991) Recombinant human interferon-α in the treatment of angioimmunoblastic lymphadenopathy. Results in 12 patients. Leukemia 5: 892–895

Silvestrini R, Piazza R, Riccardi A, Rilke F (1977) Correlation of cell kinetic findings with morphology of non-Hodgkin's malignant lymphomas. JNCI 58: 499–504

Sklar J, Cleary ML, Thielemans K, Gralow J, Warnke R, Levy R (1984) Biclonal B-cell lymphoma. N Engl J Med 311: 20–27

Slater DN (1987) Recent developments in cutaneous lymphoproliferative disorders. J Pathol 153: 5–19

Sohn CC, Blayney DW, Misset JL, Mathé G, Flandrin G, Moran EM, Jensen FC, Winberg CD, Rappaport H (1986) Leukopenic chronic T cell leukemia mimicking hairy cell leukemia: association with human retroviruses. Blood 67: 949–956

Sorg C, Bröcker E-B, Zwadlo G, Redmann K, Feige U, Ax W, Feller AC (1985) A monoclonal antibody to a formaldehyde-resistant epitope on the nonpolymorphic constant part of the HLA-DR antigens. Transplantation 39: 90–93

Spencer J, Finn T, Pulford KAF, Mason DY, Isaacson PG (1985) The human gut contains a novel population of B lymphocytes which resemble marginal zone cells. Clin Exp Immunol 62: 607–612

Spencer J, Cerf-Bensussan N, Jarry A, Brousse N, Guy-Grand D, Krajewski AS, Isaacson PG (1988) Enteropathy-associated T cell lymphoma (malignant histiocytosis of the intestine) is recognized by a monoclonal antibody (HML-1) that defines a membrane molecule on human mucosal lymphocytes. Am J Pathol 132: 1–5

Spencer J, Diss TC, Isaacson PG (1990) A study of the properties of a low-grade mucosal B-cell lymphoma using a monoclonal antibody specific for the tumour immunoglobulin. J Pathol 160: 231–238

Spier CM, Lippman SM, Miller TP, Grogan TM (1988) Lennert's lymphoma. A clinicopathologic study with emphasis on phenotype and its relationship to survival. Cancer 61: 517–524

Spiro S, Galton DAG, Wiltshaw E, Lohmann R (1975) Follicular lymphoma: A survey of 75 cases with special reference to the syndrome resembling chronic lymphocytic leukaemia. Br J Cancer 31 [Suppl II]: 60–72

Stansfeld AG (ed) (1985) Lymph node biopsy interpretation. Churchill Livingstone, Edinburgh

Stansfeld AG, Diebold J, Kapanci Y, Kelényi G, Lennert K, Mioduszewska O, Noel H, Rilke F, Sundstrom C, Van Unnik JAM, Wright DH (1988) Updated Kiel classification for lymphomas [Letter to the Editor] Lancet i: 292–293 and 603

Stark AN, Limbert HJ, Roberts BE, Jones RA, Scott CS (1986) Prolymphocytoid transformation of CLL: a clinical and immunological study of 22 cases. Leuk Res 10: 1225–1232

Stein H (1978) The immunologic and immunochemical basis for the Kiel classification: In: Lennert K et al. (eds) Malignant lymphomas other than Hodgkin's disease. (Handbuch der speziellen pathologischen Anatomie und Histologie, vol I/3 B) Springer, Berlin Heidelberg New York, pp 529–657

Stein H, Bonk A, Tolksdorf G, Lennert K, Rodt H, Gerdes J (1980) Immunohistologic analysis of the organization of normal lymphoid tissue and non-Hodgkin's lymphomas. J Histochem Cytochem 28: 746–760

Stein H, Gerdes J, Schwab U, Lemke H, Mason DY, Ziegler A, Schienle W, Diehl V (1982a) Identification of Hodgkin and Sternberg-Reed cells as a unique cell type derived from a newly-detected small cell population. Int J Cancer 30: 445–459

Stein H, Gerdes J, Mason DY (1982b) The normal and malignant germinal center. Clin Hematol 11: 531–559

Stein H, Lennert K, Feller AC, Mason DY (1984a) Immunohistological analysis of human lymphoma: correlation of histological and immunological categories. Adv Cancer Res 42: 67–147

Stein H, Lennert K, Mason DY, Liangru S, Ziegler A (1984b) Immature sinus histiocytes. Their identification as a novel B-cell population. Am J Pathol 117: 44–52

Stein H, Mason DY, Gerdes J, O'Connor N, Wainscoat J, Pallesen G, Gatter K, Falini B, Delsol G, Lemke H, Schwarting R, Lennert K (1985) The expression of the Hodgkin's disease associated antigen Ki-1 in reactive and neoplastic lymphoid tissue: evidence that Reed-Sternberg cells and histiocytic malignancies are derived from activated lymphoid cells. Blood 66: 848–858

Stein H, Dienemann D, Sperling M, Zeitz M, Riecken E-O (1988) Identification of a T cell lymphoma category derived from intestinal-mucosa-associated T cells. Lancet ii: 1053–1054

Sterry W (1985) Mycosis fungoides. Curr Top Pathol 74: 167–223

Stewart ML, Felman IE, Nichols PW, Pagnini-Hill A, Lukes RJ, Levine AM (1986) Large noncleaved follicular center cell lymphoma. Clinical features in 53 patients. Cancer 57: 288–297

Stiller D, Katenkamp D, Fritzsche V (1980) Lymphoepitheloidzellige Reaktion – lympho-epitheloides Lymphom. Zentralbl Allg Pathol 124: 424–440

Strauchen JA, Young RC, DeVita Jr VT, Anderson T, Fantone JC, Berard CW (1978) Clinical relevance of the histopathological subclassification of diffuse "histiocytic" lymphoma. N Engl J Med 299: 1382–1387

Strickler JG, Medeiros LJ, Copenhaver CM, Weiss LM, Warnke RA (1988) Intermediate lymphocytic lymphoma: an immunophenotypic study with comparison to small lymphocytic lymphoma and diffuse small cleaved cell lymphoma. Hum Pathol 19: 550–554

Stroup RM, Sheibani K, Moncada A, Purdy LJ, Battifora H (1990) Angiotropic (intravascular) large cell lymphoma. A clinicopathologic study of seven cases with unique clinical presentations. Cancer 66: 1781–1788

Suchi T (1974) Atypical lymph node hyperplasia with fatal outcome. A report on the histopathological, immunological and clinical investigations of the cases. Recent Adv RES Res 14: 13–34

Suchi T (1987) Malignant lymphomas in Japan: The geographic features. In: Wada T, Aoki K, Yachi A (eds) Current status of cancer research in Asia, the Middle East and other countries. University of Nagoya Press, Nagoya, pp 17–25

Suchi T, Tajima K, Nanba K, Wakasa H, Mikata A, Kikuchi M, Mori S, Watanabe S, Mohri N, Shamoto M, Harigaya K, Itagai T, Matsuda M, Kirino Y, Takagi K, Fukunaga S (1979) Some problems on the histopathological diagnosis of non-Hodgkin's malignant lymphoma. A proposal of a new type. Acta Pathol Jpn 29: 755–776

Suchi T, Lennert K, Tu LY, Kikuchi M, Sato E, Stansfeld AG, Feller AC (1987) Histopathology and immunohistochemistry of peripheral T cell lymphomas: a proposal for their classification. J Clin Pathol 40: 995–1015

Suzuki H, Namikawa R, Ueda R, Obata Y, Suchi T, Kikuchi M, Ota K, Takahashi T (1987) Clonal T cell population in angioimmunoblastic lymphadenopathy and related lesions. Jpn J Cancer Res 78: 712–720

Swerdlow SH, Murray LJ (1988) Low-grade lymphomas. In: Habeshaw JA, Lauder I (eds) Malignant lymphomas. Churchill Livingstone, Edinburgh, pp 127–168

Swerdlow SH, Habeshaw JA, Murray LJ, Dhaliwal HS, Lister TA, Stansfeld AG (1983) Centrocytic lymphoma: a distinct clinicopathologic and immunologic entity. A multiparameter study of 18 cases at diagnosis and relapse. Am J Pathol 113: 181–197

Swerdlow SH, Habeshaw JA, Rohatiner AZS, Lister TA, Stansfeld AG (1984) Caribbean T-cell lymphoma/leukemia. Cancer 54: 687–696

Swerdlow SH, Murray LJ, Habeshaw JA, Stansfeld AG (1985) B- and T-cell subsets in follicular centroblastic/centrocytic (cleaved follicular center cell) lymphoma: an immunohistologic analysis of 26 lymph nodes and three spleens. Hum Pathol 16: 339–352

Symmers WStC (1978) The lymphoreticular system. In: Symmers WStC (ed) Systemic pathology, 2nd edn, vol 2. Churchill Livingstone, Edinburgh, pp 504–891

Tajima K, Kuroishi T (1985) Estimation of rate of incidence of ATL among ATLV (HTLV-I) carriers in Kyushu, Japan. Jpn J Clin Oncol 15: 423–430

Tajima K, Tominaga S, Suchi T, Kawagoe T, Komoda H, Hinuma Y, Oda T, Fujita K (1982) Epidemiological analysis of the distribution of antibody to adult T-cell leukemia-virus-associated antigen: possible horizontal transmission of adult T-cell leukemia virus. Gann 73: 893–901

Tajima K, Tominaga S, Suchi T (1986) Malignant lymphomas in Japan: epidemiological analysis on adult T-cell leukemia/lymphoma. Hematol Oncol 4: 31–44

Takácsi-Nagy L, Tarkovács G, Szende B, Gráf F (1978) A clinicopathological study of non-Hodgkin's malignant lymphomas in terms of the Kiel classification. Folia Haematol (Leipz) 105: 79–92

Takatsuki K, Sanada I (1983) Plasma cell dyscrasia with polyneuropathy and endocrine disorder: clinical and laboratory features of 109 reported cases. Jpn J Clin Oncol 13: 543–556

Takatsuki K, Uchiyama T, Sagawa K, Yodoi J (1976a) Adult T cell leukemia in Japan. Excerpta Medica Int Congr Ser 415: 73–77

Takatsuki K, Uchiyama T, Sagawa K, Yodoi J (1976b) Plasma cell dyscrasia with polyneuropathy and endocrine disorder: review of 32 patients. Excerpta Medica Int Congr Ser 415:454–457

Takatsuki K, Uchiyama T, Ueshima Y, Hattori T, Toibana T, Tsudo M, Wano Y, Yodoi J (1982) Adult T cell leukemia: proposal as a new disease and cytogenetic, phenotypic, and functional studies of leukemic cells. In: Hanaoka M, Takatsuki K, Shimoyama M (eds) Adult T cell leukemia and related diseases. (GANN monograph on cancer research, no 28) Japan Scientific Societies Press, Tokyo, pp 13–22

Tashiro K, Kikuchi M, Takeshita M, Yoshida T, Ohshima K (1989) Clinicopathological study of Ki-1-positive lymphomas. Pathol Res Pract 185:461–467

Taylor CR, Burns J (1974) The demonstration of plasma cells and other immunoglobulin-containing cells in formalin-fixed, paraffin-embedded tissues using peroxidase-labelled antibody. J Clin Pathol 27:14–20

Taylor CR, Chandor SB (1981) The immunohistochemical evaluation of malignant lymphomas and related conditions. In: DeLellis RA (ed) Diagnostic immunohistochemistry. (Masson monographs in diagnostic pathology, vol 2). Masson, New York, pp 179–202

The T- and B-cell Malignancy Study Group (1981) Statistical analysis of immunologic, clinical and histopathologic data on lymphoid malignancies in Japan. Jpn J Clin Oncol 11:15–38

Theml H, Burger A, Keiditsch E, Enne W, Eggert K, Dietzfelbinger H, Gräff L, Zsida L (1977) Klinische Beobachtungen zur Charakterisierung des splenomegalen Immunozytoms. Med Klin 72:1019–1032

Thiel E, Rodt H, Netzel B, Huhn D, Wündisch GF, Haas RJ, Bender-Götze C, Thierfelder S (1978) T-Zell-Antigen positive, E-Rosetten negative akute Lymphoblastenleukämie. Blut 36:363–369

Timens W (1988) The human spleen. Development and role in the immune system. Groningen: Proefschrift, Rijksuniversiteit

Timens W, Poppema S (1985) Lymphocyte compartments in human spleen. An immunohistologic study in normal spleens and noninvolved spleens in Hodgkin's disease. Am J Pathol 120:443–454

Tindle BH, Long JC (1977) Case Records of the Massachusetts General Hospital, Case 30–1977. N Engl J Med 297:206–211

Tirelli U, Vaccher E, Ambrosini A, Andriani A, Bianco Silvestroni I, Broccia G, Chisesi T, Dessalvi P, Gobbi M, Fassio F, Lambertenghi Deliliers G, Lanza F, Lazzarin A, Lombardi F, Luzi G, Malleo C, Parrinello EA, Proto R, Puppo F, Rezza G, Rossi G, Gavosto F, Monfardini S (1988) HIV-related malignant lymphoma: a report of 46 cases observed in Italy. Acta Haematol (Basel) 80:49–51

Tkachuk DC, Griesser H, Takihara Y, Champagne E, Minden M, Feller AC, Lennert K, Mak TW (1988) Rearrangement of T-cell δ locus in lymphoproliferative disorders. Blood 72:353–357

Tokunaga M, Sato E (1980) Non-Hodgkin's lymphomas in Southern Prefecture in Japan: An analysis of 715 cases. Cancer 46:1231–1239

Tokunaga M, Sato E, Tanaka S, Sakai N (1978) Malignant lymphoma occurring in Kagoshima Prefecture, Japan: Pathological and descriptive epidemiological survey based on 849 biopsy materials. Gann 69:673–678

Tolksdorf G, Stein H (1979) Acid alpha-naphthyl acetate esterase in hairy cell leukemia cells and other cells of the hematopoietic system. Blut 39:165–176

Toninai K, Minato K, Ohtsu T, Mukai K, Kagami Y, Miwa M, Watanabe S, Shimoyama M (1988) Clinicopathologic, immunophenotypic, and immunogenotypic analyses of immunoblastic lymphadenopathy-like T-cell lymphoma. Blood 72:1000–1006

Trainor KJ, Brisco MJ, Story CJ, Morley AA (1990) Monoclonality in B-lymphoproliferative disorders detected at the DNA level. Blood 75:2220–2222

Traweek T, Sheibani K, Winberg CD, Mena RR, Wu AM, Rappaport H (1989) Monocytoid B-cell lymphoma: Its evolution and relationship to other low-grade B-cell neoplasms. Blood 73:573–578

Trinkler B, Mustroph D, Hagenah H, Mönch H, v. Heyden HW (1989) Alpha-interferon for the treatment of angioimmunoblastic lymphadenopathy and B-cell prolymphocytic leukemia. Mol Biother 1 (suppl): abstract 93

Trump DL, Mann RB (1982) Diffuse large cell and undifferentiated lymphomas with prominent mediastinal involvement. A poor prognostic subset of patients with non-Hodgkin's lymphoma. Cancer 50:277–282

Uchiyama T, Yodoi J, Sagawa K, Takatsuki K, Uchino H (1977) Adult T-cell leukemia: clinical and hematologic features of 17 cases. Blood 50:481–492

Uckun FM (1990) Regulation of human B-cell ontogeny. Blood 76:1908–1923

Vadhan-Raj S, Buescher S, LeMaistre A, Keating M, Walters R, Ventura C, Hittelman W, Broxmeyer HE, Gutterman JU (1988) Stimulation of hematopoiesis in patients with bone marrow failures and in patients with malignancy by recombinant human granulocyte-macrophage colony-stimulating factor. Blood 72:134–141

Vandenberghe E, De Wolf-Peeters C, Van den Oord J, Wlodarska I, Delabie J, Stul M, Thomas J, Michaux J-L, Mecucci C, Cassiman J-J, Van den Berghe H (1991) Translocation (11;14): a cytogenetic anomaly associated with B-cell lymphomas of non-follicle centre cell lineage. J Pathol 163:13–18

Vanden Heule B, van Kerkem C, Heimann R (1979) Benign and malignant lymphoid lesions of the stomach. A histological reappraisal in the light of the Kiel classification for non-Hodgkin's lymphomas. Histopathology 3:309–320

Van den Oord JJ, de Wolf-Peeters C, de Vos R, Desmet VJ (1985) Immature sinus histiocytosis. Light- and electron-microscopic features, immunologic phenotype, and relationship with marginal zone lymphocytes. Am J Pathol 118:266–277

Van den Oord JJ, de Wolf-Peeters C, Pulford KAF, Mason DY, Desmet VJ (1986) Mantle zone lymphoma. Immuno- and enzymehistochemical studies on the cell of origin. Am J Surg Pathol 10:780–788

Van den Tweel JG, Taylor CR, Parker JW, Lukes RJ (1978) Immunoglobulin inclusions in non-Hodgkin's lymphomas. Am J Clin Pathol 69:306–313

Van der Putte SCJ, Schuurman HJ, Toonstra J (1982a) Cutaneous T-cell lymphoma, multilobated type, expressing membrane differentiation antigens of precursor T-lymphocytes. Br J Dermatol 107:293–300

Van der Putte SCJ, Toonstra J, de Weger RA, van Unnik JAM (1982b) Cutaneous T-cell lymphoma, multilobated type. Histopathology 6:35–54

Van der Putte SCJ, Schuurman HJ, Rademakers LHPM, Kluin P, van Unnik JAM (1984) Malignant lymphoma of follicle centre cells with marked nuclear lobation. Virchows Arch [B] 46:93–107

Van der Valk P, Jansen J, Daha MR, Meijer CJLM (1983) Characterization of B-cell non-Hodgkin's lymphomas. A study using a panel of monoclonal and heterologous antibodies. Virchows Arch [A] 401:289–305

Van der Valk P, Ball P, Mosch A, Meijer CJLM (1984a) Large cell lymphomas. I. Differential diagnosis of centroblastic and B-immunoblastic subtypes by morphometry on histologic preparations. Cancer 54:2082–2087

Van der Valk P, van der Loo EM, Jansen J, Daha MR, Meijer CJLM (1984b) Analysis of lymphoid and dendritic cells in human lymph node, tonsil and spleen. A study using monoclonal and heterologous antibodies. Virchows Arch [B] 45:169–185

Van der Valk P, Mullink H, Huijgens PC, Tadema TM, Vos W, Meijer CJLM (1989) Immuno-histochemistry in bone marrow diagnosis. Value of a panel of monoclonal antibodies on routinely processed bone marrow biopsies. Am J Surg Pathol 13:97–106

Van Krieken JHJM, von Schilling C, Kluin PM, Lennert K (1989) Splenic marginal zone lymphocytes and related cells in the lymph node: a morphologic and immunohistochemical study. Hum Pathol 20:320–325

Van Unnik JAM, Breur K, Burgers JMV, Cleton F, Hart AAM, Stenfert Kroese WF, Somers R, van Turnhout JMMPM (1975) Non-Hodgkin's lymphomata: clinical features in relation to histology. Br J Cancer 31 [Suppl II]:201–207

Vardiman JW, Golomb HM (1984) Autopsy findings in hairy cell leukemia. Semin Oncol 11:370–379

Veldman JE (1970) Histophysiology and electron microscopy of the immune response. Thesis, University of Groningen

Veldman JE, Keuning FJ (1978) Histophysiology of cellular immunity reactions in B-cell deprived rabbits. An X-irradiation model for delineation of an "isolated T-cell system". Virchows Arch [B] 28:203–216

Veldman JE, Keuning FJ, Molenaar I (1978a) Site of initiation of the plasma cell reaction in the rabbit lymph node. Ultrastructural evidence for two distinct antibody forming cell precursors. Virchows Arch [B] 28:187–202

Veldman JE, Molenaar I, Keuning FJ (1978 b) Electron microscopy of cellular immunity reactions in B-cell deprived rabbits. Thymus derived antigen reactive cells, their micro-environment and progeny in the lymph node. Virchows Arch [B] 28: 217–228

Visser L, Shaw A, Slupsky J, Vos H, Poppema S (1989) Monoclonal antibodies reactive with hairy cell leukemia. Blood 74: 320–325

Vollenweider R, Lennert K (1983) Plasmacytoid T-cell clusters in non-specific lymphadenitis. Virchows Arch [B] 44: 1–14

Vyth-Dreese FA, de Vries JE (1982) Human T-cell leukaemia virus in lymphocytes from T-cell leukaemia patient originating from Surinam. [Letter] Lancet ii: 993

Wacker HH, Hansmann M-L, Lumbeck H, Radzun HJ, Parwaresch MR (1990) Ein neuer Pan-Makrophagen Antikörper Ki-M1P erkennt plasmozytoide Lymphknotenzellen in Paraffinschnitten. Verh Dtsch Ges Pathol 74: 159–164

Waldmann TA, Davis MM, Bongiovanni KF, Korsmeyer SJ (1985) Rearrangements of genes for the antigen receptor on T cells as markers of lineage and clonality in human lymphoid neoplasms. N Engl J Med 313: 776–783

Waldron JA, Leech JH, Glick AD, Flexner JM, Collins RD (1977) Malignant lymphoma of peripheral T-lymphocyte origin. Immunologic, pathologic, and clinical features in six patients. Cancer 40: 1604–1617

Watanabe A, Sullivan MP, Sutow WW, Wilbur JR (1973) Undifferentiated lymphoma, non-Burkitt's type: meningeal and bone marrow involvement in children. Am J Dis Child 125: 57–61

Watanabe S, Shimosato Y, Shimoyama M, Minato K, Suzuki M, Abe M, Nagatani T (1980) Adult T cell lymphoma with hypergammaglobulinemia. Cancer 46: 2472–2483

Watanabe S, Shimosato Y, Shimoyama M (1981) Lymphoma and leukemia of T-lymphocytes. Pathol Annu 16, II: 155–203

Weeks DA, Beckwith JB, Mierau GW, Luckey DW (1989) Rhabdoid tumor of kidney. A report of 111 cases from the National Wilms' Tumor Study Pathology Center. Am J Surg Pathol 13: 439–458

Weinberg DS, Pinkus GS (1981) Non-Hodgkin's lymphomas of large multilobated cell type. A clinicopathologic study of ten cases. Am J Clin Pathol 76: 190–196

Weintraub J, Warnke RA (1982) Lymphoma in cardiac allotransplant recipients. Clinical and histological features and immunological phenotype. Transplantation 33: 347–351

Weisenburger DD, Nathwani BN, Diamond LW, Winberg CD, Rappaport H (1981) Malignant lymphoma, intermediate lymphocytic type: a clinicopathologic study of 42 cases. Cancer 48: 1415–1425

Weisenburger DD, Nathwani BN, Forman SJ, Rappaport H (1982) Noncutaneous peripheral T-cell lymphoma histologically resembling mycosis fungoides. Cancer 49: 1839–1847

Weisenburger DD, Astorino RN, Glassy FJ, Miller CH, MacKenzie MR, Caggiano V (1985a) Peripheral T-cell lymphoma. A clinicopathologic study of a morphologically diverse entity. Cancer 56: 2061–2068

Weisenburger DD, Nathwani BN, Winberg CD, Rappaport H (1985b) Multicentric angiofollicular lymph node hyperplasia: a clinicopathologic study of 16 cases. Hum Pathol 16: 162–172

Weisenburger DD, Linder J, Armitage JO (1987a) Peripheral T-cell lymphoma: a clinicopathologic study of 42 cases. Hematol Oncol 5: 175–187

Weisenburger DD, Sanger WG, Armitage JO, Purtilo DT (1987b) Intermediate lymphocytic lymphoma: Immunophenotypic and cytogenetic findings. Blood 69: 1617–1621

Weisenburger DD, Harrington DS, Armitage JO (1990) B-cell neoplasia. A conceptual understanding based on the normal humoral immune response. Pathol Annu 25/I: 99–115

Weisenburger DD, Duggan MJ, Perry DA, Sanger WG, Armitage JO (1991) Non-Hodgkin's lymphomas of mantle zone origin. Pathol Annu 26: 139–158

Weiss LM, Wood GS, Dorfman RF (1985a) T-cell signet-ring cell lymphoma. A histologic, ultrastructural, and immunohistochemical study of two cases. Am J Surg Pathol 9: 273–280

Weiss LM, Hu E, Wood GS, Moulds C, Cleary ML, Warnke R, Sklar J (1985b) Clonal rearrangements of T-cell receptor genes in mycosis fungoides and dermatopathic lymphadenopathy. N Engl J Med 313: 539–544

Weiss LM, Strickler JG, Dorfman RF, Horning SJ, Warnke RA, Sklar J (1986) Clonal T-cell populations in angioimmunoblastic lymphadenopathy and angioimmunoblastic lymphadenopathy-like lymphoma. Am J Pathol 122: 392–397

Weiss LM, Warnke RA, Sklar J, Cleary ML (1987) Molecular analysis of the t(14;18) chromo-
   somal translocation in malignant lymphomas. N Engl J Med 317:1185–1189
Weiss RL, Kjeldsberg CR, Colby TV, Marty J (1985) Multilobated B cell lymphomas. A study
   of 7 cases. Hematol Oncol 3:79–86
Willemze R, Scheffer E, Meijer CJLM (1985) Immunohistochemical studies using monoclonal
   antibodies on lymph nodes from patients with mycosis fungoides and Sézary's syndrome.
   Am J Pathol 120:46–54
Wilson JF, Kjeldsberg CR, Sposto R, Jenkin RDT, Chilcote RR, Coccia P, Exelby RR, Kersey
   J, Meadows A, Siegel S, Hammond D (1987) The pathology of non-Hodgkin's lymphoma
   of childhood: II. Reproducibility and relevance of the histologic classification of "undiffer-
   entiated" lymphomas (Burkitt's versus non-Burkitt's). Hum Pathol 18:1008–1014
Wiltshaw E (1971) Extramedullary plasmacytoma. Br Med J 1971/II:319–328
Winberg CD, Nathwani BN, Rappaport H (1979) Nodular (follicular) lymphomas in children
   and young adults: a clinicopathologic study of 64 patients. (Abstract) Lab Invest 40:292
Witkin GB, Rosai J (1989) Solitary fibrous tumor of the mediastinum. A report of 14 cases. Am
   J Surg Pathol 13:547–557
Wotherspoon AC, Pan L, Diss TC, Isaacson PG (1990) A genotypic study of low grade B-cell
   lymphomas, including lymphomas of mucosa associated lymphoid tissue (MALT). J Pathol
   162:135–140
Wright DH (1970) Gross distribution and haematology. In: Burkitt DP, Wright DH (eds)
   Burkitt's lymphoma. Livingstone, Edinburgh, pp 64–81
Wright DH (1982) The identification and classification of non-Hodgkin's lymphoma. A review.
   Diagn Histopathol 5:73–111
Wright DH, Isaacson PG (1983) Biopsy pathology of the lymphoreticular system. Chapman and
   Hall, London
Yi PI, Coleman M, Saltz L, Norton BL, Topilow AA, Adler K, Bernhardt B (1990) Chemother-
   apy for large cell lymphoma: a status update. Semin Oncol 17:60–73
York II JC, Cousar JB, Glick AD, Flexner JM, Stein R, Collins RD (1983) Three cases
   developing in follicular center cell lymphomas. (Abstract) Lab Invest 48:96A
York JC, Glick AD, Cousar JB, Collins RD (1984) Changes in the appearance of hematopoietic
   and lymphoid neoplasms: clinical, pathologic, and biologic implications. Hum Pathol
   15:11–38
Yoshida M, Miyoshi I, Hinuma Y (1982) Isolation and characterization of retrovirus (ATLV)
   and its association with adult T cell leukemia. In: Hanaoka M, Takatsuki K, Shimoyama M
   (eds) Adult T cell leukemia and related diseases. (GANN monograph on cancer research,
   no 28) Japan Scientific Societies Press, Tokyo, pp 229–237
Young RC, Longo DL, Glatstein E, Ihde DC, Jaffe ES, DeVita Jr VT (1988) The treatment of
   indolent lymphomas: Watchful waiting V aggressive combined modality treatment. Semin
   Hematol 25 (Suppl 2):11–16
Yousem SA, Weiss LM, Warnke RA (1985) Primary mediastinal non-Hodgkin's lymphomas: a
   morphologic and immunologic study of 19 cases. Am J Clin Pathol 83:676–680
Zankl H, Ludwig B, May G, Zang KD (1979) Karyotypic variations in human meningioma cell
   cultures under different in vitro conditions. J Cancer Res Clin Oncol 93:165–172
Zankowich R, Parwaresch MR, Lennert K (1984) Blood findings in lymphogranulomatosis X.
   Blut 48:99–107
Zech L, Haglund U, Nilsson K, Klein G (1976) Characteristic chromosomal abnormalities in
   biopsies and lymphoid-cell lines from patients with Burkitt and non-Burkitt lymphomas. Int
   J Cancer 17:47–56
Ziegler JL, Drew WL, Miner RC, Mintz L, Rosenbaum E, Gershow J, Lennette ET, Greenspan
   J, Shillitoe E, Beckstead J, Casavant C, Yamamoto K (1982) Outbreak of Burkitt's-like
   lymphoma in homosexual men. Lancet ii:631–633
Ziegler JL, Beckstead JA, Volberding PA, Abrams DI, Levine AM, Lukes RJ, Gill PS, Burkes
   RL, Meyer PR, Metroka CE, Mouradian J, Moore A, Riggs SA, Butler JJ, Cabanillas FC,
   Hersh E, Newell GR, Laubenstein LJ, Knowles D, Odajnyk C, Raphael B, Koziner B,
   Urmacher C, Clarkson BD (1984) Non-Hodgkin's lymphoma in 90 homosexual men. Rela-
   tion to generalized lymphadenopathy and the acquired immunodeficiency syndrome. N Engl
   J Med 311:565–570
Zur Hausen H (1979) Viral etiology of diseases of the hematopoietic system. Recent Results in
   Cancer Res 69:1–5

Subject Index

When more than one page reference is given in an entry, **bold** type is used to indicate a main account of the topic, if appropriate.

References to illustrations and tables are printed in *italics*.

Springer-Verlag
and the Environment

We at Springer-Verlag firmly believe that an international science publisher has a special obligation to the environment, and our corporate policies consistently reflect this conviction.

We also expect our business partners – paper mills, printers, packaging manufacturers, etc. – to commit themselves to using environmentally friendly materials and production processes.

The paper in this book is made from low- or no-chlorine pulp and is acid free, in conformance with international standards for paper permanency.